# Also Available From the American Academy of Pediatrics

## Common Conditions

Allergies and Asthma: What Every Parent Needs to Know

Mama Doc Medicine: Finding Calm and Confidence in Parenting, Child Health, and Work-Life Balance

My Child Is Sick! Expert Advice for Managing Common Illnesses and Injuries

Sleep: What Every Parent Needs to Know

Waking Up Dry: A Guide to Help Children Overcome Bedwetting

## Developmental, Behavioral, and Psychosocial Information

ADHD: What Every Parent Needs to Know

Autism Spectrum Disorders: What Every Parent Needs to Know

CyberSafe: Protecting and Empowering Kids in the Digital World of Texting, Gaming, and Social Media

Mental Health, Naturally: The Family Guide to Holistic Care for a Healthy Mind and Body

## Newborns, Infants, and Toddlers

Caring for Your Baby and Young Child: Birth to Age 5*

Dad to Dad: Parenting Like a Pro

Guide to Toilet Training*

Heading Home With Your Newborn: From Birth to Reality

Mommy Calls: Dr. Tanya Answers Parents' Top 101 Questions About Babies and Toddlers

New Mother's Guide to Breastfeeding*

Newborn Intensive Care: What Every Parent Needs to Know

Raising Twins: From Pregnancy to Preschool

Retro Baby: Cut Back on All the Gear and Boost Your Baby's Development With More Than 100 Time-tested Activities

Your Baby's First Year*

## Nutrition and Fitness

Food Fights: Winning the Nutritional Challenges of Parenthood Armed With Insight, Humor, and a Bottle of Ketchup

Nutrition: What Every Parent Needs to Know

A Parent's Guide to Childhood Obesity: A Road Map to Health

Sports Success $R_x$! Your Child's Prescription for the Best Experience

## School-aged Children and Adolescents

Building Resilience in Children and Teens: Giving Kids Roots and Wings

Caring for Your School-Age Child: Ages 5 to 12

Caring for Your Teenager

Less Stress, More Success: A New Approach to Guiding Your Teen Through College Admissions and Beyond

For more information, please visit the official AAP Web site for parents, www.HealthyChildren.org/bookstore.

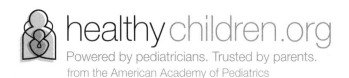
healthychildren.org
Powered by pediatricians. Trusted by parents.
from the American Academy of Pediatrics

*This book is also available in Spanish.

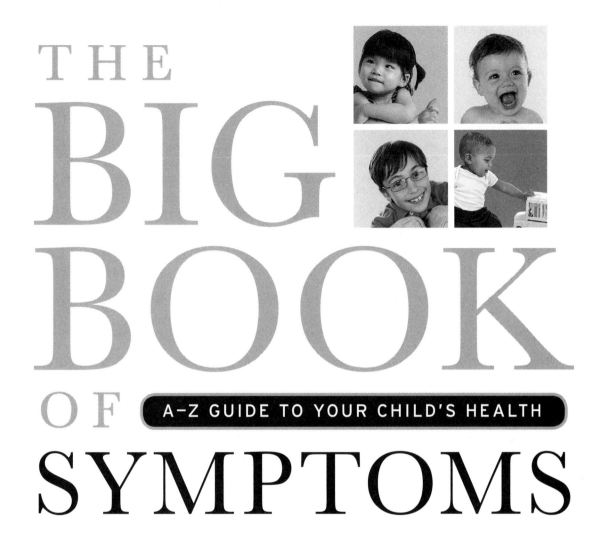

# THE
# BIG
# BOOK
## OF  A–Z GUIDE TO YOUR CHILD'S HEALTH
# SYMPTOMS

### EDITORS

Steven P. Shelov, MD, MS, FAAP    Shelly Vaziri Flais, MD, FAAP

American Academy of Pediatrics
DEDICATED TO THE HEALTH OF ALL CHILDREN™

**American Academy of Pediatrics Department of Marketing and Publications Staff**

*Director, Department of Marketing and Publications*
Maureen DeRosa, MPA

*Director, Division of Product Development*
Mark Grimes

*Project Coordinator, Product Development*
Holly Kaminski

*Director, Division of Publishing and Production Services*
Sandi King, MS

*Editorial Specialist*
Amanda Cozza

*Publishing and Production Services Specialist*
Shannan Martin

*Manager, Art Direction and Production*
Linda Diamond

*Digital Content and Production Specialist*
Houston A. Adams

*Director, Division of Marketing and Sales*
Julia Lee

*Manager, Consumer Marketing and Sales*
Kathleen Juhl, MBA

*Manager, Consumer Product Marketing*
Mary Jo Reynolds

Published by the American Academy of Pediatrics
141 Northwest Point Blvd, Elk Grove Village, IL 60007-1019
847/434-4000
Facsimile: 847/434-8000
www.aap.org

Cover design by Daniel Rembert
Book design by Linda Diamond

Second Edition–2014
First Edition–Copyright © 1997 American Academy of Pediatrics as *The Official, Complete Home Reference Guide to Your Child's Symptoms: Birth Through Adolescence*

Library of Congress Control Number: 2013945504
ISBN: 978-1-58110-840-8
eISBN: 978-1-58110-833-0
ePub: 978-1-58110-903-0
Mobi: 978-1-58110-904-7

CB0076
9-353

1 2 3 4 5 6 7 8 9 10

# About the Editors

**Steven P. Shelov, MD, FAAP,** is a professor of pediatrics at Stony Brook Medicine and associate dean of undergraduate medical education at the Winthrop University Hospital Regional Campus of Stony Brook. He received his medical doctorate from the Medical College of Wisconsin and his master's degree in administrative medicine from the University of Wisconsin. After completing his residency in pediatrics at Montefiore Medical Center, Albert Einstein College of Medicine, Dr Shelov became pediatric program director there, and over 17 years became a professor of pediatrics, director of pediatric education, and vice chairman of pediatrics. From 1997 to 2010 he was chairman of pediatrics at Maimonides Infants and Children's Hospital of Brooklyn. Author of more than 100 original publications and 15 books, he has been the founding editor in chief of the American Academy of Pediatrics guide for parents, *Caring for Your Baby and Young Child: Birth to Age 5,* since its first edition in 1991.

**Shelly Vaziri Flais, MD, FAAP,** is a board-certified practicing pediatrician and mother of 4 children. An instructor of clinical pediatrics with Northwestern University Feinberg School of Medicine and Ann & Robert H. Lurie Children's Hospital of Chicago, she is the author of the American Academy of Pediatrics *Raising Twins,* as well as a contributor for *Sleep: What Every Parent Needs to Know.* She has shared her reality-based parenting approach with national and local television, radio, Web-based, and print news outlets, as well as contributed to *Parents, Parenting, Twins,* and *Healthy Children* magazines. The first edition of *Raising Twins* was honored at both the 2010 National Health Information Awards and the 2009 Midwest Book Awards.

## About the American Academy of Pediatrics

The American Academy of Pediatrics is an organization of 62,000 primary care pediatricians, pediatric medical subspecialists, and pediatric surgical specialists dedicated to the health, safety, and well-being of infants, children, adolescents, and young adults.

# What People Are Saying

Covering over 100 childhood symptoms as well as the basics of first aid and safety, *The Big Book of Symptoms* addresses the most common ailments found in infants, children, and adolescents. This resource helps parents and other caregivers make sense of their child's physical complaints— from abdominal pain to headaches to ear infections and more—as well as behavioral and emotional issues such as anxiety, attention problems, and temper tantrums. Look no further for expert information on your child's symptoms!

— Jennifer Shu, MD, FAAP
   Pediatrician; mom; coauthor of *Heading Home With Your Newborn: From Birth to Reality* and *Food Fights: Winning the Nutritional Challenges of Parenthood Armed With Insight, Humor, and a Bottle of Ketchup*; and medical editor of HealthyChildren.org

As a mom, I've often wished I was a doctor so I would know exactly the right thing to do when my kids are hurt or sick. *The Big Book of Symptoms* saves us all the cost of medical school. It's written with real parents and their concerns in mind. It's like having your trusted pediatrician on speed dial 24/7.

— Tamara L. O'Shaughnessy
   Editor, *Chicago Parent*

Sometimes as a pediatrician I just wish I could download everything I know about children's health to a parent's brain. I still can't do that, which is probably good for my practice. But I can recommend that parents buy *The Big Book of Symptoms*. This volume should save parents an awful lot of late night phone calls while ensuring that they don't skip that one run to the emergency department if the need arises. *The Big Book of Symptoms* even includes extensive instructions on how to save a child's life. Hopefully, you'll never need to use that part, but you're still likely to call this book a lifesaver over and over again.

— David L. Hill, MD, FAAP
   Author, *Dad to Dad: Parenting Like a Pro*

# Acknowledgments

**Editors in Chief**

Shelly Vaziri Flais, MD, FAAP
Pediatric Health Associates
Naperville, IL
Instructor of Clinical Pediatrics
Northwestern University Feinberg School of Medicine
Anne & Robert H. Lurie Children's Hospital of Chicago
Chicago, IL

Steven P. Shelov, MD, MS, FAAP
Associate Dean, Undergraduate Medical Education
Winthrop University Hospital
Mineola, NY
Professor of Pediatrics
Stony Brook School of Medicine
Stony Brook, NY

**American Academy of Pediatrics Board of Directors Reviewer**

Kyle Yasuda, MD, FAAP

**Medical Reviewers and Contributors**

Leena Bhattacharya, MD, FAAP
Nathan Jon Blum, MD, FAAP
Carolyn Bridgemohan, MD, FAAP
Jane Marie Carnazzo, MD, FAAP
Manju Mathur Chandra, MD, FAAP
Earl Y. Cheng, MD, FAAP
Bernard A. Cohen, MD, FAAP
Mark Richard Corkins, MD, FAAP
James John Cummings, MD, FAAP
Elaine Donoghue, MD, FAAP
Daniel A. Frattarelli, MD
Robert W. Frenck Jr, MD
Geoffrey E. Bradford, MS, MD, FAAP
Neville Hylton Golden, MD, FAAP
Edward Goldson, MD, FAAP
Roberto Gugig, MD, FAAP
Susan M. Fuchs, MD, FAAP
Andrea Leigh Hahn, MD, FAAP
Melvin Bernard Heyman, MD, FAAP
William Paul Hitchcock, MD, FAAP
Marjorie Joan Hogan, MD, FAAP
Benjamin D. Hoffman, MD, FAAP
Anne-Marie Irani, MD, FAAP
Margaret Ikeda, MD, FAAP
Sabah Kalyoussef, DO, FAAP
Peter B. Kang, MD, FAAP
Julie P. Katkin, MD, FAAP

Leonard R. Krilov, MD, FAAP
David Matthew Krol, MD, MPH, FAAP
David Alan Levine, MD, FAAP
Sharon Levy, MD, MPH, FAAP
Michelle M. Macias, MD, FAAP
M. Jeffrey Maisels, MD, FAAP
Gerri Mattson, MD, FAAP
Juan Carlos Martinez, MD, FAAP
Rachel Y. Moon, MD, FAAP
Nancy Alice Murphy, MD, FAAP
Dennis L. Murray, MD, FAAP
Robert H. Pantell, MD, FAAP
Ian M. Paul, MD, MSc, FAAP
Georgina Peacock, MD, MPH, FAAP
Stephen J. Pont, MD, MPH, FAAP
Elizabeth C. Powell, MD, FAAP
Ritu Sachdeva, MD, FAAP
Scott R. Schoem, MD, FAAP
Richard M. Schwend, MD, FAAP
Adriana Segura, DDS, MS
Patricia D. Shearer, MD, FAAP
Irene N. Sills, MD, FAAP
Vincent Smith, MD, FAAP
Barbara K. Snyder, MD, FAAP
Edward P. Southern, MD, FAAP
Carol Cohen Weitzman, MD, FAAP

## Additional Assistance

Eileen Glasstetter
Bonnie Kozial
Jennifer McDonald

## Writer

Winnie Yu

## Associate Editor Emeritus of the Previous Edition

Donald Schiff, MD, FAAP

## Medical Reviewers/Contributors of the Previous Edition

Diane L. Barsky, MD
Robert B. Cady, MD
William J. Cochran, MD
George J. Cohen, MD
William Lord Coleman, MD
Michael K. Farrell, MD
F. Lane France, MD
Howard L. Freedman, MD
Derek Fyfe, MD
Edward M. Gotlieb, MD
Donald S. Gromisch, MD
Terry F. Hatch, MD
Jerome A. Hirschfeld, MD
Hector C. James, MD
Michael Jellinck, MD
Robert Kay, MD
Harold Koller, MD
Moise Levy, MD
Allan S. Lieberthal, MD

Jeffrey M. Maisels, MD
Douglas Moodie, MD
Edwin C. Myer, MD
William Oh, MD
Peter Pizzutillo, MD
J. Routt Reigart, MD
Anthony J. Richtsmeier, MD
Martin Sachs. DO
I. Ronald Shcnker, MD
Jack T. Swanson, MD
Katherinc C. Teets Grimm, MD
Hyman C. Tolmas, MD
Patricia A. Treadwcll, MD
Susan B. Tully, MD
David E. Tunkcl, MD
Michael Welch, MD
Robert A Wicbe, MD
Eugene S. Wiener, MD

# Foreword

The American Academy of Pediatrics (AAP) welcomes you to its newest parenting resource, *The Big Book of Symptoms: A–Z Guide to Your Child's Health.*

Designed in an easy-to-read A to Z format, this guide describes more than 100 childhood symptoms common among babies, children, and adolescents. This book helps parents distinguish minor everyday problems from more serious conditions and suggests a reasonable course of action. Also included is an illustrated first aid manual, a cardiopulmonary resuscitation (CPR) chart, and age-specific safety and injury prevention tips.

Under the direction of our medical editors, the material in this book was developed with the assistance of numerous reviewers and contributors. Because medical information is constantly changing, every effort has been made to ensure that this book contains the most up-to-date findings. Readers may want to visit the official AAP Web site for parents, HealthyChildren.org, to keep current on these findings and many other subjects.

It is the hope of the AAP that this book will become an invaluable resource and reference guide to parents. We are confident that parents will find the book extremely valuable. We encourage its use along with the advice and counsel of our readers' pediatricians, who will provide individual guidance and assistance related to the health of children.

The AAP is an organization of 62,000 primary care pediatricians, pediatric medical subspecialists, and pediatric surgical specialists dedicated to the physical, mental, and social health and well-being of all infants, children, adolescents, and young adults. *The Big Book of Symptoms: A–Z Guide to Your Child's Health* is a part of ongoing AAP educational efforts to provide parents and other caregivers with high quality information on a broad spectrum of children's health issues.

Errol R. Alden, MD, FAAP
Executive Director/CEO
American Academy of Pediatrics

# From the Editors

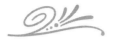

We dedicate this book to the
children, families, and colleagues
who continue to teach us on
this lifelong path of learning.

Dr Flais thanks her husband Mike
and their children, Matthew, Andrew, Ryan, and Nancy,
for steadfast and loving support.

Dr Shelov wishes to thank his wife Marsha;
his children, Josh, Danielle, and Eric;
and his grandchildren, Owen, Emma, Andrew, Henry, William, and Lydia,
for their love and devotion and for teaching him every day
how important family and children are to the
happy future of our precious world.

# Table of Contents

## Part 1 — Directory of Common Childhood Symptoms

### Chapter 1
### Common Symptoms in Babies During the First Few Months of Life

### Chapter 2
### Common Symptoms in Babies and Children

## Chapter 2
## Common Symptoms in Babies and Children *(cont)*

## Chapter 3
## Common Physical and Mental Health Symptoms in Teenagers

**Chapter 4**
**Basics of First Aid**

**Chapter 5**
**Guide to Safety and Prevention**

# Introduction

It's often said that raising a happy, healthy, well-adjusted child is one of the most demanding and challenging of all human endeavors. Fortunately, it's also one of life's most rewarding endeavors. What is more miraculous and exhilarating than the birth of a baby? Still, caring for a newborn is a demanding round-the-clock undertaking that's a learning process for both you and your baby; however, before long you will learn to interpret your baby's cries, grins, frowns, and other cues. You will gain confidence in your judgment and parenting skills. Amazingly, from the moment of birth, babies are learning at an even faster pace than their parents—not only about how to interpret cues from their parents but also about the big, new world they've entered.

Modern science is constantly confirming what parents have always known: babies thrive on love and attention. The groundwork laid for children in the first few years of life determines in large part adult values and success. But as every parent will tell you, now and then you'll come up against a situation in which you need help. It's important to realize you're not alone. For starters, your pediatrician is someone you can turn to for advice on everything from soothing a colicky baby to handling the inevitable colds, earaches, sore throats, and other common childhood ailments. Forming a solid working partnership with your pediatrician can help you get through these challenging moments and reinforce your judgment as you build confidence in your parenting skills.

Taking the lead on your child's health and well-being is among your primary responsibilities as a parent. From time to time, every parent must evaluate a child's symptoms and decide what action to take. For the first few months, it's a good idea to call your pediatrician if you're worried something is amiss. Before long you'll be able to judge whether the problem is one you can handle or whether you should seek your pediatrician's care. This book is designed to help you distinguish minor everyday problems from more serious problems. It suggests a reasonable course of action for each problem. It's important to stress, however, that no book can replace your own good judgment and your pediatrician's expertise—both very important elements in ensuring what's best for your child.

## How to Use This Book

*The Big Book of Symptoms: A–Z Guide to Your Child's Health* is divided into 2 major sections: an alphabetical directory of the most common childhood symptoms and an illustrated first aid manual and safety guide.

## Part 1

### Directory of Common Childhood Symptoms

As the bulk of the book, this section presents easy-to-follow charts for the most common childhood symptoms. The book is divided into 3 sections according to age.

 Infancy
(The First Few Months)

 Babies and Children

 Adolescence

In each section, the symptoms are listed alphabetically according to their common names. Each chart follows a similar format.

**❶ In General**

This introductory paragraph presents a brief overview of the symptom at its start and summarizes the important facts that parents should bear in mind.

**❷ Call Your Pediatrician If...**

This box lists circumstances that warrant either a conversation or a prompt call to your pediatrician. Read through it before going on to the rest of the chart.

**❸ Warning!**

This highlighted box, provides important information about specific aspects of a particular symptom.

**❹ Your Concerns**

Each chart is built on a series of concerns designed to help parents distinguish the most prominent features of an illness. The concerns begin with the most frequent characteristics of the illness and progress along the lines that your pediatrician might use.

**❺ Possible Cause**

This box gives the most likely cause of those particular symptoms.

**❻ Action to Take**

If the problem is one that you can manage at home, this box briefly outlines the action you can take. Other times you may be advised to call your pediatrician. The chart will also offer a brief summary of what your pediatrician might do to arrive at a diagnosis.

### Illustrated Boxes

In some of the charts you'll find an illustrated box that provides additional information about a particular illness.

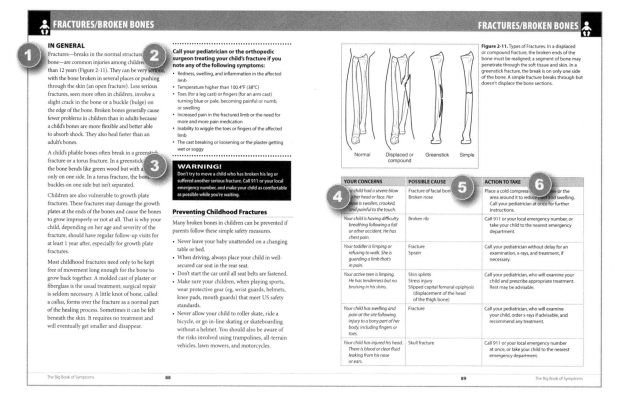

# Part 2

## Illustrated First Aid Manual and Guide to Safety and Prevention

This part of the book is designed to help you manage the unexpected—everything from minor cuts and scrapes to life-threatening emergencies. The first section, "The Basics of First Aid," is divided into parts: "Life-saving Techniques," which deals with such medical emergencies as choking and CPR (cardiopulmonary resuscitation), and "Frequently Used First Aid Measures," which covers less dire situations such as bites and stings, cuts and scrapes, bruises and sprains.

Make it a point to review this section before the need arises. When you're faced with a medical emergency, there's no time to consult this or any other books. From time to time, review this section to refresh your memory so you're ready if you're ever confronted with an emergency. Make sure that babysitters and other caregivers are also well versed in how to provide first aid. Don't forget to have an up-to-date list of all emergency numbers prominently displayed by every phone in your household.

Next comes the "Guide to Safety and Prevention." Included in this section are important measures to prevent injuries as well as a room-by-room guide to childproofing your home. We also provide safety checklists for your car, yard, playgrounds, vacation spots, and other areas you're likely to visit with a young child.

## Please Note

The information contained in this book is intended to complement, not be a substitute for, the advice of your child's pediatrician. Before starting any medical treatment or program, you should consult with your child's pediatrician, who can discuss your child's individual needs and counsel you about symptoms and treatment. If you have questions about how the information in this book applies to your child, speak with your child's pediatrician.

Products mentioned in this book are for informational purposes only. Inclusion in this publication does not constitute or imply a guarantee or an endorsement by the American Academy of Pediatrics.

The information and advice in this book apply to children of both sexes (except where noted). To indicate this, we have chosen to alternate between masculine and feminine pronouns throughout the book.

## CHAPTER 1

# Common Symptoms in Babies During the First Few Months of Life

### CARING FOR YOUR NEWBORN

Thanks to good prenatal care, serious illnesses are quite rare in babies in the first few months of life. But even healthy babies have days when they don't feel well. Germs are all around us, and infections that cause coughs and colds, stomach upsets, or eye problems are common in newborns and young infants. In general your pediatrician will want to see your baby if your baby shows any symptoms such as fever, cough, or diarrhea in her first 3 months. This is to make sure your baby doesn't have an underlying health problem that needs treatment.

Feeling a bit overwhelmed by the task of caring for a newborn is normal, especially if you haven't spent much time around babies. Family and friends are usually pleased when you ask them for help. In fact, they may give you more advice than you can handle, and some of it may not be completely up-to-date with what we currently know about newborns and young infants. Your pediatrician's main concern is to help you build your self-confidence and develop your skills as a parent. You can call on him or her for support. Together you have one goal: to see your baby grow up healthy and happy. In this you're a team, and the team leader is your baby.

Although you may feel unsure of yourself at first, your baby won't be shy about telling you what to do. Within just a few days or weeks, you'll be able to recognize the different cries that tell you your baby is hungry, happy, needing a clean diaper, or ready for play. Within months, you'll be cheering your infant's attempts to walk and listening to your infant's magical first words. This chapter is a guide to meeting your baby's needs in his first few months. It will help you recognize minor symptoms you can deal with alone as well as health problems that require your pediatrician's attention. If you have any doubts—or you just need reassurance—you can call your pediatrician. His or her advice reflects the newest information from research into babies' health and development. It also reflects your pediatrician's years of experience not just in treating children's illnesses but also in caring for children.

## IN GENERAL

All babies cry when they need something. Parents soon learn what their baby's various cries mean: hunger, a soiled diaper, fatigue, or another need. Normal, fussy crying should not be confused with *colic*—bouts of intense crying that last for hours at a time and may repeat daily. These bouts occur at about the same time each day. They begin when a newborn is 2 to 4 weeks old and usually last up to 3 or 4 months, although some infants are still colicky at 6 months of age. Babies with colic often pass a lot of gas, which is perfectly normal. No one knows for sure what causes colic, although many pediatricians believe it's a stage in the development of the nervous system. About 1 in 5 babies develops colic; interestingly, firstborn babies and boys are affected more often than later-born babies and girls.

• • • • • • • • • • • • • • • • • • • • • • • • • • • • • • •

### Talk with your pediatrician to rule out any serious medical causes if

• Your baby cries again and again for no obvious reason, or you can't seem to calm his crying.

• • • • • • • • • • • • • • • • • • • • • • • • • • • • • • •

### WARNING!

Colic can be very upsetting, especially for first-time parents. Family and friends with parenting experience know what you're going through, as does your pediatrician. Call on your pediatrician and your support network when you need to talk about your worries. Don't take your frustration out on your baby. Shaking a newborn or young infant can cause brain damage that can't be reversed. Reach out for support if you feel overwhelmed by caring for your baby.

## Coping With Colic

Many babies with colic cry at about the same time every day, for just about the same length of time. A colicky newborn or young infant often cries for 3 to 5 hours a day, beginning in the late afternoon or evening. Very often such crying stops as suddenly as it began, and the baby falls asleep. This difficult phase will pass eventually; colic rarely lasts beyond 4 or 5 months of age. Talk with your pediatrician to rule out any medical causes for your baby's crying, and ask about ways you and your baby can cope with colic, such as

• Your baby may find it soothing to be swaddled in a blanket or held close to you in an infant carrier or sling that meets current safety standards. You may need to swaddle or rock your baby for hours at a time. Some pediatricians suggest placing the baby in an infant swing.

• Offer your baby a pacifier.

• Lay your baby on his tummy and gently rub his back; your touch is soothing, and the pressure on his abdomen may relieve discomfort.

• Quietly sing or hum a repetitive, rhythmical tune. To soothe your baby you might also consider using a white noise machine, an electric fan (pointed elsewhere in the room) for white noise, or even a morning radio station turned to static.

• If you're breastfeeding, check with your pediatrician about dietary changes you can make. You may wish to try cutting out dairy products, caffeine, and gassy foods. Colic caused by sensitivity to any of these foods should disappear within a few days.

• If your baby is on a cow's milk formula, ask your pediatrician to recommend an alternative.

• Try to take regular breaks. If you haven't yet found a babysitter you can depend on, at least alternate evenings with your partner so one of you can get out of the house for a short break. At the very least, take a walk or a hot shower.

• Admit feelings of anger and frustration, and call a relative or friend at once if you feel you may lose control or harm your baby. Try taking a deep breath and counting to 10. If you're feeling at your wit's end, the safest action to take is to leave your baby in her crib or another safe place and go into another room while allowing her to cry it out alone. Getting a handle on your anger and frustration is important to prevent abusive head trauma, a serious form of child abuse that occurs mostly in infants in the first year of life.

| YOUR CONCERNS | POSSIBLE CAUSE | ACTION TO TAKE |
|---|---|---|
| *Your baby cries with great force and energy at about the same time each day, but she calms down after she's received attention.* | Fussiness | Keep giving your baby the attention she's asking for. She enjoys your company and will soon find ways to ask for it other than fussy crying. |
| *Your baby is younger than 4 months and generally content. He cries regularly throughout the day and especially hard for 1 to 3 hours in the late afternoon or evening. When he cries, he passes gas, pulls up his legs, and wriggles as if in pain.* | Colicky crying, which normally occurs between 2 weeks and 4 or 5 months of age | Make sure your baby is properly fed and burped, is comfortably clothed, and has a clean diaper. Cuddle your baby, and train yourself to put up with his crying, knowing it will stop on its own within a few weeks (see "Coping With Colic," page 2). If his crying seems unusually desperate, call your pediatrician, who may wish to examine your baby to rule out any medical causes. |
| *Your baby cries a lot at the end of a day that involved several new experiences, such as meeting new people.* | Overstimulation | Comfort your baby and make sure her needs are met. Some newborns and young infants are extremely sensitive to new experiences and simply need time to get used to them. |
| *You have tension in your family. The primary caregiver is under an unusual amount of stress.* | Emotional tension | Even newborns sense emotional changes. If a major change is taking place, one that causes a lot of conflict, confusion, or anger, try to keep your baby's routine as close to normal as possible. Give him extra attention, and try to ease your own stress. |
| *Your baby rarely cries. She is refusing her last feeding of the day. She has a runny nose or sniffles.* | Ear infection | Carefully watch and listen to your baby for 48 to 72 hours. A baby with an ear infection may appear fine during the day but experience severe pain when you lay her down or at night. Call your pediatrician if your baby doesn't improve. Your pediatrician may suggest over-the-counter pain relievers or numbing drops to lessen your baby's pain. Or your pediatrician may wish to see your baby. |
| *Your breastfed baby cries several hours after you eat a dairy product, and you can't seem to calm his crying.* | Sensitivity to cow's milk (uncommon) | Talk with your pediatrician and, if he or she agrees, eliminate all dairy products from your diet for 2 weeks. A few babies will respond, but most don't. If your baby's symptoms do disappear but recur when you start to eat dairy products again, your baby may have a sensitivity to cow's milk. If so, ask your pediatrician about changing parts of your diet. |
| *Your baby's crying is distressed but more than usual. Her abdomen is tense and distended (larger and rounder because of pressure from inside). She is vomiting yellowish-green material or passing blood in her stool.* | Intestinal blockage or other potentially serious intestinal problems | Call your pediatrician without delay. Don't feed your baby until your pediatrician has seen her. Your baby may need emergency treatment. |

It's never ok to shake, throw, hit, slam, or jerk your baby. Abusive head trauma can cause serious brain damage, blindness, damage to the spinal cord, and delay in normal development. Signs and symptoms include irritability, lethargy (trouble staying awake), tremors (shakiness), vomiting, seizures, trouble breathing, and coma.

If your baby has been shaken by a caregiver, take him to the emergency department or your pediatrician right away. He will need to be evaluated. Any brain damage that might have occurred will only get worse without treatment.

## Keeping Your Baby Happy With a Pacifier

Pacifiers should never be used to replace or delay feedings. If you give a pacifier to a hungry baby, she may get so upset that she can't feed. Properly used, pacifiers don't cause any medical or psychological problems. If you're buying a pacifier, look for a one-piece model with a soft nipple in a size that's right for your baby's age. Clean it in boiling water or in the dishwasher. Never tie a pacifier around your baby's neck or give your baby a bottle nipple in place of a pacifier.

## IN GENERAL

Diarrhea isn't just a loose stool; it's a watery stool that occurs up to 12 times a day. A breastfed baby's stools are light yellow, soft, or even runny, and they often contain small pieces that look like seeds. Breastfed babies may pass stools with every breastfeeding. Babies who are formula-fed pass stools that are yellow to tan and about as firm as peanut butter. Whether you breastfeed or formula-feed your baby, as he grows it's normal for you to see stools less frequently. For diarrhea in older infants and young children, see "Diarrhea in Infants and Children," page 70.

A greenish tinge to the stools is normal. As long as your baby is feeding and growing normally, you should not be concerned unless her stools are whitish and clay-like, watery and filled with mucus, or hard and dry. They should also not be black or bloody. If they are, call your pediatrician.

### Call your pediatrician right away if your baby has diarrhea and

- Is 3 months or younger
- Has a rectal temperature of 100.4°F (38°C) or higher
- Is vomiting
- Lacks energy or is irritable and doesn't want to feed
- Has signs of dehydration, such as dry mouth, or has not passed urine for 3 or more hours

### WARNING!

A baby can become dehydrated quickly. If your baby is younger than 3 months and has a fever (see "Fever in Babies Younger Than 3 Months," page 8) as well as diarrhea, call your pediatrician at once. If your baby is older than 3 months and has had mild diarrhea with a slight fever for more than a day, check whether he's passing a normal amount of urine. Also check his temperature with a thermometer. Then call your pediatrician.

## Coping With Diarrhea in Babies

A viral infection that causes vomiting and diarrhea may make your baby irritable for 1 or 2 days. If your baby is otherwise healthy, symptoms should clear up on their own. Your pediatrician will advise giving fluids to your baby to make up for the fluids and electrolytes (eg, sodium, potassium) lost with the diarrhea. If you're breastfeeding, your pediatrician will probably recommend that you keep breastfeeding as usual. If your baby is formula-fed, your pediatrician may instruct you to give your baby a special drink that contains electrolytes and sugar. Pharmacies carry premixed drinks with the right balance of electrolytes for newborns and young infants; homemade solutions may not have the correct electrolyte balance and therefore should not be used.

| YOUR CONCERNS | POSSIBLE CAUSE | ACTION TO TAKE |
|---|---|---|
| Your baby passes several stools every day. | Normal digestion | As long as your baby is happy and feeding well, you don't need to take action. Her number of stools will decrease eventually. |
| Your baby suddenly starts passing more stools than usual. His stools are watery. He is vomiting, feverish, or irritable. | Diarrhea<br>Viral gastroenteritis (inflammation of the stomach and intestinal lining caused by a virus) | Call your pediatrician, who may wish to examine your child and recommend treatment. |

## IN GENERAL

During the first year of life, a baby's main food is human milk, formula, or a combination of both foods. (Pediatricians advise introducing solids when your infant is 4 to 6 months of age or doubles her birth weight.) Your concern is to make sure your baby is getting enough calories. You can do this by laying down a regular schedule for feedings. This doesn't mean setting a rigid schedule and insisting that your baby eat a certain amount of food at each feeding. Paying attention to your baby's signals and working around her needs is more important (also see "Spitting Up," page 16).

Early on your baby should be fed about every 2 to 3 hours on demand, with your attempts to feed him occurring 8 to 12 times a day. If your baby sleeps longer than 4 to 5 hours and starts missing feedings, wake him up and offer a bottle or breast. In fact, if your baby is younger than 2 to 3 months and sleeping through the night without feeding, he may not be getting enough to eat. On the other hand, some babies may "cluster feed" every 1 to 2 hours, which helps increase your milk supply.

Growth spurts may make your baby hungrier than usual. These occur around 3 weeks, 6 weeks, 3 months, and 6 months of age, although they may vary from baby to baby. Even if you can't see a change in the rate of growth, be prepared to let your baby feed more often if she's breastfed, or offer her more formula at bottle feedings. For feeding problems in older children and teenagers, see "Eating Disorders," page 184.

• • • • • • • • • • • • • • • • • • • • • • • • • • • • • • • • • •

### Talk with your pediatrician if your baby

- Is losing or unable to gain weight
- Continues to have wrinkled or yellow skin after the first week of life
- Has loose, very watery stools 8 or more times a day
- Vomits forcefully after every feeding

• • • • • • • • • • • • • • • • • • • • • • • • • • • • • • • • • •

**WARNING!**
Many parents worry that their baby isn't feeding properly. Visiting your pediatrician to check your baby's weight gain during the first 2 months of life can be reassuring.

### Giving Your Baby the Right Amount of Food

Knowing if you're giving your baby the correct amount of human milk or formula is never easy. But keep in mind that your baby's stomach is small, about the size of his tiny fist. After the first few days of life, your formula-fed newborn will take 2 to 3 ounces (60–90 mL) of formula per feeding. During his first few weeks, he'll eat every 3 to 4 hours on average. Breastfed newborns usually take smaller, more frequent feedings. By the end of their first month, they will be up to at least 4 ounces (120 mL) per feeding, with a fairly predictable schedule of feedings about every 4 hours. By 6 months of age, your infant will consume 6 to 8 ounces (180–240 mL) at each of his 4 or 5 feedings in a 24-hour period.

On average your baby should take about 2.5 ounces (75 mL) of formula a day for every pound (453 g) of body weight; however, she will regulate her intake from day to day to meet her unique needs. Rather than going by fixed amounts, let your baby tell you when she's had enough. Most babies are satisfied with 3 to 4 ounces (90–120 mL) at each feeding during the first month of life. They will increase that amount by 1 ounce (30 mL) per month until they reach a maximum of about 7 to 8 ounces (210–240 mL) when they are 7 to 8 months of age. If your baby consistently seems to want more or less than this amount of food, talk with your pediatrician.

| YOUR CONCERNS | POSSIBLE CAUSE | ACTION TO TAKE |
|---|---|---|
| *Your baby is sometimes slow to take the breast or nipple. Sometimes she goes back to sleep after a few mouthfuls.* | Not yet really hungry Sleepy (very common in a baby's first week of life) | Stroke your baby's cheek and mouth next to the breast or bottle to stimulate the rooting reflex and make her seek the nipple. If your baby isn't hungry, wait a few minutes. If you find your baby tends to fall back asleep, undress her down to her diaper. |
| *Your baby gets too frantic and upset to feed.* | Temperament Over-hungry Colic (See "Crying/Colic," page 2.) | Have everything ready before your baby becomes overly upset. Feed him in a quiet place. Your baby will outgrow colic. Test out shorter times between feedings. |
| *Your baby spits up after most feedings but is gaining weight normally (see "Spitting Up," page 16).* | Normal behavior or possible overfeeding | Your baby will outgrow spitting up. Protect yourself with a towel, and keep your baby calm after feedings. Ask your pediatrician if you may be overfeeding your baby. |
| *Your baby vomits after every feeding. She is losing or unable to gain weight.* | Pyloric stenosis or other digestive blockage, gastroesophageal reflux disease (backward flow of the stomach contents into the esophagus) | Call your pediatrician for evaluation and management. |
| *Your baby's stools are watery, bloody, or full of mucus. He passes 8 or more stools in a day.* | Infectious diarrhea Food sensitivity or allergy | Call your pediatrician. |
| *Your baby isn't gaining weight as you think she should.* | Failure to thrive | Call your pediatrician promptly. Your baby may need only simple measures, but your pediatrician should examine her to rule out any serious health problems. Your pediatrician can also go over your baby's growth chart with you. |

## IN GENERAL

Many parents are uneasy to learn that their baby has a fever; however, most fevers are harmless. In fact, a fever turns on our immune system and helps our body fight infection. You should treat a fever only if it causes your baby discomfort. Keep in mind too that how your baby appears is more important than the number on a thermometer.

Normal human body temperature ranges within about 1°F higher or lower than the average temperature of 98.6°F (37°C). Few babies get through infancy without at least 1 or 2 mild infections. These infections are signaled by any number of symptoms, which may include an increase in body temperature.

If you suspect your baby has a fever and you want to take his temperature, take a rectal temperature with a digital thermometer. This will give you the best reading (if your baby is younger than 12 months). Call your pediatrician right away if your baby›s temperature is 100.4°F (38°C) or higher. In addition, call your pediatrician for further advice if your infant's fever continues longer than 24 or 48 hours. Your infant may be at risk of dehydration due to increased fluid losses due to the fever. This danger is made worse if your baby is also vomiting or has diarrhea.

### Call your pediatrician right away if

- Your baby is younger than 3 months and has a temperature higher than 100.4°F (38°C).
- You can't comfort your baby, and he has symptoms such as trouble breathing, little energy, diarrhea, or vomiting, or he seems to be getting progressively sicker.

### WARNING!

Never give aspirin to your baby to reduce his fever. The use of aspirin has been linked to an increased risk of Reye syndrome. Reye syndrome is a rare but serious illness, associated with viral infections, that affects the brain and liver. While acetaminophen (eg, Tylenol) can help reduce a fever and relieve discomfort, never give it or any other medications to a baby younger than 3 months without your pediatrician's advice. If your pediatrician advises giving a medication, be careful not to exceed the recommended dose (eg, by giving your baby cold medication that also contains acetaminophen). Also make sure you use the measuring device that comes with the medication.

| YOUR CONCERNS | POSSIBLE CAUSE | ACTION TO TAKE |
|---|---|---|
| *Your baby's face looks flushed. She is restless and sweaty, although she doesn't seem ill. Her hair is damp, and she has a heat rash.* | Overheating | Keep the temperature of the room comfortable and on the cool side. Check to make sure your baby isn't overdressed. If your baby is sweating or has damp hair, flushed cheeks, or heat rash, she is getting too hot. |
| *Your infant's temperature is 100.4°F (38°C) or higher, and he's younger than 3 months.* | Infection or another health problem that may require evaluation and treatment | Call your pediatrician. A fever in a baby younger than 3 months is potentially serious. Your pediatrician will want to examine your baby to rule out any serious infections or illnesses. |

## How to Take a Rectal Temperature

If your baby is younger than 12 months and you suspect he has a fever, taking a rectal temperature will give you the best reading. To take a rectal temperature, follow these 6 steps (Figure 1-1).

1. Always use a digital thermometer to check your baby's temperature.

2. Clean the end of the thermometer with rubbing alcohol or soap and water. Rinse it with cool water. Don't rinse it with hot water.

3. Put a small amount of lubricant, such as petroleum jelly, on the end of the thermometer.

4. Place your baby belly-down across your lap or on a firm surface. Hold him by placing your palm against his lower back, just above his bottom. Or place your baby faceup and bend his legs to his chest. Rest your free hand against the back of his thighs.

5. With the other hand, turn the thermometer on and insert it half an inch to an inch into the anal opening. Don't insert it too far. Hold the thermometer in place loosely with 2 fingers, keeping your hand cupped around your baby's bottom. Keep it there for about 1 minute, until you hear the "beep." Then remove it and check the digital reading.

6. Be sure to label the rectal thermometer so it's not accidentally used in the mouth.

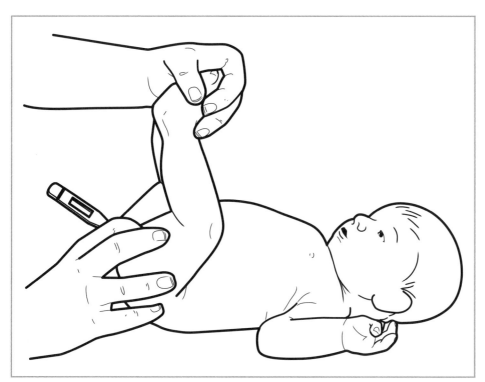

**Figure 1-1.** Baby lying on back getting rectal temperature taken.

## IN GENERAL

Jaundice is a yellow-green discoloration in the skin and usually the whites of the eyes. It is caused by higher than normal levels of bilirubin in the blood. Bilirubin is a pigment that forms when red blood cells break down at the end of their natural cycle or are damaged. It is normally processed through the liver and passed in the stools. Jaundice is seen in 4 out of 5 newborns because their immature livers can't keep up with the amount of bilirubin being produced (see "Treating Jaundice in a Newborn"). Many breastfed babies develop jaundice that continues past the first week of life. This isn't a cause for alarm; your pediatrician can examine your baby to rule out unusual and serious causes of jaundice.

In older children, teenagers, and young adults, jaundice signals that an infection or another health problem is getting in the way of the liver's function. A child of any age with jaundice must be seen by a pediatrician who will determine the cause of it and recommend treatment.

### Call your pediatrician right away if

• Your child develops a yellow color in her skin or the whites of her eyes.

## Treating Jaundice in Newborns

Many healthy babies develop a yellowish tinge in their skin and the whites of their eyes during the first few days of life. This health problem, called *physiologic jaundice,* shows that the blood has an excess of bilirubin, a chemical that's released during the normal breakdown of old red blood cells. Everyone's blood contains bilirubin, but newborns often have higher levels of it. This is because they have extra red blood cells at birth, and the life span of these cells is shorter than it is in adults. Bilirubin is processed and cleared through the liver. The livers of newborns, however, aren't yet working at full capacity. Babies with mild jaundice regain their healthy pink color without special treatment.

Normal bilirubin levels are harmless in a healthy baby, but if the bilirubin level becomes unusually high, it may cause brain injury. Depending on your baby's bilirubin level and degree of prematurity, or if your baby is ill, your pediatrician may prescribe phototherapy. In this treatment exposure to special lights helps eliminate bilirubin until the baby's liver is more mature. These lights don't produce ultraviolet light. Even with this treatment, the bilirubin level may remain mildly higher than normal for several days or weeks. How your pediatrician treats your baby with phototherapy depends on your baby's bilirubin level. Your baby may receive treatment at home or in the hospital where he can be continually monitored by health care professionals. Sometimes doctors prefer to treat babies with mild jaundice by using more frequent feedings of human milk or formula. This helps them pass the bilirubin in their stools.

| YOUR CONCERNS | POSSIBLE CAUSE | ACTION TO TAKE |
|---|---|---|
| *Your baby is older than 1 day but younger than 1 week and has jaundice.* | Physiologic jaundice | Talk with your pediatrician. He or she will examine your baby and prescribe any necessary treatments. (Usually treatment isn't required.) |
| *Your breastfed baby is older than 1 week and is still yellow in appearance.* | Breastfeeding jaundice or another health problem that requires evaluation and treatment | Call your pediatrician. He or she will examine your baby and determine the cause of the jaundice. Three-fourths of breastfed babies remain mildly affected by jaundice for at least 1 week, which isn't harmful. |
| *Your breastfed baby is older than 2 weeks and still has jaundice. His stools are unusually pale.* | Breast milk jaundice | Call your pediatrician. If the jaundice persists for a few more days, further testing might be necessary. |
| *Your formula-fed baby is older than 2 weeks and still has jaundice. Her stools are unusually pale.* | Biliary atresia (blockage of the bile ducts) Another blockage that makes bile flow difficult | Call your pediatrician. Further testing will be necessary for him or her to determine the cause and recommend treatment. |

## IN GENERAL

A baby's skin is protected before birth by a cheese-like coating, called *vernix*. Vernix is produced toward the end of pregnancy. Once it's washed off (after birth), the baby's skin may peel a little as it's exposed to air. This is normal and doesn't require treatment.

In addition, many babies have birthmarks that fade away slowly over time without treatment. But some birthmarks may grow larger before they disappear, and others are permanent. Your pediatrician will advise whether a birthmark should be treated or left alone. Newborns and young infants may develop many different rashes in the first few months of life. Like birthmarks, these rashes generally disappear without treatment. But if your baby has a persistent (won't go away) or widespread rash, bring it to your pediatrician's attention.

A baby usually doesn't need powders, oils, and lotions to keep the skin smooth, no matter what baby product advertisements may claim. If your baby's skin seems very dry, rub a little non-perfumed baby lotion or ointment on the dry patches. Avoid using baby oil, which contains fragrance and doesn't lubricate as well as lotion. Use only soaps and skin-care products that are made especially for babies; other products may contain perfumes, dyes, alcohol, and other chemicals that can cause irritation.

A daily bath is fine for your baby, and while unnecessary, it can be part of a consistent bedtime routine. Just make sure the water temperature is warm against the inside of your wrist or elbow, and limit the time length of the bath. Use fragrance-free moisturizers. Cream or ointments applied after a bath can help skin stay hydrated. Keep your baby clean by washing all traces of food from his face and hands, and wash the diaper area thoroughly during changes.

. . . . . . . . . . . . . . . . . . . . . . . . . . . . . . . . . .

### Talk with your pediatrician if your baby has

- A persistent (won't go away) or widespread rash
- An birthmark that's becoming larger

. . . . . . . . . . . . . . . . . . . . . . . . . . . . . . . . . .

### WARNING!

Use plain water and absorbent cotton or a fresh washcloth for cleaning your baby—Using commercial wipes is unnecessary. But if you do, choose ones made for babies; those made for adults contain alcohol, which may dry and irritate the skin.

## Coping With Diaper Rash

Many babies have a mild rash in the diaper area at some point during infancy. Common causes of this rash include a diaper that has been left on for too long or irritation from diarrhea or loose stools. Chemicals that form in the wet or soiled diaper irritate the skin, making it vulnerable to infection. The rash usually appears as redness or bumps on skin surfaces that are in direct contact with a wet or soiled diaper. These surfaces include the lower abdomen, the buttocks, the genitals, and the folds of the thighs. If you promptly attend to your baby's rash, it usually improves in 3 or 4 days. Treating diaper rash is important because damaged skin becomes more easily irritated by contact with urine and stools.

Diaper rash is more likely if babies are not changed frequently. It is also common in babies who have very frequent bowel movements. In addition, babies tend to get diaper rashes when they are being treated with antibiotics, which kill friendly bacteria and allow an increase in loose stools and an overgrowth of yeasts normally found on the skin.

Try to reduce your baby's risk of diaper rash by changing his diaper as soon as possible after his bowel movements. Also clean his diaper area with plain water and absorbent cotton or a soft cloth. Change wet diapers to keep your baby's skin from being exposed to moisture and chemicals in his urine. Let your baby go without a diaper whenever you can. If you use disposable diapers that close tightly around the thighs and abdomen, make sure they are loose enough so that air can circulate inside of them.

If your baby gets a diaper rash, apply a zinc oxide–based cream or petroleum jelly to the rash, and change her diaper frequently. Talk with your pediatrician if you don't see an improvement in 2 to 3 days.

| YOUR CONCERNS | POSSIBLE CAUSE | ACTION TO TAKE |
|---|---|---|
| Your baby has 1 or more pinkish, brown, red, or purple patches on her body. | Nevus flammeus (birthmarks), hemangiomas (blood vessels or growths) or port-wine stains (dark red to purple birthmarks) acquired in the first few weeks of life | Evaluation and treatment, if necessary, depends on the type of birthmark. Pink, patchy flat marks in certain locations (ie, nape of the neck, mid-forehead, midline upper lip, around the sides of the nose, eyelids) are known as salmon patches or stork bites. They usually fade on their own in 12 to 18 months. Bright red hemangiomas ("strawberry marks") first grow quickly and then hold steady. They disappear slowly by the time your child is about 5 to 7 years of age. If a hemangioma develops an ulcer in its center, interferes with your baby's vision, or causes other concerns, it may require treatment. Your pediatrician may need to evaluate port-wine stains for possible treatment. |
| Your baby has a large bluish-gray mark like a bruise on his back or buttocks. | Mongolian spot | This mark is common. It will fade, probably before your child reaches 5 years of age. |
| Your new baby has lots of little yellow-white spots on her nose, upper lip, cheeks, and forehead. | Sebaceous hyperplasia Milia (tiny whiteheads) Miliaria (prickly heat) | The first 2 conditions are caused by enlarged oil glands, which require no treatment and will disappear. Prickly heat will clear up without treatment; in the meantime, avoid overdressing your baby. |
| Your baby is getting blackheads, whiteheads, or another acne-like blemish. | Neonatal acne | Acne is common in newborns and young infants, possibly due to the mother's or baby's hormones. It should clear up without treatment, but if it persists, talk with your pediatrician. |
| Your baby has developed greasy, yellow-brown patches on his scalp and behind his ears. | Seborrheic dermatitis (cradle cap; see "Hair Loss," page 94) | Wash your baby's scalp often with a mild shampoo and pat it dry; rubbing his scalp with baby lotion or petroleum jelly before washing it may soften the crusts. Your pediatrician may recommend a cream. |
| Your baby has a red, spotty rash in her diaper area. | Diaper rash (irritation by urine or stools, or complicated with a yeast or bacteria infection) Seborrhea (skin glands secrete an excess of fatty matter) Psoriasis (rare; skin becomes rough and red, and falls off) | Change wet or soiled diapers promptly. Clean your baby with plain water, and pat her dry. Petroleum jelly or a zinc oxide–based cream can protect her affected skin. If the rash doesn't improve or gets worse, call your pediatrician. |
| Your baby has red, scaly patches on his cheeks, diaper area, or elsewhere. | Eczema | Talk with your pediatrician. If the eczema is severe, your pediatrician may talk with a dermatologist (see "Allergic Reactions," page 26). |
| Your baby has developed fluid-filled blisters on her body. | Bullous impetigo (a staphylococcal infection) | Call your pediatrician at once. This is a potentially serious health problem and requires prompt medical treatment. |

## IN GENERAL

Newborns and young infants sleep when their stomachs are full and wake up when it's time for a feeding; however, even at this stage, you can begin to teach your baby that daytime is for play and interaction, whereas nighttime is for sleeping. During nighttime feedings, keep lights dim, speak quietly, and avoid taking longer than necessary to change your baby's diaper. Put your baby right back to bed after feeding, changing, and quietly cuddling her.

By the time a baby reaches 12 or 13 pounds, his stomach can hold enough milk to tide him through the night. In fact, by 3 months of age most babies are sleeping 6 to 8 hours without waking for most nights. But try not to be upset when the pattern changes; sleep can be broken by colds and other illnesses, separation anxiety (see "Fears," page 84), and many other factors. Even after you've established a routine, your baby may get mixed up by oversleeping during the day and sleeping less at night. He will return to his old sleep patterns if you're patient and keep to the schedule.

Ending your baby's day with a bath, changing her into sleep clothes, and following a regular going-to-bed routine also help divide the hours into waking and sleeping. If you set a regular schedule, you'll find it easier to cope with those few exceptions to the rule.

Babies sometimes need a little help to get back to sleep, mostly in the first few months of life. Newborns fall asleep more easily in a soothing environment. For many infants a pacifier is helpful. Many babies also do well with a relaxing and consistent evening routine that includes a bath, changing into pajamas, and a bedtime story. Listening to soft music can help too. Once your baby is drowsy, place him into his crib while he's still awake. (For more tips on calming a restless baby, see "Crying/Colic," page 2.) While babies can often sleep through a surprisingly high level of steady noise, such as the sounds of street traffic or older siblings playing, a sudden, different sound—crinkling paper or a key in a lock—can wake them up at once.

### Call your pediatrician if

- Your baby is waking at night and has a fever.
- Your baby sleeps almost all the time and is never fully alert.

### WARNING!

Try not to rush to your baby every time you hear a sound. She may be fussing or even crying during a phase of very light sleep. This is normal for some babies as they learn to resettle back to sleep. Of course, if her crying tells you she's hungry, in pain, or wants her diaper changed, give her the attention she needs and then put her back to bed.

## Positioning Your Baby for Sleep

When it comes time to put your baby down to sleep, make sure to place her on her back on a firm mattress. Studies suggest that infants who sleep on their backs are less likely to experience sudden infant death syndrome (SIDS). Exceptions to this practice include babies with facial malformations that could cause an airway blockage when they are lying on their back, babies who are vomiting, and babies with upper airway anatomic problems, such as a laryngeal cleft. Vomiting does not mean the same thing as spitting up. For more information on spitting up, please see page 16. For more information on vomiting, refer to "Vomiting," page 168.

Also important is clearing the crib of toys and any kind of soft bedding, including blankets and bumpers. These items can impair sleep if they are close to your baby's face.

Sudden infant death syndrome occurs for many reasons, and sleep position may be only a minor one. Still, pediatricians feel these 2 things are possibly linked, so as of now the safest action is to follow their advice. Once a baby can roll over and find a comfortable position for himself—most often between 4 and 7 months of age—he's usually past the highest-risk time for SIDS.

| YOUR CONCERNS | POSSIBLE CAUSE | ACTION TO TAKE |
| --- | --- | --- |
| *Your baby twitches, jerks, and moves his eyes when asleep. He sleeps with his eyes partly open.* | Normal sleep behavior for a newborn or young infant | None. The movements are probably occurring during rapid eye movement sleep, when the baby is dreaming. In time, he will close his eyes completely when asleep. |
| *Your baby is 3 months of age and still not sleeping through the night. She is feeding well and growing normally.* | Normal behavior | Your baby will settle eventually. Try to establish a bedtime routine. Consider testing out earlier bedtimes. |
| *Your baby cries as if in pain when you lay him in his crib. He is feverish and has a runny nose.* | Illness such as a respiratory or ear infection (See "Fever in Babies Younger Than 3 Months," page 8.) | Call your pediatrician. |
| *Your baby breathes noisily whether asleep or awake.* | Laryngotracheal malacia (normal softness of airway tissues) | If your baby is feeding, sleeping, and growing normally, the noisy breathing just shows that the tissues are not yet firm. She will outgrow this noisy breathing by about 18 months of age, but bring it to your pediatrician's attention. |
| *Your baby's breathing is labored. He seems to be having trouble breathing.* | Respiratory distress | Call your pediatrician right away, or go directly to the emergency department. |
| *Your baby has become more wakeful at night during the latter half of his first year.* | Separation anxiety (See "Fears," page 84.) | Discuss your concerns with your pediatrician. |

## IN GENERAL

If a baby's stomach is full or the baby's position is all of a sudden changed after a feeding, the stomach contents can force the sphincter open and flood back up the esophagus. In contrast to vomiting (see "Vomiting," page 168), spitting up doesn't involve forceful muscle contractions, brings up only small amounts of milk, and doesn't distress your baby or make him uncomfortable.

Many babies spit up after gulping down air with milk or formula. The best way to prevent this is to feed your baby before she gets very hungry. Hold her at an angle that prevents air from entering her mouth while she feeds. Gently burp her when she takes breaks during feedings (see "Tips to Reduce Spitting Up"). Limit active play after meals, and hold your baby in an upright position for at least 20 minutes. If spitting up is happening more than usual, some pediatricians advise thickening the formula with a small amount of rice cereal. To do this, add 1 to 3 teaspoons of cereal to each ounce of formula. Spitting up usually stops once your baby learns to pull herself into a sitting position, but a few babies continue to spit up until they are weaned to a cup or can walk. Until the spitting up stops, try to get in the habit of protecting yourself with a towel or cloth diaper during feedings and burpings.

### Talk with your pediatrician if
- Your baby vomits forcefully after every feeding.
- Your baby is losing or unable to gain weight.
- There is blood in your baby's vomit.

### WARNING!

Don't persist with feeding once your baby has turned away from the bottle. He knows how much his stomach can handle, and the extra milk you urge him to take may only cause him to spit up.

## Tips to Reduce Spitting Up

Spitting up is almost impossible to prevent. But you can use feeding techniques to keep your baby from swallowing air she doesn't need. The following tips may help you reduce the amount of food your baby spits up and the number of times it happens:

- Feed your baby before he becomes famished.
- Keep feeding times calm, quiet, slow, and relaxed.
- Avoid interruptions, sudden noises, bright lights, and other distractions during feedings.
- Burp your baby every 3 to 5 minutes or when she pauses or changes over from one breast to the other.
- Your breastfed baby will be frustrated and upset if he's not getting a good flow of milk. You can help by positioning him correctly. Hold him so his entire body—not just his head—faces your body. Hold your breast with your thumb above the areola (the pink area around the nipple) and your fingers and palm beneath it. Gently press your breast and guide it into the baby's mouth so he can grasp the entire nipple.

- Feed your baby in a comfortable sitting position, and keep her upright on your lap or in her stroller or infant seat for about 20 minutes after feedings. Avoid feeding her while she's lying down.

- Try not to jostle your baby or play too actively right after a feeding.

- If your baby has a bottle, make sure the nipple is in good condition and the hole is not too big (which causes the formula to flow too fast) or too small (which frustrates your baby and causes him to gulp air). If the hole is the proper size, a few drops should come out when you invert the bottle and then stop.

| YOUR CONCERNS | POSSIBLE CAUSE | ACTION TO TAKE |
|---|---|---|
| *Your baby spits up a little after most feedings.* | Gastroesophageal reflux (normal if mild) | None. The spitting up will grow less frequent and stop as your baby's muscles mature. |
| *Your baby gulps her feedings and seems to have a lot of gas.* | Aerophagia (swallowing more air than usual) | Make sure your baby is positioned properly (see "Tips to Reduce Spitting Up," page 16; also see "Feeding Problems in Babies," page 6). |
| *Your baby spits up when you bounce him or play after meals.* | Overstimulation | Keep mealtimes calm, and limit active play for about 30 minutes afterward. |
| *Your baby's spitting up has changed to vomiting with muscle contractions that occur after every feeding. The vomit shoots out with force.* | Pyloric stenosis or another health problem that requires diagnosis and treatment | Call your pediatrician, who will examine your baby to determine the cause of the vomiting. |
| *You are finding blood in your baby's spit-up or vomit.* | Esophagitis or another health problem that requires diagnosis and treatment | Call your pediatrician right away so he or she can examine your baby. |

CHAPTER 2

# Common Symptoms in Babies and Children

## RAISING A HEALTHY CHILD

As babies grow older they come into more and more frequent contact with people and objects that spark their curiosity and stimulate their development. Exciting as parents find this new phase, it worries them too. As your baby's circle of contacts widens, he can be exposed to infectious diseases and hazardous situations.

Even when you take all possible precautions to protect your child from illness and harm, at some point your child, even at her healthiest, is sure to develop symptoms. Some symptoms may signal temporary discomfort, such as those of the common cold; others may point to a more serious illness that demands your pediatrician's immediate attention. The charts in this chapter cover the most common symptoms seen from infancy through the teenage years. These charts will help you recognize the differences between symptoms that are likely to clear up on their own and those that require your pediatrician's attention. If your child's symptoms don't quite match those presented in this chapter, or you have any doubts about what to do, call your pediatrician for advice.

## IN GENERAL

Children have abdominal pain for any number of physical and emotional reasons. When the pain comes on suddenly, it's known as *acute* abdominal pain (for information about *chronic* pain, which lasts for a week or more and comes and goes, see page 22). Luckily, most stomachaches disappear on their own without special treatment. That being said, parents should be familiar with the symptoms that indicate unusual or possibly serious causes.

## Treating Appendicitis

Appendicitis is an infection or inflammation of the appendix (Figure 2-1). The appendix is a worm-shaped pouch near the place in the body where the large and small intestines join. When a child's abdominal pain, other symptoms, and tests signal appendicitis, the appendix should be removed as soon as possible; otherwise, it may burst, causing peritonitis, a dangerous infection that spreads throughout the abdomen. After surgery, children almost always recover quickly with no aftereffects.

**WARNING!**

Don't force your child with abdominal pain to eat, but make sure she has plenty of clear fluids to drink if she wishes. Don't give her a pain reliever (eg, acetaminophen if older than 3 months and not vomiting or dehydrated) unless your pediatrician has seen her and says it's OK.

### Call your pediatrician right away if

- Your baby under age 1 shows signs of distress that might suggest abdominal pain (such as unusual crying, legs pulled up toward his abdomen).
- Your child has continuous pain for 3 or more hours.
- Your child has pain along with swelling in his groin or testicles.
- Your child still has pain 3 hours after vomiting or passing diarrhea.
- Your child vomits greenish material or passes blood in his vomit or stools.

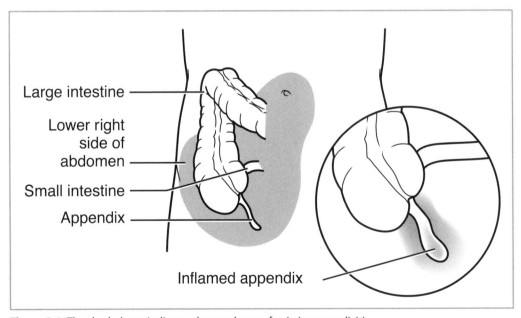

**Figure 2-1.** The shaded area indicates the usual area of pain in appendicitis.

| YOUR CONCERNS | POSSIBLE CAUSE | ACTION TO TAKE |
|---|---|---|
| Your child has diarrhea or is vomiting along with the pain. | Gastroenteritis (inflammation of the stomach and intestinal lining) | If your child is younger than 6 months, continue feeding her breastmilk or formula. Give an older child electrolyte drinks and small servings of a normal diet. If your child's symptoms don't improve in 48 hours, call your pediatrician. |
| Your child is unwilling to let you gently press on his abdomen. | Gastroenteritis or, if the pain persists for more than 3 hours, early appendicitis (For a definition of appendicitis, see page 20.) | If your child's symptoms improve, give him clear liquids and a normal diet as soon as he can tolerate food. If diarrhea develops, treat as for gastroenteritis, above. If your child's pain lasts for more than 3 hours, call your pediatrician. |
| Your child has had continuous pain for at least 3 hours. It began near her navel and is now toward her lower right abdomen. | Appendicitis | Call your pediatrician; you should not give your child anything to eat or drink until after your pediatrician examines her. Your pediatrician may suspect appendicitis or another serious condition. If so, your child will be tested for those problems and may be hospitalized. |
| Your child older than 3 years has a sore throat and other symptoms such as a headache. | Viral infection or streptococcal throat infection (strep throat) | Call your pediatrician so he or she can examine your child and recommend treatment. Give your child drinks he enjoys and acetaminophen to relieve his pain and discomfort. |
| Your child has tender swelling in his groin or testicles. | Strangulated hernia (a hernia that cuts off the blood supply to the intestines) Torsion (twisting) of the testicles | Call your pediatrician right away. Your child may be hospitalized for treatment. |
| Your child has at least 2 of the following symptoms: temperature higher than 101°F (38.3°C), bedwetting (after having been dry for months), or urination with pain, frequency, or odor. | Urinary tract infection | Talk with your pediatrician, who may order tests to diagnose the infection. He or she may also prescribe an antibiotic. |
| Your child has vomited greenish material. | Intestinal blockage | Call your pediatrician at once. You should not give your child anything to eat or drink until after your pediatrician examines him. |
| Your child frequently complains of pain but has no symptoms between bouts. She is at least 4 years of age. | Nonspecific abdominal pain often related to stress (See page 22.) | Let your child rest with a heating pad, and offer her fluids. Watch for danger signals (see warning on page 20). Talk with your pediatrician, who will examine your child to rule out disease and discuss possible pain triggers. |
| Your child has abdominal pain associated with constipation. | Constipation | Encourage scheduled toileting and fluid intake. For acute symptoms, call your pediatrician, who may prescribe an enema or stool softener. |

## IN GENERAL

Chronic abdominal pain is common but not usually serious in children. Unlike acute pain, chronic pain lasts for a week or more and comes or goes (for information about acute abdominal pain, which comes on suddenly, see page 20). Often in the case of chronic abdominal pain, stomachaches disappear within 1 or 2 hours. In many cases, no physical cause is found and the symptom is described as *functional pain* (ie, nonspecific pain, most often related to stress). The pattern and site of symptoms may reveal the reason for the pain (eg, school phobia, emotional upset due to problems at home). As long as your child's growth and physical examination are normal, his pain isn't limited to a specific site, and he has no associated symptoms, a stomachache is unlikely to signal a serious condition that would require immediate treatment. Even when no cause is found, your child's pain is real, and his distress requires attention. For feeding difficulties in newborns and young infants, see page 6.

### Call your pediatrician if

- Your child has very severe pain that does not improve with time.
- Pain wakes your child from sleep.
- Your child is 4 years or younger and has pain in her abdomen that occurs again and again.
- Your child has a decreased appetite and weight loss.
- Your child is vomiting severely with abdominal pain.
- Your child has blood in his stools, urine, or vomit.

### WARNING!

If your child has pain in her abdomen that's occurring again and again, it can be upsetting. However, thorough testing and treatment efforts aren't always helpful; they may only increase your child's anxiety.

| YOUR CONCERNS | POSSIBLE CAUSE | ACTION TO TAKE |
|---|---|---|
| Your child has had fewer bowel movements than usual (for him) over the past 2 or 3 days. | Constipation | If your child is generally well, increase his fluid and fiber intake. If his bowels still don't move, call your pediatrician, who may prescribe a stool softener (see "Constipation," page 54). |
| Your child's pain occurs at times of stress, such as school tests or problems at home. | Functional pain | Consult your pediatrician, who will examine your child, order tests if necessary, and discuss pain triggers. These triggers may be physical, emotional, or dietary. |
| Your child also has bloating, cramping, and diarrhea. She gets rashes or swelling. Some attacks occur after she's eaten certain foods—even hours or days later. | Food allergy or intolerance | Talk with your pediatrician, who will examine your child. He or she may suggest you keep a food diary, eliminate or bring back certain foods, or take other measures to identify and avoid the problem food (see "Allergic Reactions," page 26). |
| Your child's pain occurs when he drinks milk or eats ice cream. His bouts of pain include bloating, gas, cramps, and diarrhea. | Lactose intolerance (sometimes seen in children aged 2 to 3 years and of African or Asian ancestry) | If your pediatrician agrees, use fortified soy or rice substitutes in place of dairy products for 1 to 2 weeks. Bring back milk slowly over time to see if your child's symptoms recur. (A breath test can also reveal if your child has lactose intolerance.) Ask your pediatrician about diet and enzyme supplements to replace your child's missing lactase. If you remove milk from your child's diet, make sure he has enough alternative adequate sources of vitamin D and calcium in his diet. |

| YOUR CONCERNS | POSSIBLE CAUSE | ACTION TO TAKE |
|---|---|---|
| *Your child's pain occurs when she eats foods that contain wheat, barley, or rye. She is irritable and is gaining weight slowly. Sometimes she vomits and has pale or foul-smelling stools.* | Celiac disease (small intestine is hypersensitive to gluten, which causes digestive problems) | Call your pediatrician, who will order blood tests before diagnosing any illnesses. Your pediatrician will refer your child to a registered dietitian for nutritional guidance and information on how to eat a gluten-free diet. |
| *Your child complains about vague abdominal pain. Your family lives in an older home that has peeling paint or is being renovated.* | Lead poisoning (common in urban areas and in regions with older housing) | Call your pediatrician, who will order blood tests to determine the level of lead in your child's blood. Your child may require treatment, and measures must be taken to remove the source of lead. |
| *Your child's bouts of pain occur with bloating, gas, cramps, and diarrhea. You live where fresh water may be contaminated, or your child has recently vacationed in such an area.* | Parasitic infection, possibly giardiasis (an infection of the small intestine) | Consult your pediatrician, who may order tests for giardia and other parasites. If the results are positive, your pediatrician will prescribe medication. |
| *Your child has bloating, gas, and diarrhea, and he recently consumed a large amount of apples, juice, or sugarless candy or gum.* | Excessive consumption of fructose or sorbitol (sugars) | Reduce your child's intake of apples and fruit juice, and withhold candy and gum. If your child's symptoms don't improve in 2 days, talk with your pediatrician. |
| *Along with the pain, your child also has frequent headaches with nausea or vomiting. Sleep helps stop a bout of pain, and each bout is often preceded by symptoms related to vision (eg, blurring, blind spots, flashes of light). Your family has a medical history of migraines.* | Migraine with associated nausea or vomiting (uncommon in children) | Help your child rest in a quiet, darkened room. Talk with your pediatrician, who may recommend anti-migraine treatment or medication for severe nausea and vomiting (see "Vomiting," page 168, for more information). |
| *Your child is passing bloody stools. She has pain in her abdomen and joints. She has lost her appetite and has nausea and fatigue.* | Inflammatory bowel disease such as ulcerative colitis or Crohn disease | Talk with your pediatrician without delay; diagnostic tests and appropriate treatment are necessary. |
| *Your child is passing bloody stools. He has pain in his abdomen and joints and has lost his appetite. He also has nausea and fatigue with constipation or diarrhea that lasts for a week or more and comes and goes.* | Inflammatory bowel disease such as ulcerative colitis or Crohn disease Irritable bowel syndrome | Consult your pediatrician without delay; diagnostic tests and appropriate treatment are necessary. Treatment recommendations might include increased fiber, stool softeners, or referral for further evaluation and consideration of prokinetic and antispasmotic medications. |

## IN GENERAL

Toddlers usually look as if they have a potbelly (ie, a large abdomen that sticks out) balanced by a swayback (ie, an inward curving of the lower back). This is perfectly normal. By your child's third birthday, however, she will probably have a longer, leaner look. She will have a flatter stomach, straighter back, and longer, slimmer legs. If you feel that your child's posture is wrong, or you worry that she's not growing normally, check with your pediatrician.

## Swelling Around the Navel

If your baby's navel looks as if it's pushing outward when he cries, he may have an umbilical hernia (Figure 2-2). This condition occurs when intestinal tissue bulges through a small weak spot in the muscular abdominal wall; pressure inside the abdomen causes the bulging. An umbilical hernia isn't serious and usually closes up by the time a child is between 3 and 4 years of age. When the condition doesn't heal itself, your pediatrician may advise a consultation with a surgeon.

••••••••••••••••••••••••••••••••••••••••••••••

**Call your pediatrician right away if**

- Your child's abdominal swelling is hard or painful.
- Your child is vomiting or has diarrhea or severe constipation.
- Your child's temperature is higher than 101°F (38.3°C).

••••••••••••••••••••••••••••••••••••••••••••••

**WARNING!**
Swelling of your child's abdomen can indicate a problem in the digestive tract or other organs. It may be caused by a buildup of fluid or gas, or an intestinal blockage.

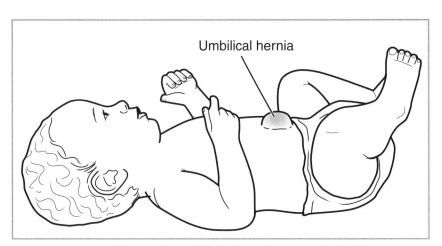
Umbilical hernia

**Figure 2-2.** An umbilical hernia is a bulge of intestinal tissue on the umbilicus (navel) due to a small weak spot in the muscular abdominal wall. This fairly common hernia is usually more noticeable when a baby cries. It is not serious and usually heals on its own by the time the child is 3 to 4 years of age. If it doesn't heal on its own, which is rare, it can be treated with surgery.

| YOUR CONCERNS | POSSIBLE CAUSE | ACTION TO TAKE |
|---|---|---|
| *Your child is constipated but otherwise well.* | Constipation | Make sure your child is getting enough fluids and fiber. If this health problem persists, talk with your pediatrician (see "Constipation," page 54). |
| *Your child's abdominal swelling and very severe pain come on suddenly.* | Intestinal blockage | Call your pediatrician, who will examine your child, order tests, and start treatment to remove the blockage. |
| *Your child's stools are pale, bulky, and unusually foul smelling. Your child often passes gas and has a persistent (won't go away) cough. He is underweight, and his skin tastes salty.* | Malabsorption problem, such as celiac disease; cystic fibrosis (an inherited condition that affects the cells that produce mucus, sweat, and digestive juices, and causes lung problems) | Consult your pediatrician, who will examine your child and order tests. Using the results, your pediatrician may recommend a treatment program and refer you to a dietitian for guidance in adapting your child's diet. |
| *Your child recently had a streptococcal infection such as a sore throat or impetigo (a contagious skin illness). Her urine is smoky or reddish brown in color. Her face is swollen, and she has a headache or fever.* | Poststreptococcal glomerulonephritis (kidney inflammation) | Call your pediatrician right away. This kidney condition can follow a streptococcal infection and may lead to chronic kidney disease if not treated promptly. |
| *In addition to abdominal swelling, your child has generalized swelling, especially around his eyes and face. His urine looks normal, but the amount of it is very small.* | Nephrotic syndrome (a kidney disorder that causes the body to excrete too much protein in the urine) | Talk with your pediatrician at once. This kidney condition (more common in boys between 1 and 6 years of age) may become chronic. It requires prompt diagnosis and treatment. |
| *Your child's swelling is very noticeable in her upper abdomen. Your child also has unexplained bruising or fever. She has lost weight.* | Uncommon blood disorder such as leukemia | Talk with your pediatrician right away. |

## IN GENERAL

Our body's immune system is on constant alert against threats from the environment. When a foreign substance tries to break through the body's defenses, the immune system fights back with inflammation; symptoms such as heat, redness, and swelling affect areas of the body that are in direct contact with the environment. These areas include the skin, nose, eyes, throat, lungs, and digestive tract. Sometimes the immune system overreacts by trying to defend the body against substances that are harmless or even beneficial. The result is an allergic reaction.

Allergies tend to run in families; if one or both parents have allergies, odds are high that their children will also develop them; however, children may not be allergic to the same substances as their parents. But allergic rhinitis and conjunctivitis (environmental allergies), eczema, asthma, and food allergies often occur together within the same child or family.

Many allergens (allergy-causing substances) can be identified. This is because a reaction to an allergen usually occurs shortly (within minutes to a few hours) after exposure to it. Based on information about your child's exposures and reactions, your pediatrician will look for a pattern that reveals allergies; some environmental allergies result in seasonal symptoms, and others cause problems year-round.

Skin tests or blood tests can be useful for diagnosing allergies. While environmental allergies may result in missed school days or trigger an asthma attack (exacerbation), food allergies can potentially be life-threatening. A child with a known food allergy must have immediate access to auto-injectable epinephrine (adrenaline) in case of exposure to the problem food.

Treatment includes efforts to avoid known allergens in order to prevent symptoms. When exposure to allergens can't be avoided, such as with airborne tree or grass pollens, medications can help control your child's symptoms. In severe cases your pediatrician may refer you to an allergy specialist, who may recommend allergy shots—a series of injections in which small amounts of the problematic substance are given to your child to make him less sensitive to it.

**Call 911 or your local emergency number right away if your child has any symptoms of anaphylaxis (a severe allergic reaction), such as**

- Dizziness
- Weakness
- Confusion
- Faintness
- Pale or blue skin
- Sweating
- Difficulty breathing
- Wheezing
- Significant coughing
- Tightness in the throat
- Difficulty swallowing
- Significant swelling
- Widespread hives
- Vomiting
- Diarrhea
- Abdominal cramping

> **WARNING!**
> Discuss over-the-counter products with your pediatrician before treating your child's rash, runny nose, or respiratory symptoms. Except for nasal saline sprays, some commercial decongestant nasal sprays can actually worsen nasal congestion over time. Older generation antihistamines can cause side effects such as drowsiness, dry mouth, constipation, change in appetite, and sometimes, a change in behavior. Newer, longer-acting, nonsedating antihistamines may help your child, but use them only as instructed by your pediatrician.

## Food Allergies Versus Sensitivities

In the United States food allergies affect 1 in 13 children younger than 18 years. They are most common in infants and children younger than 6 years. Food allergies occur when we eat a food that triggers an allergic reaction in our body's immune system. If your child has a food allergy, she will have a reaction to it every time she eats a specific food, usually within 20 to 30 minutes.

A food sensitivity or intolerance, on the other hand, tends to be a digestive problem; it doesn't always occur when the specific food is eaten. Food intolerances are actually more common than food allergies. People with lactose intolerance, for example, lack an enzyme in their intestines, called *lactase*. This enzyme is needed to digest the sugar in milk, called *lactose*.

Together your pediatrician and an allergy specialist can evaluate your child to determine if he has a food sensitivity or a true food allergy.

Keeping a food diary can often help you identify foods that cause your child's symptoms. Record all of the foods and beverages your child consumes, along with the time they are eaten. Note any symptoms and when they occur. The pattern of symptoms may point to the problem food. Eliminate any suspect foods, and discuss what you find with your pediatrician or an allergy specialist.

| YOUR CONCERNS | POSSIBLE CAUSE | ACTION TO TAKE |
|---|---|---|
| *Your child has a runny nose with clear discharge, itchy eyes, tearing, sneezing, and coughing. Her symptoms are worse at certain times of the year.* | Seasonal allergic rhinitis (environmental allergy) | Talk with your pediatrician if your child's symptoms start to interfere with school and other activities. Your pediatrician may prescribe medication to relieve acute symptoms. He or she may also recommend measures you can take to lessen your child's exposure to problem substances. |
| *Your child has dry patches of irritated, red skin. Other family members have eczema.* | Atopic dermatitis (eczema) | If your child's rash is mild, no medical treatment is necessary. Use unscented skin moisturizers regularly. Give your child brief daily baths in warm (not hot) water. Right after the bath, apply a moisturizing cream or ointment to your child's skin to lock in moisture. Your child should avoid wearing woolen clothing next to his skin. |
| *Your child has an irritated red rash in a specific area of her body.* | Contact dermatitis (inflammatory reaction in the skin) | Consult your pediatrician, who will need to examine your child for a proper diagnosis. Identifying and avoiding the problem substance is critical. It can help prevent the reaction from happening again. A common cause of contact dermatitis is sensitivity to nickel in jewelry or the button snap-closures on clothing. Poison ivy is another cause. |
| *Your child's breathing is fast and noisy. He is wheezing and coughing, and he has hay fever or eczema. Asthma runs in your family.* | Asthma, perhaps triggered by environmental allergies or an upper respiratory infection | Call your pediatrician, who will examine your child and prescribe treatment to improve symptoms and prevent attacks. Allergy testing may be necessary to find the asthma triggers, and your pediatrician may recommend changes in your home and lifestyle (see "Keeping Asthma Under Control," page 50). |
| *Your child's rash is made up of red, raised spots that might look similar to mosquito bites. The spots vary in size and location.* | Hives, sometimes due to an allergic reaction to medication or food | Hives sometimes disappear without treatment, although your child may need an over-the-counter antihistamine. Call your pediatrician if you suspect a drug or food reaction; if your child has trouble breathing, difficulty swallowing, or repeated attacks; or if your child's rash lasts more than 4 hours. |
| *Both of your child's eyes are red with tearing, itching, and puffiness. This might occur seasonally.* | Allergic conjunctivitis (environmental allergy) | Ask your pediatrician about treatment that can relieve your child's acute discomfort. Avoid known irritants. |
| *Your child has one or more of the following symptoms: rash, swelling, nausea, vomiting, diarrhea, difficulty breathing, wheezing, or coughing shortly after eating a specific food.* | Food allergy | Talk with your pediatrician, and report any suspect food. Allergy testing may identify the culprit allergens and guide you in avoiding the problem food. The most common food allergies are to cow's milk, eggs, peanuts, tree nuts (such as almonds), soy, wheat, fish, and shellfish. |

## IN GENERAL

Many parents worry whether their children are eating enough (or too much), but most children eat what they need to make up for energy spent in growth and play. It's perfectly normal for children's appetites to vary just as those of adults do. Your child may ask for second helpings one day and turn up his nose at food the next. Parents of toddlers may wish to take note: after the rapid growth that occurs in the first year of life, your child's rate of growth slows down. This is sometimes made clear by a decrease in your child's appetite.

Young children's changing food likes and dislikes can be frustrating for parents. A 2 year old, for example, may suddenly refuse all foods of a certain color or insist that one food on the plate not touch another. But when parents get upset, children quickly learn that food can be used to get their own way. If parents take these whims in stride, children even-tually lose interest in food as a means of control.

As long as they have access to nourishing foods, children won't starve themselves, and they rarely lose weight. An exception is an older child or teen with the eating disorder anorexia nervosa (see "Eating Disorders," page 184).

• • • • • • • • • • • • • • • • • • • • • • • • • • • • • • • • • • • • • •

### Talk with your pediatrician if your child

- Has a noticeable loss in appetite (ie, for more than 1 week)
- Refuses fluids
- Has lost or been unable to gain weight over a 3- to 4-month period

• • • • • • • • • • • • • • • • • • • • • • • • • • • • • • • • • • • • • •

### WARNING!

Children should drink plenty of fluids, ideally mostly milk and water. Infants younger than 6 months should not be given any fruit juices. After 6 months, juice intake should be limited, if given at all. Children between 1 and 6 years of age should not drink more than 4 to 6 ounces (120–180 mL) of fruit juice each day. Make sure your child doesn't fill up on fluids. Children who drink excessive amounts of milk (ie, more than 24 ounces in a day) may lose their appetite for solid foods. As a result their diet may not be nutritionally complete.

## Fostering Good Eating Habits

Eating habits that are established early in life often become a lifelong pattern. Many adults bear the consequences of having been urged to clean their plates when they weren't hungry or bribed with treats for good behavior. Such behavior teaches children to eat for reasons other than hunger.

The best thing you can do is to trust your child's instincts. Left to themselves, children will eat as much as they need to keep up their energy stores. Encourage your child's dawning independence— and make allowances for her natural likes and dislikes—by ensuring that she has a moderate array of healthy foods to choose from. Parents should also model good eating habits themselves. Children know how much they need; it's up to you to provide wholesome foods for healthy eating.

| YOUR CONCERNS | POSSIBLE CAUSE | ACTION TO TAKE |
|---|---|---|
| Your child aged 1 to 2 years is healthy with normal growth and energy but no interest in eating. | Normal change in appetite due to slowing of growth rate | None. A decrease in appetite is normal at this age; however, be sure to provide a varied diet based on ChooseMyPlate.gov (see "Eating Problems," page 80). |
| Your child has a sore throat, cough, runny nose, and fever. | Upper respiratory tract infection (viral) | Provide cold drinks, ice cream, or yogurt to soothe your child's inflammation. Provide chicken soup for comfort. Give her acetaminophen or ibuprofen to relieve her discomfort. |
| Your child has swollen glands in his neck and is feverish. He has a sore throat that's getting worse. He has developed other symptoms, such as difficulty with swallowing. | Streptococcal throat infection<br>Infectious mononucleosis ("mono," a viral infection that causes sore throat, fever, and fatigue) | Visit your pediatrician, who will examine your child and prescribe treatment. |
| Your child has diarrhea. | Gastroenteritis (inflammation of the stomach and intestinal lining) | If her diarrhea is mild, continue feeding her a normal diet. If it's severe, give her rehydrating fluids (see "Diarrhea in Babies," page 5). Call your pediatrician if your child's vomiting persists for more than 12 hours or her diarrhea is bloody or lasts for more than 48 hours. |
| Your child has been urinating frequently. Her urination is painful or urgent. She may also have a stomachache. | Urinary tract infection | Consult your pediatrician, who will test your child's urine and prescribe an antibiotic, if such treatment is appropriate. |
| Your child is passing large volumes of urine. He has lost weight and seems unusually tired. | Diabetes mellitus (a deficiency of the pancreatic hormone insulin, which results in a failure to metabolize sugars) | Call your pediatrician without delay; if diagnostic tests indicate diabetes, your child must start insulin injections and other measures to control the disease. |
| Your child has pain that began around her navel and has moved to her lower right abdomen. She has nausea or is vomiting. | Acute appendicitis | Call your pediatrician without delay (see "Abdominal Pain, Acute," page 20). |
| Your child has been unusually pale, lethargic (lacking energy), or irritable over a period of weeks. | Systemic illness (illness that affects the body as a whole) | Consult your pediatrician, who will examine your child for anemia, lead poisoning, or other illnesses. |

## IN GENERAL

Children have a range of what pediatricians and other experts consider normal behavior. Most children will act restless and fidgety once in a while. Some children can be impulsive and, at times, may find it hard to concentrate fully on a task. What's different about children with attention-deficit/hyperactivity disorder, or ADHD, is that their behavior is more intense than it is in other children who are the same age. They rarely sit still. They are impulsive and distracted almost all of the time, and frequently disturb others with their disruptive behavior. Children with ADHD often have a hard time paying attention. Because they are easily distracted, they find it difficult to finish a task they have started. Their behavioral problems (see page 38) are so frequent and intense that they can interfere with functioning at home, at school, and with peers. Teachers may have trouble managing children with ADHD, and other children may reject them. Often children with ADHD struggle with criticism, failure, and disappointment.

Attention-deficit/hyperactivity disorder affects 6% to 9% of all school-aged children; boys are diagnosed 3 times more often than girls. Researchers believe ADHD may have a number of causes. Studies reveal that the brain of a child with ADHD may function differently from that of a child without the condition. Many families have a history of similar attention difficulties in a close relative (eg, parent, sibling); this suggests that the condition may be at least partly genetic. Whatever the causes may be, ADHD isn't due to poor parenting; however, you and your child can develop special techniques for coping with ADHD. Behavioral modifications and approaches are the first-line of intervention for children who have ADHD. If necessary, your child may also be prescribed a medication.

If your child has ADHD, you may feel overwhelmed by his boundless energy 24 hours a day. Don't hesitate to talk about your worries with your pediatrician. Ask for help finding a support group where you can hear how others cope.

### Talk with your pediatrician if your child generally

- Gets overexcited and loses control
- Is falling behind in schoolwork
- Fights with others or has trouble keeping friends
- Doesn't complete tasks

### WARNING!

The first-line of intervention for attention issues is behavioral, nonmedical modifications. If used, medication doesn't cure ADHD, but it helps control symptoms and lets your child make the best use of his abilities.

## Recognizing Warning Signs of ADHD

Experts agree that the tendency to develop ADHD is present from birth. Yet parents, teachers, and other caregivers often don't notice ADHD behaviors until children enter elementary school. One reason for this delay is the fact that nearly all preschool aged–children, as part of their normal development, frequently exhibit the core behaviors or symptoms of ADHD—inattention, impulsivity, and hyperactivity. As children without ADHD begin to grow out of such behaviors, children with ADHD don't. This difference becomes increasingly clear as the years pass. The school setting can highlight a child's inattention, impulsivity, and hyperactivity because classroom activities demand more focus, patience, and self-control. These kinds of demands aren't as common at home or in playgroups, so in those settings, the child may have fewer problems.

| YOUR CONCERNS | POSSIBLE CAUSE | ACTION TO TAKE |
|---|---|---|
| *Your child is overly fearful. Her laughs or cries can't be controlled. She has experienced frightening events. She has friends and does fairly well at school.* | Anxiety | Talk with your pediatrician, who may recommend a plan to help your child deal with her fears and control her behavior. |
| *Your school-aged child still has temper tantrums. He gets overexcited and overtired. Yet other times he sticks to tasks and gets along with other family members and friends.* | Temper tantrums (Also see page 156.) | Keep to a schedule for sleep, play, and meals so your child doesn't get overtired or hungry. Anticipate situations that are likely to trigger a tantrum, and avoid them when possible. Reward his positive behavior with praise and attention. Offer brief, simple reasons for your rules. If these measures don't help, discuss your concerns with your pediatrician. |
| *Your school-aged child's behavior is making everyday life difficult for himself and others at home, at school, and in social activities. He is often on the move. He sleeps very little.* | Hyperactivity; ADHD; learning problems; family stress; temperamental mismatch; inappropriate expectations | Talk with your pediatrician, who may recommend evaluation and treatment. |
| *Your child is impulsive and easily distracted. He has a short attention span.* | ADHD | Discuss your concerns with your pediatrician, who may advise evaluation. |
| *Your child daydreams at school. She struggles with completing tasks and prefers to be alone. She is being picked on.* | ADHD; learning disorder; lack of social skills; emotional problems; inappropriate expectations | Talk with your pediatrician, who may advise evaluation and recommend a plan for treatment. |
| *Your child often disobeys you, and his behavior is hard to manage. He resists or fights you when you correct him.* | Testing which behaviors are and aren't normal; temperamental problems; school problems; family stress; unreasonable expectations | When both of you are calm, review problem areas with your child. Agree on a plan of action that involves working together to improve specific areas. Set up a reward chart system. If a 2-month trial is unsuccessful, ask your pediatrician to evaluate the situation. |
| *Your child is always on the move. He is impulsive, reckless, and unable to concentrate. He was slow in reaching developmental milestones.* | Neurologic or physical condition requiring medical evaluation | Talk with your pediatrician, who will examine your child and may refer your child to another specialist. |
| *Your child is frequently tired, despite sleeping through the night. He snores loudly. During the day he has trouble paying attention and doing his schoolwork.* | Sleep apnea (moments of being unable to breathe during sleep) | Consult your pediatrician, who will evaluate your child and may refer your child for a sleep study. |
| *Your child falls asleep at her desk and has trouble concentrating at school.* | Sleep problems | Find ways to help your child get more sleep by improving her sleep hygiene. Make sure she goes to bed at a reasonable hour and stays on schedule. Help her avoid caffeinated foods and drinks (eg, chocolate, cola, tea). If necessary, talk with your pediatrician. |

Pediatricians will look for hyperactivity, impulsivity, and inattention in their effort to diagnose ADHD; however, many children with attention deficits aren't hyperactive. They may primarily act distracted or forgetful, and these behaviors can be equally difficult to manage. Diagnosing ADHD is important because similar symptoms may accompany other conditions, such as depression (see Chapter 3, page 182), stress, or learning problems (see page 110). In these cases, the approach to treatment will be different.

Attention-deficit/hyperactivity disorder can be difficult to diagnose because different standards of behavior apply at different ages. For example, a preschooler should not be expected to show the same level of concentration as a fifth grader. To diagnose ADHD, your pediatrician doesn't rely on what he or she has observed during a single office visit because, during that visit, your child may be on his best behavior or even a bit fearful; instead; your pediatrician sifts out a pattern of behavior from what he or she observes over time, school reports, and the comments of parents, teachers, and other caregivers.

To create a uniform process for diagnosing ADHD in school-aged children, the American Academy of Pediatrics has created a list of standard guidelines for pediatricians in evaluating a child reported to be inattentive, hyperactive, impulsive, underachieving academically, or having behavioral problems. Pediatricians also rely on criteria from the latest edition of the *Diagnostic and Statistical Manual of Mental Disorders.* Many pediatricians also use rating scales like the Vanderbilt Scales to organize what parents, teachers, and other care-givers observe. The scales ask parents and teachers to assess a child on a number of measures, including attentiveness, listening, organization, physical aggression, and moods.

In order to make a diagnosis, the symptoms must be present for 6 months or more, and are more pronounced than in most children at the same developmental level. Some symptoms must have been present before age 7. The symptoms have been observed to interfere with the child's functioning in 2 or more major settings. The behaviors must significantly impair the child's ability to function in academic or social situations. And the symptoms cannot be accounted for by another condition, either physical or mental, such as head trauma, physical or sexual abuse, or a major psychological stress in the family or at school.

Only a physician or psychologist can diagnose ADHD. Teachers can't diagnose ADHD, although they can identify problems that should be evaluated by your pediatrician. Attention deficits and learning problems are often present together, and each problem can make the other worse.

**Talk with your pediatrician if your child displays several of the following behaviors and they are interfering with his progress at school or his relationships with other children:**

- Can't keep his mind on a task
- Is easily distracted
- Is often impulsive
- Is easily frustrated and often impatient
- Constantly fidgets with his hands and feet
- Is often restlessness and can't control his energy
- Constantly interrupts
- Talks excessively
- Performs below grade level on schoolwork
- Lacks organization
- Disobeys
- Has mood swings and is often irritable
- Has difficulty completing instructions
- Has trouble making and keeping friends

## Coping With ADHD

Many parents can't understand why the same parenting techniques that worked on their other children don't work on their child with ADHD. In reality, children with ADHD comprehend and retain what you tell them; they just aren't able to perform in a way they know is appropriate. One of the most effective ways to guide a child with ADHD toward appropriate behavior is with behavior therapy and parent training. Parent training can provide you with the tools and procedures you need to help your child manage his behavior. Although behavior therapy works best on younger children who haven't developed long-standing habits, it can also work on older children and even teens. The process is also designed to enhance relationships between you and your child.

Helping your child change his behavior is necessary in treating ADHD. But many pediatricians will also recommend medications to control the symptoms of ADHD. Treatment usually involves educational measures too. These include tutoring and psychological counseling. Your pediatrician will guide you to other programs for support. Some families benefit from family therapy. Successful treatment of ADHD depends on cooperation among you, your pediatrician, other specialists, teachers, and your child. The ultimate goal of treatment is to give your child a sense of feeling in control and prepared to face life's challenges. Doing so will build his self-esteem and self-confidence.

All children function best in a structured environment. Children with ADHD have more trouble than most with organization and rules, and they need a consistent schedule. Give your child extra attention to help her focus on tasks such as getting dressed or doing homework. Social events and outings may be easier if you let your child know beforehand how you expect her to behave. But don't expect your child, hyperactive or not, to sit still throughout events that are far beyond her capacity to understand or enjoy.

Controversial treatments such as additive-free diets, sugar restriction, and megadose vitamins haven't held up when tested scientifically. Talk with your pediatrician before trying any treatments.

## IN GENERAL

Problems that affect a child's back are most often due to injuries from sports or play, falls, or unusual strain, such as that caused by wearing a heavy backpack. Back pain and stiffness are most often caused by a pulled muscle, a strained ligament, or bruising. Symptoms of back pain usually disappear within a week without special treatment.

Although regular exercise is beneficial for all children, intensive training may lead to overuse injuries with back pain in some young athletes. For example, dancers and gymnasts, are especially prone to back pain due to overuse. On the other hand, children who are overly sedentary (ie, don't move much) may have back pain from weak core muscles, back strain from being overweight, or poor posture.

Scoliosis (a severe curvature of the spine) is a possible cause of back pain, especially in adolescent girls. Your pediatrician evaluates your child's posture during regular well-child visits to make sure her back is straight and she's growing normally.

Spondylolysis is a weakness in the bony bridges of the vertebral bones, usually in the lower spine. It can cause low back pain aggravated by activity and is frequently accompanied by minimal or no physical findings. Radiographs may be helpful if spondylolysis is suspected.

**Consult your pediatrician if your child with back pain is younger than 10 years or has**

- Pain that won't go away or is getting worse
- Fever or weight loss
- Difficulty in moving a limb
- Numbness or tingling in a limb
- Loss of bladder or bowel control
- A change in gait or posture

### WARNING!

Back pain in a young child who hasn't been injured is concerning and needs to be evaluated by your pediatrician.

## Curvature of the Spine

About 1 in 25 adolescent girls and 1 in 200 adolescent boys have, to some degree, curvature of the spine, called scoliosis (Figure 2-3). Some schools now have screening programs to detect scoliosis in children as they approach puberty and before their bone growth is complete. If an abnormality is detected, your school health authority will contact you and advise talking with your pediatrician. If your child's spine has a mild curvature, your pedia- trician may just closely observe it. More severe, worsening scoliosis may require your child to wear a special brace or surgery to straighten her spine. Scientific studies haven't shown any benefits from manipulation therapy (kneading of muscles and joints) in children with scoliosis. Spinal deformity in a child younger than 10 years is abnormal; so is spinal deformity associated with any neurologic symptoms or findings. Both abnormalities require prompt evaluation.

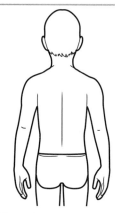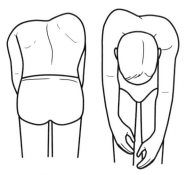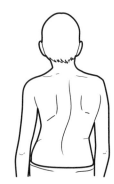

**Normal**
- Head centered over buttocks
- Shoulders level
- Shoulder blades level and equally prominent
- Hips level and symmetrical
- Equal distance between arms and body

**Possible scoliosis**
- Upper back, lower back, or possibly both, assymetrical

**Possible scoliosis**
- Head over to one side of mid buttocks
- One shoulder higher
- One shoulder blade higher, possibly more prominent
- One hip more prominent
- Unequal distance between arm and body

**Figure 2-3.** Detecting scoliosis.

| YOUR CONCERNS | POSSIBLE CAUSE | ACTION TO TAKE |
|---|---|---|
| *Your child has recently been involved in sports or very active play. He had a minor fall or another injury.* | Pulled muscle, strained ligament, or bruise | Apply a cold compress to your child's injury right away; a warm bath may be comforting to him later. Give your child acetaminophen or ibuprofen to relieve his pain. |
| *Your child fell from a considerable height.* | Spinal or head injury | Call 911 or your local emergency number at once. Don't try to move your child unless her life is in danger (see "Fractures," page 226). |
| *Following an apparently minor back injury, your child has difficulty in moving, numbness or tingling in one of his limbs, or loss of bladder or bowel control.* | Spinal injury | Call your pediatrician, or take your child to the nearest emergency department. |
| *Your child is complaining of a sharp, one-sided pain in the middle of her back. She has painful or frequent urination, a fever, or nausea.* | Acute kidney infection | Call your pediatrician without delay. |
| *Your child has lower back pain that is aggravated by physical activity.* | Spondylolysis, a weakness in the bony bridges of the vertebral bones of the lower spine | Consult your pediatrician, who will examine your child, order tests or x-rays, and refer your child to another specialist, if necessary. |
| *Your child has back pain that wakes him from a sound sleep at night.* | Diskitis (inflammation of a spinal disk) Infection Tumor | Consult your pediatrician, who will examine your child, order tests or x-rays, and refer your child to another specialist, if necessary. |

## IN GENERAL

Children vary widely in the order and timing at which they achieve daytime bladder control and nighttime dryness. Most are fully toilet trained between 3 and 4 years of age; they can control nighttime urination about 6 months to 1 year after gaining daytime control. But many children—up to 15%—continue to wet the bed regularly until 5 years of age or even later. This is known as *primary nocturnal enuresis,* which is more common in boys than in girls; often their family has a history of bedwetting. Some children will wet the bed after having been dry previously. This usually is associated with an identifiable cause and is referred to as *secondary nocturnal enuresis.* In any event, most children with primary nocturnal enuresis outgrow bedwetting by puberty.

### Talk with your pediatrician if your child

- Continues bedwetting at night beyond 5 years of age
- Resumes regular nighttime bedwetting after months of dryness
- Has bladder control problems during the day and at night
- Has other symptoms such as more thirst than usual, pain or burning during urination, or daytime wetting

### WARNING!

Be wary of claims for bedwetting treatments in mail- order advertisements or on the Internet. Your pediatrician is your most reliable source for information; don't enroll in or pay for any bedwetting treatment without your pediatrician's advice.

## Steps to Toilet Training

Children gain control of bladder and bowel function when they are physically ready. You can't speed up the process, but you can bolster your child's confidence and encourage his efforts. Pushing your child into toilet training before he's ready may only prolong the process. Often in a toddler's early months, the toddler is likely to resist toilet training. Toilet training isn't likely to succeed until your toddler is past this stage of resistance. Your toddler must want to take on the independence that comes with this major step forward. This stage of independence usually occurs between 18 and 24 months of age, but it's quite normal for it to happen a bit later.

When your toddler is ready to start, toilet training should go fairly smoothly as long as you both stay relaxed about it. Praise your toddler for his efforts, and don't dwell on his accidents. Showing displeasure will add an element of tension that may hinder progress. Here are 5 steps for training your toddler to use the toilet.

1. Let your toddler become familiar with a potty-chair (or the toilet fitted with a toddler seat), but don't expect her to use it for some time.

2. Look for signs that your toddler is uncomfortable when wetting or soiling his diaper during the day. Once he's able to stay dry for about 2 hours, suggest—but don't insist—that he use the potty-chair or toilet from time to time. Your toddler should also know the difference between wet and dry, be able to pull his pants up and down, and show an interest in learning how to use the potty-chair.

3. Help your toddler learn about using the toilet. Read child-directed, age-appropriate books about potty training with your child. Take your toddler into the bathroom with the appropriate-sex parent or older sibling to learn the routine. Praise her attempts to sit on the potty-chair.

4. When your toddler is confident with the potty-chair, fit a child's seat and step stool to the toilet and let him become familiar with the new arrangement. He can alternate use of the potty-chair and toilet until eventually he's using just the toilet.

5. Many children don't achieve nighttime control until after they have mastered daytime control. Don't be surprised if your child still requires overnight diapers for a while after she has gained daytime control. If you have questions about your child's overnight control and whether it's age appropriate, talk with your pediatrician (see "Urinary Incontinence," page 160).

| YOUR CONCERNS | POSSIBLE CAUSE | ACTION TO TAKE |
|---|---|---|
| *Your child is younger than 3 years and does not stay dry overnight.* | Age-appropriate bladder control | The mechanisms for controlling bladder and arousal are still developing. Your child will achieve control as these mechanisms mature. |
| *Your child is younger than 5 years. He wears a diaper at night or still wets the bed.* | Immature bladder size or arousal mechanism | Many children have nighttime dryness that may lag behind their daytime control. This situation isn't a cause for concern and will eventually resolve itself. |
| *Your child is older than 6 years and still wetting the bed.* | Primary nocturnal enuresis | Consult your pediatrician, who will evaluate your child's condition and your family history. Your pediatrician may recommend treatment such as a nighttime alarm, behavior modification, counseling, or a medication. |
| *Your child who has been dry for months wets the bed during a time of stress (eg, starting school, parental discord).* | Emotional stress | Reassure your child, and protect his mattress with a waterproof sheet. If his bedwetting lasts for longer than 2 weeks, or if the source of his stress isn't clear, talk with your pediatrician. |
| *Your child complains of burning or pain during urination. She is urinating frequently during the day.* | Urinary tract infection | Consult your pediatrician, who may order tests and prescribe an antibiotic, if appropriate. |
| *In addition to bedwetting, your child passes large volumes of urine during the day. He has lost weight and seems unusually tired.* | Diabetes mellitus (a deficiency of the pancreatic hormone insulin, which results in a failure to metabolize sugars) | Consult your pediatrician at once. |

## IN GENERAL

Infants and young children express themselves through behavior long before they can talk. Behavior is formed partly out of your child's temperament, and his ability to adapt. Behavior is modified by your responses to your child, your family's situation and any stressors, positive and negative reinforcements, genetics, and other life experiences. Good discipline is a framework that teaches your child how to express her feelings and how to behave properly. Secure, nurturing relationships and safe environments help foster resilience and develop strengths to overcome challenges.

Children learn to behave largely by copying others and watching how adults and other children resolve their differences. Parents provide a good example when they treat their family and outsiders with kindness and respect. But parents are also showing a way to behave when they act aggressively, allow destructiveness, or promote stereotypes and prejudices, as well as violence on television and in films.

Keep in mind that behavior that's acceptable at one developmental stage may cause concern at another. For example, temper tantrums are normal during the "terrible twos" but worrisome in your school-aged child; see page 156. What's never acceptable is behavior that can harm your child, your family, and others, including animals and property. If your child is acting up, he may be sending out a cry for help. Often overlooked, however, is the excessively compliant child whose self-control and eagerness to please may also be signs of trouble.

"Normal" behavior also varies according to family customs. For example, some cultural groups let children be outspoken in a way that other groups may find inappropriate. Some children struggle with self-control because their parents don't set limits. Still, other children may behave in ways that reflect a developmental delay or problem (see page 64). At the very least children should be taught to respect the rights and feelings of others. Give your child specific guidelines on how to behave. But don't make unreasonable demands and place her in situations she's not ready to handle. Don't be in a hurry to label your child's behavior. Labels tend to become self-fulfilling prophecies. What's important is the overall pattern of your child's behavior, not an occasional lapse when she's tired or overexcited.

### Talk with your pediatrician if your child

- Acts younger than other children who are the same age
- Resists or fights you and doesn't respond to reasonable requests and discipline
- Often overreacts to events and can't be calmed down
- Acts without regard to safety
- Threatens others, is cruel to animals, plays with fire, or harms property
- Has mood swings, school problems, loss of friends, alcohol or drug use, or self-esteem issues

### WARNING!

The earlier a behavioral problem in your child is recognized and dealt with, the greater the likelihood of success. Without help, a child with a behavioral problem may eventually develop a conduct disorder and potentially emotional problems.

## Using Positive Reinforcement to Discipline

Helping your child develop skills to regulate her emotions and actions more effectively requires consistent and effective discipline. One of the best ways to encourage more displays of a desired behavior is to use positive reinforcement. Positive parenting builds strong relationships through activities such as regular one-on-one time (sometimes called "time-in") to reinforce appropriate behaviors. Unlike negative reinforcement, which involves taking something away from your child to discourage unwanted behavior, positive reinforcement uses praise and other incentives to reward your child for displaying good behavior.

As your child gets older, it's also important to communicate the behavior you expect by using positive phrases such as "I like it when you play nicely with your sister," or "You picked up your toys—thank you for helping keep our home clean."

As angry as you may feel, never spank your child when she misbehaves. A better alternative is a time-out: when your child misbehaves, put her in a quiet place for a few minutes, away from people, television, or books. When the time-out is over, explain to your child why her behavior was unacceptable.

Although time-outs have their place in disciplining children, the most effective tool is still positive reinforcement. Remember, the goal of discipline is to teach, not to punish.

| YOUR CONCERNS | POSSIBLE CAUSE | ACTION TO TAKE |
|---|---|---|
| Your child usually disobeys the rules you've set. He is defiant when you correct him. | Testing behavior<br>Trouble with temperament, school, or family<br>Unreasonable expectations | When both of you are calm, agree on a plan of action to change behavior in specific areas. For a school-aged child, set up a scoring system. If a 2-month trial doesn't work, see your pediatrician. |
| Your school-aged child is aggressive at home. Teachers at her school and other parents have complained of her bullying her peers. | Lack of self-control<br>Seeking attention<br>Stress<br>Sibling rivalry<br>Jealousy | Children should be able to control their aggressive impulses by the time they are in kindergarten. Your pediatrician may advise therapy and parent-effectiveness training. |
| Your child is being bullied at school. He is anxious and insecure. He lacks good social skills. | Social, emotional, or developmental factors | Your pediatrician may refer your child to a therapist. Victims of bullying tend to stay anxious and insecure unless they get help with finding new ways of thinking and acting. |
| Your child is almost too well behaved. She is shy. She avoids other children and seeks adult company instead. | Normal behavior<br>Anxiety<br>Shyness | Encourage your child to take part in hobbies or sports that let her mix with other children. If she has anxiety attacks with rapid breathing, talk with your pediatrician. |
| Your child frequently uses profanity. He swears at people or calls them names. | Lack of self-control<br>Mimicking adult behavior or media<br>Disrespect for others | Let your child know that while a mild curse word may do no harm, foul words and swearing at others aren't tolerated. Set a good example. |
| Your child has money or possessions she can't account for. You're worried she may have stolen or shoplifted goods. | Unacceptable but not abnormal phase of development<br>Stress<br>Peer pressure<br>Need for attention | Ask your child where she got the goods. If she stole them, insist she return them with an apology; go with her, if necessary. Let her know that stealing is never tolerated. If it seems to become a pattern, or you find a hoard of stolen goods in your child's possession, your child may need urgent help. Talk with your pediatrician. |
| You have caught your school-aged child lying. | Awareness of having done something wrong<br>Fear of punishment or disappointing parents<br>Peer behavior | Tell your child that lying isn't acceptable and he'll be in less trouble if he tells the truth. Change your behavior if you're setting a double standard with "white lies" and partial truths. If your child's lying lasts for a long time, or he can't tell fact from fiction, see your pediatrician. |

## IN GENERAL

Animal bites may appear minor, but they carry a high risk of infection. In contrast, most insect bites and stings cause minor redness, irritation, and itching that soon disappear without special treatment. In some people, however, insect venom causes an allergic reaction ranging from mild to life-threatening in severity. It is important to remove an insect stinger quickly and completely. Bites or stings that result in a break in the skin may become infected. A few insects can transmit infections; for example, ticks can transmit Lyme disease, Rocky Mountain spotted fever, or tularemia (Figures 2-4 and 2-5). Mosquitos can transmit disease-causing viruses, such as arboviruses. International travelers may encounter mosquitoes that carry malaria, a serious parasitic infection. Make sure your children know and can identify dangerous insects, plants, and animals common in your area.

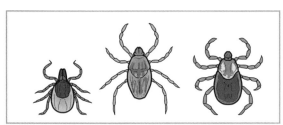

**Figure 2-4.** Tick identification. The deer tick carries Lyme disease; the brown dog tick and the wood tick carry Rocky Mountain spotted fever. (These renderings are greatly enlarged; the deer tick is only about the size of a poppy seed.)

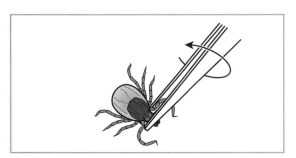

**Figure 2-5.** Tick removal. Use tweezers to remove a tick, taking care to pull out the entire insect. Grab as close to the head as possible, and pull the tick away from where it's attached.

### Call your pediatrician right away if your child

- Is bitten by a snake, a wild animal, or an unknown dog or animal
- Develops a rash or hives in a location away from that of the original bite or sting
- Develops a rash and other symptoms following a tick bite
- Develops signs of infection (eg, red streaks, warmth, increased swelling) around a bite
- Is feverish, vomiting, stiff in his neck or behaving differently

### WARNING!

Keep an auto-injectable epinephrine pen with your child if she has allergies to bites and stings. Learn how to use it, and teach other caregivers how to use it too. Always check the expiration date of the pen, and make sure the dosage is appropriate for children. Call 911 or your local emergency number right away if signs of a severe allergic reaction, known as anaphylaxis, develop following an insect bite or sting. Symptoms include swelling of the mouth, tongue, and throat; clammy skin and paleness; weakness or confusion; and difficulty breathing.

## Keeping Bugs at Bay

- Apply insect repellent to your child's skin, avoiding areas with cuts or abrasions. Read the label to make sure the repellent contains no more than 30% of diethyltoluamide, called *DEET*. This liquid is effective and has a good safety profile, but it can be harmful if ingested or used in excess. Permethrin is another repellent that can be applied to clothing, but it's not as easy to find as DEET.
- Oil of citronella and peppermint are natural insect repellents that can be diluted with vegetable oil and applied to clothing.
- Keep window screens in good repair to prevent bugs from entering your home.
- Before venturing outside where there may be ticks, dress your child in light-colored clothing with long sleeves and pants. Apply an insect repellent to his clothing. When you return home, look for ticks and use tweezers to remove them completely.

| YOUR CONCERNS | POSSIBLE CAUSE | ACTION TO TAKE |
|---|---|---|
| Your child has minor pain, swelling, redness, and itching. | Minor bite or sting from an insect such as a mosquito, fly, or ant | Apply a cold compress to your child's skin to reduce his discomfort. For a child younger than 2 years, use a cold, wet cloth but not an ice pack. |
| Your child was stung by an insect, and the location of the sting is red, itchy, swollen, and sore. | Bee, hornet, or wasp sting | If you can see the stinger, use a credit card to scrape it out. Wash the affected area with soap and water. Apply an ice pack or cold compress. |
| Your child was stung and is showing signs of a severe reaction, such as weakness, paleness, and shortness of breath. He also has a rash and widespread swelling. | Severe, generalized allergic reaction | If your child has swelling around his mouth or other signs of anaphylaxis, call 911 or your local emergency number right away. If your child has no pulse, start cardiopulmonary resuscitation right away after calling for help (see pages 215–216). |
| Your child's bite is red, swollen, and painful, and you suspect a spider inflicted the bite. | Spider venom, which can be especially dangerous from a black widow, brown recluse, or tarantula | If you think the spider was one of the highly poisonous species, call 911 or your local emergency number, or go to the nearest emergency department; otherwise, clean the site of the bite with soap and water, and apply a cold compress. If the site becomes inflamed or develops an ulcer, call your pediatrician at once. |
| Your child has a mark resembling a bull's-eye (a dark central blotch surrounded by a light halo and a red ring). | Lyme disease caused by deer tick bite, which may have occurred days earlier | Inspect your child's skin for the tick. Use tweezers to grasp the tick as closely as possible to its head. Pull the tick away from where it's attached; use of your fingers or another method of tick removal isn't recommended. Call your pediatrician, who will examine your child and prescribe antibiotics if he or she suspects or diagnoses Lyme disease. |
| Your child's skin has been punctured by an animal or human bite. | Bite with risk of infection, including tetanus or rabies | Wash the bite with soap and water, and call your pediatrician right away for help in preventing infection. Your child may need a tetanus booster. Capture the animal if you can do so without risk (or keep the animal if it's dead) for rabies testing (see Chapter 4, "Animal Bites," page 219). |
| Your child was stung while swimming in saltwater. | Jellyfish venom Stingray | Apply a cold compress. If your child is short of breath or faint, call 911 or your local emergency number. In the meantime, use clothing or sand to brush off tentacles from your child's skin. |
| Your child came into contact with nettles or another "stinging" plant. | Allergy-type reaction to plant toxin | The hives-like rash caused by nettles disappears without special treatment. If your child touched poison ivy, oak, or sumac, remove her clothing and wash her exposed skin with soap and water. Also wash her clothing. Keep your child from scratching the area of her skin with the rash. If the rash is severe, affects your child's face or genitals, or infection develops, call your pediatrician. |
| Your child was bitten by a snake (in particular, a rattlesnake, cottonmouth, coral, or copperhead). | Snake venom | Call 911 or your local emergency number, or take your child to the emergency department at once. Don't apply ice or a tourniquet; use a splint to keep the bitten area from moving. If the bite came from a coral snake, call emergency medical services, and keep your child very still. |

## IN GENERAL

Bleeding (hemorrhage) refers to the flow of blood from the body's tissues, such as the skin, and from the body's cavities, such as the mouth, the nose, or the rectum. Bruising (ecchymosis) is the leakage of blood under the skin. Bleeding and bruising in children may come from injury (intentional or unintentional), infections, certain medications, conditions that affect the immune system, clotting factor deficiencies, and, rarely, cancer.

In a healthy child with an injury that breaks the skin, bleeding stops, and clots form within a few minutes. These clots eventually form a protective cover over the wound, called a *scab*. Scalp wounds may be especially prone to bleeding because the scalp has a rich supply of blood vessels (see Chapter 4, "Cuts and Scrapes," page 222). Children with cuts or scrapes on any parts of the body that bleed longer than a few minutes, especially after they receive first aid, should be seen by a pediatrician. If your child experiences changes in her level of alertness, has severe pain (including headache), has difficulty moving any part of her body, develops paleness, is sweating, or is swelling, she should be evaluated right away by your pediatrician. These signs may mean a child is bleeding internally.

Bruises after an injury appear as black-and-blue-areas in the skin. They change color slowly over time as the tissue underneath them heals. Bruises on the shins, especially in active toddlers, and bruises that develop after a traumatic event, such as a sports injury, aren't usually a cause for con-cern; however, bruises that can't be explained by your child or his caregiver, or bruises on his buttocks, face, shoulders, or back, require prompt evaluation.

### Talk with your pediatrician if your child has

- Unexplained bruising or bruising in unusual sites
- Blood in his stools or urine
- Prolonged bleeding from trivial cuts
- Unusual paleness, fatigue, and other symptoms along with bruising easily
- Heavy menstrual flow

### WARNING!

Persistent (won't go away) bleeding or bruises in unexpected places should be seen by your pediatrician. Don't overlook the possibility of abuse, especially if your child doesn't want to tell you how she got the bruises.

## Leukemia

Leukemia is the most common form of childhood cancer; it accounts for one-third of all childhood cancers. Most children who develop leukemia will have a fever and paleness, and many will develop petechiae and purpura. Petechiae are small, pinpoint-sized red lesions that don't turn white when pressed. The bleeding occurs within the layers of the skin. Purpura are larger, raised lesions that also don't turn white when pressed. Their color can vary, which depends on the age of the lesion. Both types of lesions can occur anywhere on the body. If you see what you think is petechiae or purpura on your child's body, contact your pediatrician right away.

| YOUR CONCERNS | POSSIBLE CAUSE | ACTION TO TAKE |
| --- | --- | --- |
| *Your child's bruises are mainly on his shins. He is otherwise healthy and energetic.* | From minor bumps and falls during physical activity | No medical treatment is necessary. |
| *Your child has nosebleeds but is generally healthy.* | Childhood epistaxis (nosebleeds) Von Willebrand disease (See page 122.) | Apply firm, continuous pressure to the soft part of your child's nose. Have your child sit leaning forward until her bleeding stops. If her nose bleeds often and with large amounts of blood, discuss with your pediatrician ways to prevent future nosebleeds. Your pediatrician may order blood tests to further evaluate your child's nosebleeds. |

| YOUR CONCERNS | POSSIBLE CAUSE | ACTION TO TAKE |
|---|---|---|
| Your child is bleeding from the rectum. She has blood in her stools. | Anal fissure (ulcer at the margin of the anus)<br>Gastroenteritis (inflammation of the stomach and intestinal lining)<br>Intussusception juvenile polyps (small, benign nodules of the large intestine) | Talk with your pediatrician; further tests may be necessary. |
| Your child has multiple pinpoint-sized bruises, called petechiae, or large, expanding bruises. He has had a recent illness. | Idiopathic thrombocytopenic purpura (fewer platelets after a recent illness) | Call your pediatrician, who will order appropriate tests and may refer your child to a pediatric hematologist. Go to the emergency department if your child has severe headache or changes in his level of alertness. |
| Your child has expanding bruises with fever and vomiting. He is sleepy, dazed, or irritable. | Serious bacterial infection<br>Child abuse | Call your pediatrician right away, and go to the emergency department. |
| Your child has developed pinpoint-sized bruises and is vomiting while taking a medication such as an antibiotic. | Reaction to medication | Call your pediatrician without delay; he or she may need to prescribe an alternative medication. |
| Your child has unexplained bruises on her legs and ankles. She also has a stomachache and joints that are swollen and tender. | Allergy problem<br>Henoch-Schönlein purpura (a disorder that causes inflammation and bleeding in the small blood vessels in skin, joints, intestines, and kidneys) | Call your pediatrician, who will examine your child and order diagnostic tests. |
| Your child is bleeding from a minor cut in the mucous membranes, and his bleeding has persisted for hours or days. | Bleeding disorder or clotting factor deficiency, such as hemophilia or von Willebrand disease | Talk with your pediatrician about diagnostic tests and management of the deficiency. Von Willebrand disease and hemophilia run in families. |
| Your child returns from child care or a babysitter with an unusual number of bruises or oddly-shaped bruises. Your child is fearful or withdrawn too. | Child abuse | Call your pediatrician right away; if abuse is confirmed, the proper authorities will be notified, and steps will be taken to protect your child. |
| Your child bruises easily. She is pale, lethargic (lacking energy), or irritable. | A generalized disorder, which may include leukemia | Call your pediatrician right away. |

## IN GENERAL

A bluish tinge to the skin (cyanosis) shows that the underlying tissues are not getting enough oxygen. When the blue color occurs in just one part of the body, such as a hand or foot, it may mean that blood flow has been reduced by tight clothing or a bandage. Exposure to the cold can cause the lips, fingers, or toes to turn blue too. Skin returns to its normal color when it's warmed.

Very young babies often develop a blue-white ring around the mouth during feedings. This is perfectly normal and disappears after the feeding. However, if blue discoloration covers a large part of the body, it may be a sign that the baby is starved for oxygen and requires medical attention right away.

Some children with congenital heart disease will normally have a low oxygen saturation and may appear cyanotic all of the time. Discuss acceptable limits for oxygen saturation and methods for monitoring your child with your cardiologist.

Methemoglobinemia is a rare condition that can run in families. Affected children have an abnormal amount of a protein called *methemoglobin* inside red blood cells. Its presence limits the ability of the red blood cells to carry oxygen to the body. Skin deprived of oxygen often appears bluish. Because bluish skin can have other causes, talk with your child's pediatrician for advice about diagnosis and management.

### Call your pediatrician right away if your child has bluish discoloration of the

- Entire body
- Lips and tongue, together with noisy breathing
- Face, with fever

### WARNING!

If your child turns blue and cannot breathe, speak, or cough, call 911 or your local emergency number right away and follow procedures on page 215 or 216, depending on your child's age.

## Dealing With Breath-holding

It's a frightening scene: your normally loving child screams and cries so hard—usually during a temper tantrum but also when he's frightened or in pain—that he can't catch his breath and inhale. His face may go from scarlet to a grayish blue; some children fall to the floor and seem to pass out or go into a convulsion. While the scene looks alarming, it's probably not as bad as it appears. Most parents are more frightened by a breath-holding episode than the child is himself. So resist the temptation to restrain your child or force him to breathe; it's physically impossible for even the most determined and angry toddler to hold his breath long enough to cause any harm. If the youngster loses consciousness, his natural reflexes take over and he soon breathes normally again.

Even so, if your child faints or has a convulsion during a breath-holding episode, call your pediatrician. Your pediatrician may want to examine your child to make sure there is not a physical cause for the loss of consciousness or seizure. If your pediatrician suspects an emotional problem, he or she may refer you to a mental health professional. Most episodes, however, are harmless, and your child eventually finds more constructive ways to vent his anger. In the meantime, don't overreact to breath-holding. Stay calm, make sure your child is safe, but resist the temptation to play up the incident or give in to his demands. Such responses simply set the stage for future incidents. (For more guidelines, see "Temper Tantrums," page 156.)

| YOUR CONCERNS | POSSIBLE CAUSE | ACTION TO TAKE |
|---|---|---|
| Your child has been outdoors in the cold or swimming or playing in the water. She is shivering and cold to the touch. | Reaction to cold temperature (hypothermia) | Dry your child and wrap her in a blanket or move her to a warm room. If she is very cold, put her in a tub of tepid (moderately warm or lukewarm) water. Prevent hypothermia by dressing children according to the temperature. |
| Your child has a barking cough, and his breathing is labored and noisy. | Croup | Call 911 or your local emergency number or go to the nearest emergency department. (See "Dealing With Croup," page 58.) |
| Your child is blue around the mouth and wheezing. | Respiratory problem, possibly asthma | Call 911 or your local emergency number at once. (Also see "Allergic Reactions," page 26, and "Breathing Difficulty/Breathlessness," page 50.) |
| Your baby's skin looks blue. He has had a worsening cold and cough for the last day or two. He's breathing rapidly and with difficulty. He refuses to eat and is irritable and generally unwell. | Bronchiolitis (Also see "Breathing Difficulty/ Breathlessness," page 50.) | Call 911 or your local emergency number or your pediatrician at once. Your baby needs prompt evaluation and treatment. |
| Your child cries, holds his breath, passes out, then quickly comes to. | Breath-holding spell | Talk with your pediatrician, who will examine your child to rule out physical problems and recommend ways to deal with upsets and tantrums. (See "Dealing With Breath-holding," page 44, and "Temper Tantrums," page 155.) |
| Your child looks bluish, especially around the lips. She is feverish, feels poorly, and is breathing rapidly. She recently had symptoms of a cold or other viral illness. | Bronchopneumonia | Call your pediatrician right away. Your pediatrician will examine your child and may prescribe treatment or advise admission to the hospital. |
| Your child turns blue while eating, playing, or exercising. Her nails, lips, tongue, and mucous membranes are blue. | Heart, lung, or circulatory disorder | Call your pediatrician, who will examine your child and may refer her to another specialist for evaluation. |
| Your child has passed out and lost bladder control. She has previously had a seizure. | Seizure disorder (See page 134.) | Talk with your pediatrician, who will order tests and may prescribe an anticonvulsant medication. |

## IN GENERAL

A baby usually has bowleg (far-apart knees but close-together ankles) and intoeing (toes pointing toward each other [Figure 2-6]). These curvatures straighten out slowly over the first 3 years of life, so few toddlers have very straight legs. In fact, as they begin to walk, they sometimes develop tibial torsion (an inward curve of the shins). Tibial torsion often turns into mild knock knee (close-together knees but far-apart ankles) between 2 and 3 years of age. This curvature corrects itself by about 10 years of age; braces and corrective shoes are unhelpful. Most children have straight legs by adolescence (ie, 13 to 17 years of age), although having bowleg, knock knee, or intoeing as an adult runs in some families. Surgery may correct severe curvature of the knees or toes.

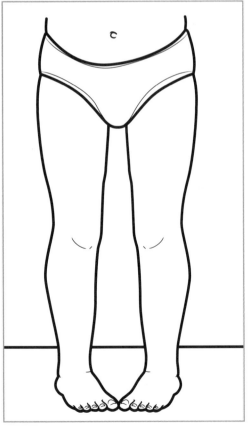

### Talk with your pediatrician if your child has

- Extreme curvature of a limb
- Curvature of a limb on one side
- Bowleg getting worse after 3 years of age
- Severe knock knee after 11 years of age
- Bowleg or knock knee and is extremely short for her age

**WARNING!**
Make sure to talk with your pediatrician if your child's bowleg seems to be getting worse after 3 years of age.

## Preventing Rickets

Rickets is poor mineralization of the bones (so the bones become soft). Once a leading cause of deformities, rickets has become less common with better nutrition. Your child needs vitamin D to help her bones form and stay strong. Children at risk for rickets include those with absorption problems, those who are on long-term treatment that prevents or relieves convulsions, and older infants and toddlers who are only breastfed and don't get enough nutrition. If you're unsure if your child is getting enough vitamin D in her diet, discuss your concern with your pediatrician.

**Figure 2-6.** The typical bowleg and intoeing of the early months gradually straighten out over the first 3 years. As the child begins to walk, however, the inward curve of the lower leg may turn to mild knock knee between ages 2 and 3. The legs generally straighten out by about 10 years without treatment. Braces and corrective shoes are rarely helpful. Most youngsters have straight legs by adolescence, although a tendency to intoeing or out-toeing may run in some families.

| YOUR CONCERNS | POSSIBLE CAUSE | ACTION TO TAKE |
|---|---|---|
| *Your child is younger than 3 years, and his legs look bowed (bent downward and forward).* | Genu varum (bowleg) | The bowed appearance is normal. The legs usually straighten by 3 years of age. |
| *Your child is between 12 and 24 months of age, and her lower legs are turned inward and bowed. Her feet point inward.* | Tibial torsion (a turning of the shin bone) | This problem is normal. It may be very noticeable at 18 to 24 months of age but usually corrects naturally by 3 years of age. |
| *Your child is unable to make his ankles meet when standing with his knees together.* | Genu valgum (knock knee) | If the problem is very severe, or if it interferes with your child's walking or running, talk with your pediatrician. |
| *Just one of your child's legs is bowed. She is older than 2 years and severely bowed.* | Tibia vara, also called *Blount disease* (a growth disorder of the tibia that causes the lower leg to angle inward) | Talk with your pediatrician. |
| *Your child is older than 10 years, and his feet still turn in when he runs.* | Femoral anteversion (thigh bone turning inward) | Check with your pediatrician. |
| *Your child's bowleg developed after a fracture.* | Injury to growth plate Poor healing | Talk with your pediatrician. |

## IN GENERAL

If you're concerned about breast swelling in your child, talk with your pediatrician. The presence of breast tissue may be normal, but this depends on your child's age and developmental stage.

Newborns sometimes have breast swelling. Their breasts may even secrete small amounts of milk. This happens because some of the mother's estrogen is passed on to her newborn while he's in the uterus. The newborn's breasts will decrease in size as the effect of the mother's hormones fades in him during the first few weeks of life. Older infants who are girls and toddlers may have a "mini-puberty" with short-lived swelling underneath their areola and nipple. This may also be normal. School-aged children who show signs of breast enlargement before 8 years of age (if girls) or 9 years of age (if boys) should be evaluated by their pediatrician for precocious puberty (earlier than usual puberty). Older girls and boys who are overweight may have breasts that appear enlarged because of fat that has accumulated in their upper chest. For more information about breast development in preteen and teenaged boys who are midway in puberty, see "Puberty," page 202.

### Call your pediatrician if

- Rather than general swelling, your child has a lump separate from her breast tissue and outside of her areola (the central pink area).
- Your child's breast swelling is inflamed and tender, and he has a fever.

### WARNING!

In a child of any age, tender breast swelling with redness on it may mean infection. Talk with your pediatrician because antibiotics may be required.

### Premature Breast Growth

Sometimes a young girl's breasts begin to enlarge when there are no other signs of sexual development. This condition, called *premature thelarche*, is common in girls younger than 3 years. It is due to some low level activity of the hormones that will bring her through puberty later in childhood; however, breast development may be the first sign of puberty and requires your pediatrician's attention and advice. Your pediatrician will help you recognize the differences between true breast enlargement and excess fat tissue.

| YOUR CONCERNS | POSSIBLE CAUSE | ACTION TO TAKE |
|---|---|---|
| Your newborn has breast swelling but is otherwise healthy. | Effect of mother's hormones | None. Newborn breast swelling and enlargement is due to the short-lived presence of the mother's hormones in her newborn's system. The swelling will subside as the hormonal effects fade over several weeks. |
| Your older infant who is a girl or your toddler aged 6 months to 2 years has enlarged breasts. | Premature thelarche, a benign development in some girls | Discuss your concerns with your pediatrician. Your child's growth chart and physical examination will help your pediatrician determine if this is a benign development or if talking with a specialist is necessary. |
| Your daughter is younger than 8 years and has breast development. | Precocious puberty (earlier than usual puberty) | Your pediatrician will examine your child and her growth charts. Breast development is often the first sign of puberty. Consultation with an endocrinologist may be necessary. |
| Your son is midway in puberty, and he has some breast enlargement. | Normal pubertal stage | Discuss your concerns with your pediatrician, who will examine your child and growth charts. Breast enlargement on only one side of the body happens quite frequently in boys. |
| Your school-aged child or teen, boy or girl, is over-weight and has breast enlargement. | Fat accumulation | Discuss this health problem with your pediatrician. Obesity is a major health risk, and a new nutrition and exercise plan should be started. |
| One of your baby's breasts is red or swollen. Your baby is in her first few months of life. | Breast infection or abscess (collection of pus) | Talk with your pediatrician, who will examine your newborn. Your newborn may need antibiotic treatment or placement in a hospital. |
| Breast swelling is occurring in your daughter younger than 8 years or your son younger than 9 years. | Accidental exposure to hormones In a girl, premature breast development In a boy, an adrenal tumor (hormone-producing tumor) | Talk with your pediatrician. Your child may have taken a family member's hormone medication, such as contraceptive pills, or used a lotion with estrogen in it. Premature breast development or an adrenal tumor may also be the cause. |

## IN GENERAL

Shortness of breath, called *dyspnea,* or trouble breathing often means that a child needs medical attention. Feeling short of breath occurs in many conditions, from respiratory diseases such as asthma and pneumonia to less common disorders such as defects in the lung or heart failure. These defects cause fluid buildup in the lungs. Fluid buildup in the lungs may also be caused by a blockage or infection in the airways. Sometimes anxiety may cause a child to hyperventilate (breathe too fast), which can lead to a change in the body's chemistry that, in turn, spurs more overbreathing.

### WARNING!

Don't put off seeking emergency treatment if your child's breathing gets more and more labored, if he's not making sounds or speaking, or if he's turning blue. These are signs that the respiratory tract is blocked, and your child is in danger of suffocating (see Chapter 4, "Basics of First Aid," pages 215–216).

### Call your pediatrician if your child

- Has severe shortness of breath
- Makes a whistling or barking noise when he breathes in
- Wheezes when he breathes out or in

### And has any of the following symptoms:

- Fever and chills and is vomiting
- Chest pain
- Thick, discolored, or bloody sputum (liquid that comes up from the lungs during illness)
- Bluish skin and tongue
- Unusual drowsiness
- Inability to swallow or speak
- Drooling
- An odd sitting posture

## Keeping Asthma Under Control

Asthma affects 6% to 10% of American children. The number of cases of asthma in the United States in children older than 5 years has increased 160% in the last 2 decades. Most children have mild asthma, but some experience frequent flare-ups; even severe asthma can usually be controlled by avoiding any substance or activity that triggers an attack.

Asthma occurs when tightened muscles in all airways, as well as inflamed bronchial tubes (the larger airways), prevent air from flowing properly into and out of the lungs. Attacks are often set off by viral infections, allergies, exercise, cold air, and smoke. The rate at which attacks occur is rising; experts believe exposure to cockroaches and an indoor lifestyle may be a trigger of attacks in children who live in urban areas. Although stress can also trigger attacks, asthma is a lung problem, not an emotional one.

Identifying your child's asthma triggers is important. Your pediatrician may recommend skin tests to identify allergens (allergy-causing substances). Or he or she may recommend you keep a diary to see what activities are related to your child's attacks. Most pediatricians advise a combined approach—avoidance of triggers, preventive medication, and lifestyle changes—to control asthma. When your child's asthma is properly controlled, she should be able to fully enjoy active sports and playtime. If you find she's having symptoms with activity, talk with your pediatrician so that the symptoms can be appropriately treated. Good asthma control doesn't restrict your child's physical activity.

| YOUR CONCERNS | POSSIBLE CAUSE | ACTION TO TAKE |
|---|---|---|
| *Your child has a stuffy nose, a sore throat and cough, and a mild fever.* | Common cold (Also see "Cough," page 58.) | Encourage your child to rest, and offer him fluids to thin his secretions. If he has a fever, give him a single-ingredient ibuprofen or acetaminophen. Call your pediatrician if your child's symptoms worsen or last for a week. If your baby has a stuffy nose, ask whether you should use saline nasal drops or spray and nasal suction. |
| *Your child has a barking cough, hoarseness, low fever, and chest discomfort. The symptoms worsen at night. Your child recently had a viral infection.* | Laryngotracheobronchitis (croup, or inflammation of the larynx, trachea, or bronchi) | Talk with your pediatrician. Use a cold-water vaporizer or humidifier at night (see "Dealing with Croup, page 58). If breathing is labored or your child begins to turn blue, go to the nearest emergency department or call 911 or your local emergency number. |
| *Your child is suddenly gasping, and her face is turning blue. She is unable to speak or make normal sounds.* | Choking on a foreign object or food | This is an emergency. Do the Heimlich maneuver while someone else calls 911 or your local emergency number (see Chapter 4, "Basics of First Aid," pages 215–216). |
| *Your child wheezes and coughs, especially at night or during or after exercise.* | Asthma | Call your pediatrician, who will examine your child and confirm if asthma is the cause. If it is, your pediatrician will recommend ways to control your child's disease. |
| *Your child is having an asthma attack, with bluish skin and difficulty speaking. She is confused and/or agitated.* | Sudden and severe asthma attack | If your child has a bronchodilator (medication that opens the airways), try it right away. Go to the nearest emergency department, or call 911 or your local emergency number at once. |
| *Your child is sitting up, gasping noisily, and has her mouth wide open and chin pushed down. Her skin and nails are bluish. She has a fever above 101 F° (38.3 C°).* | Epiglottitis (swelling of the tissue at the back of the throat that protects the windpipe from foreign objects) | This is a medical emergency. Call 911 or your local emergency number right away, or take your child to the nearest emergency department. Epiglottitis is now a rare infection, thanks to the Hib vaccine. It usually occurs only in children 3 years and older. |
| *Your infant or young child is breathing fast and hard. Has he had a cold and cough for 1 or 2 days. He is refusing to eat and is irritable and unwell.* | Bronchiolitis (inflammation of the smallest breathing airways of the lungs) | Call your pediatrician at once to examine your child. If he or she diagnoses bronchiolitis, your infant or young child needs prompt treatment. |
| *Your child is breathing fast and noisily, and she has a cough and chest pain. She is feverish and recently had a respiratory illness.* | Pneumonia | Call your pediatrician. You can frequently manage pneumonia at home with rest and medication as prescribed by your pediatrician. Some children need oxygen either at home or in the hospital. |
| *Your young child has developed noisy breathing over hours or days. He is coughing with or without a fever.* | Aspiration pneumonia (pneumonia caused by an inhaled object or food) | Call your pediatrician, who will order x-rays and, if necessary, arrange treatment. |
| *Your child is suddenly having trouble breathing. Her skin is clammy with widespread swelling, and her pulse is racing. She has allergies and has she been stung by an insect.* | Anaphylaxis (severe allergic reaction) | Call emergency medical services right away, or take your child to the nearest emergency department. This is a medical emergency. Your child needs urgent attention. |
| *Your preteen or teenager is having trouble breathing. She is lightheaded and has numbness or tingling in her hands and feet.* | Hyperventilation (overbreathing caused by anxiety; also see Chapter 3, page 180) | Try to identify and eliminate causes of your child's anxiety. Your pediatrician may wish to examine your child to rule out physical conditions that produce symptoms similar to those of anxiety. He or she will recommend a treatment plan. |

## IN GENERAL

Chest pain that starts, stops, and starts again is common in children and not usually caused by a serious health problem. The most common cause of chest pain is chest muscle strain—usually caused by increased physical activity or a new sport. Chest pain may also be caused by muscle tension that stems from emotional stress at school or home, or just from your child's inner anxiety. Pain in the chest wall may be due to inflammation of the cartilage between the ribs and the sternum, called *costochondritis*. This health problem can be treated with an anti-inflammatory medication such as ibuprofen. Pain caused by heart and lung problems needs to be checked for and, if found, treated appropriately. Serious but unusual causes of chest pain in children include illnesses that can cause infection, such as pneumonia; problems in the digestive tract, such as esophagitis (an inflamed esophagus) or ulcers; hyperventilation (in older children); and pneumothorax (a collapsed lung).

### Call your pediatrician right away if your child

- Has persistent (won't go away) or unusually severe chest pain, even when resting
- Complains of unusual thumping or racing sensations in her chest
- Has difficulty breathing

### WARNING!

If your child has chest pain that persists and gets worse during exercise, see your pediatrician. Chest pain that develops after an injury requires prompt medical attention to rule out a broken rib, a collapsed lung, and other injuries.

## Collapsed Lung as a Cause of Chest Pain

Sometimes a collapsed lung, called *pneumothorax,* causes sharp chest pain and sudden and severe shortness of breath in a child; however, pneumothorax is more common in men between 20 and 40 years of age. Children with chronic illnesses, such as cystic fibrosis, are most often affected by pneumothorax, but it can also occur in healthy children—usually thin teenaged boys—for no apparent reason.

Pneumothorax occurs when a small patch of lung tissue ruptures, which allows air to leak out of the lung and accumulate between it and the chest wall. If the leak is small, your child will have pain but no other symptoms; your pediatrician should evaluate your child, but specific treatment may be unnecessary. This is because the leak will seal itself, and the free air will be absorbed slowly over time. But if a large accumulation of air causes part of your child's lung to collapse, your child may have sharp chest pain; a dry, hacking cough; and difficulty breathing. Treatment may involve a minor procedure to remove the air, but most children recover under the careful watch of medical professionals.

| YOUR CONCERNS | POSSIBLE CAUSE | ACTION TO TAKE |
|---|---|---|
| Your child is growing at a normal rate and has a healthy appetite. He is breathing normally and has recently increased his level of athletic activity or taken up a new sport. He has had a recent injury. | Muscle strain<br>Bruise<br>Costochondritis (inflammation of the chest wall) | Give your child ibuprofen to relieve his pain. Talk with your pediatrician if your child's pain doesn't improve in 2 to 3 days. |
| Your child feels pain while resting but not for longer than 1 to 2 minutes at a time. His health is generally good, but he's academic and social difficulties at school. There is some unusual tension at home. Your child is also a worrier. | Nonspecific chest pain | Call your pediatrician, who will examine your child to rule out serious causes. Using sensitive questioning, your pediatrician may be able to identify sources of your child's anxiety. He or she may suggest treatment. In the meantime, help your child concentrate on a hobby, which may divert his attention from his physical symptoms. |
| Your child has a cough or respiratory illness. Her temperature is elevated (101°F [38.3°C] or higher). | Pneumonia or another infectious disease | Call your pediatrician, who will examine your child; your child may require treatment. Your pediatrician will advise on pain relief and prescribe other medications as appropriate. |
| Your child sometimes awakens with pain in his chest or upper abdomen. He complains of heartburn or a sour taste in his mouth. He sometimes vomits, but he's growing normally. | Digestive problem, such as gastro-esophageal reflux, esophagitis, or peptic ulcer | Talk with your pediatrician, who may prescribe medication. Cut out caffeine, such as in colas or chocolate. Raise the head of your child's bed, which may help prevent nighttime reflux of stomach acid into his esophagus. |
| Your child complains of a pounding heart or unusual changes in his heart rhythm (other than normal increases during exercise). These changes last longer than 1 or 2 minutes. She gets chest pain when exercising and feels dizzy, light-headed, or faint. When this happens, she appears pale, ill, or sweaty. | Heart disorder (rare) | Call your pediatrician without delay. Your child may require an extensive examination and diagnostic tests. These actions will help your pediatrician rule out serious causes of your child's chest pain; they will also help your pediatrician identify the source of the pain. |
| Your child's chest pain occurs while she's resting. She has swelling and tenderness of her joints along with a rash on her face or body. | Autoimmune disorder such as juvenile idiopathic arthritis or lupus | Talk with your pediatrician, who will examine your child and refer her, if necessary, to a health specialist for evaluation. |

## IN GENERAL

Many parents mistakenly think that a child who doesn't have a daily bowel movement is constipated. The fact is, children's bowel patterns vary widely: some children have several bowel movements daily, while others may go 2 or 3 days before passing a stool of normal consistency. In contrast, constipation involves passing a hard, dry stool, may require straining, and even causes pain.

Don't be alarmed if your infant gets red in his face, grimaces, and grunts during his bowel movements. This is perfectly normal and simply means your child's coordination is developing. If his stool is soft, he isn't constipated or in pain.

Children's diets should include plenty of fluids and high-fiber foods such as fruits, vegetables, and whole-grain products. Regular exercise is important for regularity too. Make sure your child sits on the toilet once or twice a day so he can develop a healthy bowel habit. A regular toilet schedule can help set good bowel habits for life.

### Talk with your pediatrician if your child

- Complains of painful bowel movements
- Passes hard, dry stools
- Has abdominal pain that is relieved by bowel movements
- Has blood in or on his stools
- Is leaking fluid between bowel movements

### WARNING!

Don't use laxatives or enemas to treat your child's constipation unless your pediatrician says it's OK. Unwarranted use of laxatives can disrupt your child's normal bowel function.

## Anxiety and Stool Withholding

Conflicting emotions about independence and control often emerge when toilet training is introduced, and some youngsters express these feelings through reluctance to move their bowels on the potty or toilet. When they withhold stools, the result is that retained feces become dry and compacted, and bowel movements are painful. A vicious cycle of stool withholding and pain can lead to severe anxiety and a situation in which your family's attention is focused on the child's bowel movements. Sometimes newer liquid stool leaks out around the compacted stool, and parents mistake this soiling for diarrhea.

Your pediatrician will approach this problem with a step-by-step program of bowel retraining, which usually involves giving your child a stool softener and keeping a regular toileting schedule. Increasing fiber in your child's diet with more fruits, vegetables, and cereals may be helpful. You should also encourage your child to drink plenty of water, juices, and other fluids, especially in hot weather and after exercise. Regular physical activity also promotes smooth bowel function (also see Chapter 2, page 150).

| YOUR CONCERNS | POSSIBLE CAUSE | ACTION TO TAKE |
|---|---|---|
| *Your breastfed infant who is 4 to 6 months of age has changed her bowel pattern; she's passing fewer and harder stools.* | Mild constipation during the transition to solid foods<br>Child's own bowel rhythm | Some breastfed infants become mildly constipated when introduced to solid foods, but they soon return to normal. If your infant's stool is hard, your pediatrician may suggest a change in your infant's diet. |
| *Your formula-fed infant is passing hard, dry stools.* | Composition of the formula | Consult your pediatrician, who may recommend treatment that softens your infant's stools |
| *Your child has a normal bowel movement at least every 3 days. She is otherwise healthy and in no discomfort.* | Child's own bowel rhythm | Make sure your child gets plenty of fluids and high-fiber foods, including fruits and vegetables. Cut back on low-fiber foods such as bananas, rice, cereals, or breads. |
| *You have weaned your infant from breastmilk or formula to cow's milk.* | The switch to cow's milk and dairy products, which may have a binding effect | Limit cow's milk to 16 to 24 ounces per day. Ask your pediatrician for dietary suggestions. |
| *Your infant is passing infrequent, hard stools. He cries in pain when he has a bowel movement.* | Tight anal sphincter (tight band of muscles around his anus) | Talk with your pediatrician, who will examine your infant and may recommend treatment. |
| *Your newborn or young infant has passed only a few, hard stools since birth, despite being given a stool softener. Her abdomen is swollen.* | Hirschsprung disease, an *uncommon* inborn absence of the nerves needed for bowel movements | Talk with your pediatrician, who will examine your baby to determine whether retained stool is causing her abdomen to expand while her rectum is empty. If Hirschsprung disease is diagnosed, it can be treated with surgery. |
| *Your child has become constipated since you started toilet training him.* | Not ready to be trained | Hold off on toilet training for now; try again when your child takes the initiative and is no longer constipated. |
| *Your child is complaining of discomfort because he can't move his bowels. His stools are small and dry pellets.* | Constipation, which may have many causes, including not enough fiber and fluid in the diet or stress | Call your pediatrician, who will help with a course of treatment. Increase the fiber and liquids in your child's diet. Encourage your child to eat fresh fruits and vegetables and to take part in regular physical activity. Try to eliminate or reduce your child's sources of stress. |
| *Your child complains of pain during or after a bowel movement. She has blood on or in her stools. She has a rash around her anus.* | Anal fissure (a painful line-shaped ulcer at the margin of the anus)<br>Perianal dermatitis (skin inflammation in the anal area) | Talk with your pediatrician, who will examine your child and recommend treatment. He or she may recommend giving your child a stool softener. |
| *Your constipated child is vomiting greenish-yellow material, and his abdomen is distended (also see "Abdominal Swelling," page 24).* | Intestinal blockage (rare) | Call your pediatrician right away. Don't give your child anything to eat or drink until your pediatrician has examined your child. If your pediatrician diagnoses intestinal blockage, your child may be hospitalized for treatment. |

## IN GENERAL

Children develop coordination (ability to move different parts of the body at the same time) and dexterity (ability to use the hands) at different rates. While a few children are naturally graceful and agile, others have more difficulty with motor development. Your infants' fine motor skills (ability to move small muscles) develops similarly to and at the same time as her gross motor skills (ability to move large muscles). But gross motor skills develop more than fine motor skills in her first 6 months of life. Some preteens and teens go through an awkward phase as they adjust to the physical changes and growth spurt of puberty.

You can help your child improve coordination with crafts and sports. Encourage your child to take part in recreational activities at a level he finds physically and emotionally rewarding.

### Talk with your pediatrician if

- Your coordinated child becomes clumsy.
- Your child develops clumsiness with headaches, vomiting, or vision problems.
- Your child becomes increasingly clumsy.

### WARNING!

If clumsiness is making your child self-conscious or preventing him from being part of certain activities, talk with your pediatrician. He or she may recommend physical, movement, or occupational therapy to improve your child's coordination.

## Clumsiness and Hyperactivity

Impulsive, fidgety, overactive: if this sounds like your child, see your pediatrician. Often these and other behaviors point to attention-deficit/hyperactivity disorder (page 30), especially if a close relative (ie, parent or sibling) had similar difficulties in childhood. Only specialists can diagnose ADHD and recommend necessary treatment. If your family is under stress because your child acts clumsy, restless, and unpredictable, seek professional help.

| YOUR CONCERNS | POSSIBLE CAUSE | ACTION TO TAKE |
|---|---|---|
| *Your child is younger than 3 years and seems clumsy.* | Normal motor development | Discuss your concerns with your pediatrician. Play movement games to help your child develop coordination and hone her fine motor skills. |
| *Your school-aged child is clumsy, and the clumsiness gets worse when he's under stress.* | Slow motor development | Your pediatrician will examine your child to rule out physical problems, and he or she may recommend further evaluation and therapy. |
| *Your school-aged child finds it hard to tell right from left or to recognize words, letters, and numbers.* | Developmental problems (central processing disorder) | Your pediatrician will examine your child and, if necessary, refer him for psychological and educational evaluation. |
| *Your child is taking a medication and develops poor coordination.* | Side effect of the medication | Your pediatrician will determine whether the medication can cause coordination problems. He or she will change the dosage or order tests. |
| *Your child has developed muscle weakness and a tendency to stumble. He has headaches or vomits.* | Disorder of the muscles or nervous system | Call your pediatrician without delay to arrange an examination. She will refer your child to a health specialist, if necessary. |

## IN GENERAL

Coughing is our body's way of keeping our airways clear. When your child has a cold or other minor illness, the coughing and other symptoms disappear slowly over time. But when your child has a more serious illness, such as asthma or whooping cough, the coughing doesn't slow down, stop, or grow weaker, and it can tire your child. Your child may need medical help to cure the underlying cause of the coughing, open her airways, clear away her secretions, and help her get the rest she needs to regain her health.

• • • • • • • • • • • • • • • • • • • • • • • • • • • • • • • • •

### Call your pediatrician right away if your child is coughing and

- Has noisy, rapid, difficult breathing
- Has a temperature of 101°F (38.3°C) or higher that lasts longer than 24 to 48 hours
- Is sluggish or drowsy
- Has bluish discoloration around her lips, mouth, and fingernails
- Refuses to drink

• • • • • • • • • • • • • • • • • • • • • • • • • • • • • • • • •

## WARNING!

Don't give your child over-the-counter cough medicines without talking with your pediatrician. Cough suppressants aren't recommended for children younger than 6 years and should not be given to older children unless coughing is interfering with their sleep.

## Dealing With Croup

Croup attacks usually ease when a child breathes in a steamy bathroom or next to an opened window that lets in cool air. Medical treatment may be necessary, however, if your child's symptoms are severe or prolonged. Children should not be exposed to second-hand tobacco smoke, particularly if they are prone to croup. Placing a cool-mist humidifier in your child's bedroom can often prevent croup attacks, especially if the air in her bedroom is normally dry.

Boys get croup more often than girls. Attacks often follow a viral infection, such as the common cold or influenza, so antibiotics are rarely helpful. Croup that happens again and again is thought to be caused by an allergy rather than an infection. Children generally outgrow croup by about 5 years of age.

| YOUR CONCERNS | POSSIBLE CAUSE | ACTION TO TAKE |
|---|---|---|
| *Your child has a runny nose and sore throat.* | Common cold | Make sure your child gets extra rest, and give her clear fluids to help thin her secretions. If she has irritated lips and nostrils, soothe them by applying salve to them. If your child is older than 12 months, offer her honey to relieve coughing. Cold symptoms should clear up in about a week (also see "Breathing Difficulty/Breathlessness," page 50, and "Runny/Stuffy Nose," page 132). |
| *Your child wakes up at night with a barking cough and difficulty breathing. He is younger than 5 years and recently had a cold. You may hear a high-pitched sound when he breathes in, called* stridor. | Croup | Ease your child's breathing in a steamy bathroom (see "Dealing With Croup"). |
| *Your baby is younger than 12 months and has been coughing hard for at least 2 hours. She recently had a cold or sniffles.* | Bronchiolitis (a viral lung infection that sometimes follows a cold) | Call your pediatrician for advice and care. This infection usually clears up within a week (see "Breathing Difficulty/Breathlessness," page 50). |

| YOUR CONCERNS | POSSIBLE CAUSE | ACTION TO TAKE |
|---|---|---|
| Your child's temperature is higher than 100.4°F (38°C). She has a runny nose, sore throat, and cough. She also has joint and muscle pains and generally doesn't feel well. | Influenza | Make sure your child drinks lots of fluids; give her acetaminophen or ibuprofen to lower her temperature and ease her discomfort. Call your pediatrician if her symptoms don't improve within 2 days, she develops a rash or has difficulty breathing (see "Breathing Difficulty/Breathlessness," page 50), or she seems sicker. Influenza is largely preventable with annual vaccination for all children 6 months and older. |
| Your child coughs and sneezes throughout the day but rarely at night. He has a constantly runny nose with clear discharge. | Allergic rhinitis (hay fever; any allergic reaction of the nasal lining) Tracheobronchitis (inflammation of the airways) | Talk with your pediatrician, who may recommend a medication (see "Allergic Reactions," page 26). |
| Your child has a persistent (won't go away) cough and a yellowish nasal discharge for 10 or more days following a cold. | Sinusitis (inflammation of a sinus) | Talk with your pediatrician, who will examine your child and prescribe an antibiotic if he or she confirms a sinus infection (see "Treating Sinusitis," page 132). |
| Your child has a persistent (won't go away) daytime cough with no other symptoms. The cough usually stops once your child is asleep. | Habit cough or a tic | Try to identify and remove sources of your child's anxiety. Talk with your child's teachers if school difficulties are causing emotional problems in your child. Ask your pediatrician whether counseling might help your child. |
| Your child has a persistent (won't go away) cough and throat irritation. There is a source of air pollution nearby, and someone in your household smokes. | Environmental irritant | Ask your pediatrician how to lessen your child's exposure to the irritant. Test out ways of filtering household air or minimizing the effects of pollutants. Encourage family members to stop smoking. At the very least, forbid smoking inside of your house or apartment. |
| Your child's coughing is worse at night. He coughs when exercising or in cold air. He also wheezes. You have family members with allergies and asthma. | Asthma | Your pediatrician will examine your child and evaluate his lung function. If your pediatrician confirms asthma, your child will need treatment; you'll need to take measures to lessen your child's exposure to her asthma triggers (see "Breathing Difficulty/Breathlessness," page 50). |
| Your young child suddenly starts coughing but has no other symptoms. You suspect he's choking on a small object or piece of food. | Foreign object in the airways | If your child can't speak and is turning blue, start help for choking (see Chapter 4, "Basics of First Aid," pages 215–216) and call 911 or your local emergency number. Otherwise, call your pediatrician at once. Your child needs treatment to remove the object and prevent further health problems. |
| Your child has a chronic cough and frequent colds. Her sputum (liquid from the respiratory tract) is hard to cough up and may be discolored. Physically she seems to be growing slowly. Her stools are very large in number, greasy, and foul smelling. Her sweat tastes salty. | Cystic fibrosis (an inherited condition that affects the cells that produce mucus, sweat, and digestive juices) | Your pediatrician will examine your child and order tests. This inherited disorder is usually diagnosed in babies, but a cough, poor growth, and other symptoms may point to cystic fibrosis in an older child. If your pediatrician confirms this diagnosis, your child will need lifelong treatment and a special diet. |

## IN GENERAL

A baby's eyes normally tend to wander off and on during the first few months of life; however, babies soon learn to use both eyes together, and they are able to coordinate their eye movements between 3 and 6 months of age.

If your child's eyes continue to wander at times, cross, or move in different directions after early infancy, he may have an eye muscle imbalance called *strabismus.* Strabismus causes misaligned eyes. Eyes can wander outward, called *exotropia;* cross inward, called *esotropia;* and misalign in other ways (Figure 2-7). Strabismus makes it impossible for both eyes to focus on the same object.

Sometimes young children may appear to have cross-eye when they don't; they have a wide nasal bridge and broad skin folds that distort the appearance of their eye alignment. This eye problem is known as *pseudostrabismus.* As their face matures and the bridge of their nose becomes narrower, the alignment of their eyes starts to look normal; however, a child whose eyes are truly crossed needs medical attention. Children with strabismus won't outgrow it, and it can negatively affect their vision in the future.

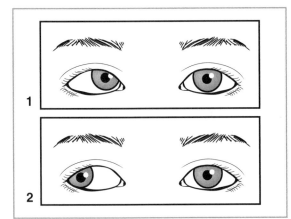

**Figure 2-7.** When one eye is lazy and not tracking correctly, as shown here in the child's left eye, it may move inward (1) or outward (2). A young child with this condition may need to wear eyeglasses and/or a patch to correct a lazy eye. Glasses, exercise, or surgery can help correct the misalignment.

### Talk with your pediatrician if

- Your infant's eyes appear crossed or don't work together after she's 4 months of age.
- Your child often holds her head in an abnormal or tilted position.
- Your child regularly squints in an effort to see more clearly.
- A drooping eyelid makes one of your child's eyes appear smaller than the other.
- Your child often closes one eye.
- Your child's eyes shake or appear to bounce.
- Your child's eyes reflect light differently from each other in photographs.

> **WARNING!**
> If strabismus isn't diagnosed and treated early, your child will have poor depth perception and risk a loss of vision in her misaligned eye.

## Correcting Eye Problems

Eye problems in children must be treated early; certain conditions can't be corrected once the visual system is fully developed by mid-adolescence (ie, 14 to 16 years of age). That's why your pediatrician checks your young child's eyes at every regular well-child visit. He or she looks for signs of eye disease and makes sure that both eyes are working together. Formal vision testing is often done when your child is 3 years of age—old enough to follow directions and describe what she sees. If you have a family history of serious eye problems, amblyopia (lazy eye), or cross-eye, or you're concerned about specific problems, your pediatrician will examine your young child and refer her (even if she's a very young infant) to a pediatric ophthalmologist (eye specialist) for more thorough testing.

Children born prematurely are more likely than other children to develop eye problems, including problems inside the eye, cross-eye, and very blurred vision.

Strabismus may be present from infancy, appear later in childhood, or be caused by poor focusing. It can also result from disease or injury of the eye or brain. Treatment usually involves eyeglasses, eyedrops, exercises, or surgery. Surgery, if necessary, is best performed when the pediatric ophthalmologist feels the eye misalignment isn't improving, even as early as 6 to 18 months in babies and young children who were born with strabismus. Many children still need eyeglasses and patches, at least for a while, after undergoing corrective surgery.

Amblyopia (lazy eye) is the loss of vision, usually in one eye, due to strabismus, high refractive errors (usually astigmatism or farsightedness), ptosis (a very droopy upper eyelid), or other problems that affect one eye more than the other. Treatment of amblyopia may involve consistent use of eyeglasses, treatment of strabismus or ptosis, a patch over the stronger eye, or eyedrops in the stronger eye. These treatments can greatly improve the vision in your child's amblyopic eye. Treatment works best in young children. Without good enough treatment, amblyopia becomes permanent in children as young as 8 years.

| YOUR CONCERNS | POSSIBLE CAUSE | ACTION TO TAKE |
|---|---|---|
| Your child is 6 months or older. His eyes still move independently, at least part of the time. One eye looks out or in when the other is focused on an object; both eyes are turned in; or both eyes were normal but suddenly developed into cross-eye or wandering eye. | Strabismus (crossed or misaligned eyes) | Talk with your pediatrician, who will examine your infant or young child and refer him to an eye doctor (pediatric ophthalmologist) for complete evaluation and treatment. |
| One of your child's eyes appears much smaller than the other because of a drooping upper eyelid. This eyelid appears to interfere with your child's vision. She lifts her chin or face to see. | Ptosis (drooping of the upper eyelid) | Talk with your pediatrician, who will determine if referral to another specialist is advisable. Severe ptosis may interfere with your child's vision development and should be treated. |
| Your child has strabismus, or his results on a vision screening reveal potential vision problems. Your family has a medical history of amblyopia (lazy eye). | Amblyopia (lazy eye) | Talk with your pediatrician, who will determine if referral to a pediatric ophthalmologist (eye specialist) is appropriate. Amblyopia doesn't improve without treatment. If amblyopia persists in a child after about 5 to 6 years, the vision in the child's unused eye may be permanently damaged (see "Correcting Eye Problems," page 60). |
| Your child's eyes appear to bounce or wiggle. | Nystagmus (involuntary, rapid, rhythmic movement of the eyes) | Talk with your pediatrician without delay; your child may need to be evaluated by a neurologist or pediatric ophthalmologist (eye specialist), who will determine the cause of this eye problem. |

## IN GENERAL

Healthy teeth are essential to clear speech and proper nutrition. The primary teeth must be well cared for if the permanent teeth are to be sound and well positioned. Your baby's teeth should be cleaned regularly with a soft toothbrush. You should be brushing your child's teeth twice a day. After your child is 8 years of age, you can supervise her brushing. Most children need close supervision and help with brushing and flossing. But even long afterward, you may have to remind your child to brush her teeth every night and morning until the act becomes second nature.

Sugar directly damages the teeth; sugars that linger on the teeth—such as sticky dried fruits or sugars produced from starchy cereal residues in the mouth—are especially damaging. Your child's diet should emphasize water intake as well as non-cariogenic (don't produce tooth decay) snacks such as raw vegetables.

Dentists use an array of approaches, including sealants and fluoride treatments, to prevent tooth decay. Orthodontic treatment, when necessary, is most effective while the bones are young and pliable. It can help promote lifelong dental health.

Don't ignore a child's complaint of mouth pain (see page 118). While some minor causes of discomfort clear up by themselves, severe or nagging pain may signal a serious problem that could have lasting effects on your child's health and appearance if left untreated.

**Call your child's dentist right away if one of your child's permanent teeth has been knocked loose. A tooth can often be re-implanted if**

- You rinse it under running tap water right away, don't touch the root, and place it in cow's milk for transport to your child's dentist.
- Your child is seen by his dentist as soon as possible. The re-implantation of a tooth is most successful if done within 30 minutes.

> **WARNING!**
> Never put your child to bed with a bottle of milk, formula, juice, or similar sweet drinks. Prolonged contact with sugar in these beverages can cause serious dental decay, called *early childhood caries*. If your child can't settle down without a bottle, fill it with plain water. Similarly, never dip a pacifier in honey or another sweet.

## Coping With Drooling and Biting

A baby entering the teething phase usually drools more and may keep several fingers or a fist constantly in her mouth. Many people believe that fever, diarrhea, and other symptoms are caused by teething, but they aren't. If your baby has these symptoms, talk with your pediatrician. A fussy, teething baby may be comforted by chewing on a teething ring or a hard, unsweetened teething cracker. Don't use frozen teething toys; the extreme cold may injure your baby's mouth tissues and cause more pain. The pain relievers you rub on her gums are not necessary or helpful.

| YOUR CONCERNS | POSSIBLE CAUSE | ACTION TO TAKE |
|---|---|---|
| *Your baby is drooling more than usual. She keeps her fist or finger constantly in her mouth.* | Teething, a normal developmental stage | Comfort your baby and ease her soreness by rubbing her gums with your clean finger or a clean, cold washcloth (see "Coping With Drooling and Biting," page 62). If she's unusually upset or has a temperature higher than 100.4°F (38°C), call your pediatrician; your baby's symptoms may be due to another condition. |
| *Your child has throbbing tooth pain that comes and goes. His teeth (or a tooth) are sensitive to heat and cold.* | Early childhood caries (tooth decay) | Schedule an appointment with your child's dentist as soon as possible. Treatment may require a filling. |
| *Your child's recently filled tooth hurts when she bites on it. Her tooth feels as though it doesn't fit properly in her mouth.* | Temporary sensitivity following treatment | Sensitivity that lingers after a filling will eventually grow weaker. If your child's tooth doesn't feel right, talk with your child's dentist, who may adjust the filling for a better fit. |
| *Your child's gums are red and swollen. They bleed easily on brushing.* | Gingivitis or periodontal disease (inflammation of the gums, especially in preteens and teens) | Talk with your pediatrician, who will refer you to your child's dentist if treatment is needed for gum disease. |
| *Your child grinds his teeth while asleep. He complains of jaw pain when he wakes.* | Bruxism (tooth grinding), usually due to stress | Talk with your pediatrician and your child's dentist. Tooth grinding may damage your child's teeth or gums, but a nighttime mouth guard may help break his habit. |
| *Your child older than 6 still sucks her thumb. You're concerned that thumb-sucking may distort her permanent teeth.* | Thumb-sucking | If she sucks her thumb briefly to get to sleep, treatment is unnecessary. If her habit is more severe, ask your pediatrician or your child's dentist for advice about dealing with thumb-sucking. They may recommend a mouth appliance to remind your child not to suck her thumb. |
| *Your child has steady pain in his mouth. A tooth of his feels loose, raised, or different. It aches when your child eats sweets or cold foods.* | Tooth abscess (collection of pus) Cracked tooth Decay under a filling | Call your child's dentist right away. He or she will determine whether your child's tooth can be saved or must be extracted. Give your child acetaminophen or ibuprofen to relieve his discomfort. |
| *Your child's primary tooth apparently has been knocked out and is nowhere to be found.* | Tooth extruded (pushed out), intruded (depressed), lost, or swallowed | Call your child's dentist right away. Sometimes a tooth is forced back into the gum, but it often re-erupts on its own and remains healthy until shed at the appropriate time. Only permanent teeth are placed back into the gum. |

## IN GENERAL

Growth and development tend to follow a general pattern, but every child develops at his own pace, depending on genetics and other factors. The age at which a child reaches major milestones, such as walking and talking, varies from one child to another. If your child is reaching his milestones within a certain age range (see "Developmental Milestones for the First 3 Years," page 66), his progress is probably quite typical.

About 1 in 88 children, however, have a hereditary or inborn condition that may be associated with development delay, such as an autism spectrum disorder see page 68). In other children, a severe illness or injury can lead to developmental delay. Other problems present themselves as these children get older, such as when a child begins school and has trouble keeping up with classmates.

In a large number of hereditary or congenital defects, the cause can be identified; new technology can detect some conditions before birth such as Down syndrome, neural tube defects, and certain genetic conditions so that parents are better prepared to deal with the extra care their child may need from the very beginning. In some cases, a developmental delay occurs with a chronic medical condition. Early detection and treatment can lessen the impact and give your child a better quality of life.

A child whose development seems delayed should have a complete medical and developmental examination. If your pediatrician is concerned that your child isn't developing typically, he or she will advise an evaluation, possibly including a consultation with a developmental specialist. Properly conducted tests show not only a child's problems but also his particular strengths and abilities. In many communities, evaluations are provided without charge or at minimal cost. Your local board of education, health department, or social services agency can provide information about services offered in your area.

Depending on the screening or assessment results, your pediatrician can recommend a plan for physical, speech, and occupational therapy. Special education may also be required. With the support of teachers and therapists, parents can set realistic goals and help their child develop his abilities. Federal and state programs provide extra help for children with developmental disabilities and their families.

Even experts find it difficult to make long-range predictions about development from tests conducted when a child is 1 or 2 years of age. This is because children affected with the same condition vary widely in their degree of developmental delay. A series of tests over time provides a broader and more accurate picture than a single assessment. Studies have confirmed that regardless of any disability detected during the early years, the environment in which a child is reared is a very important factor in helping him reach his maximum potential.

**Talk with your pediatrician if your child**

- Was making progress but is losing skills such as talking, social interaction, or walking
- Is not meeting milestones outlined on page 66

### WARNING!

Postpartum depression is a serious mood disorder that can affect both mothers and fathers. Parental depression can harm the parent-child relationship and even lead to child abuse, neglect, and discontinuation of breastfeeding. It can also cause developmental delays in your baby, as well as social and behavioral problems down the road. If you suspect that either parent has depression, seek medical attention immediately.

## Early Brain Development

The first 1,000 days of a baby's life are critical to building a healthy brain. The plasticity of the developing brain in these early years makes it extremely sensitive to early experiences, especially early relationships.

Brain development isn't about just one activity. Instead, it's an integrated process in which social, emotional, and learning skills are closely intertwined and dependent on each other. The areas supporting memory and learning are closely connected to the areas that support social, emotional, and language development.

Toxic stress such as abuse, neglect, and parental mental illness or substance abuse disrupts the developing brain and can cause lasting damage to a child's health.

Positive parenting and nurturing, on the other hand, helps buffer the brain from stress and build resilience. The family—and in particular, the parents—play a critical role in a child's early brain development. The American Academy of Pediatrics encourages parents to engage in the 5 Rs.

- Read together with your child every day.
- Rhyme, play, and cuddle with your child every day.
- Develop routines, particularly around meals, sleep, and family fun.
- Reward your child with praise for successes to build self-esteem and promote positive behavior.
- Develop a strong and nurturing relationship with your child as the foundation for their healthy development.

In addition, your child needs time to play. Play is so important to optimal child development that it's been recognized by the United Nations High Commission for Human Rights as a right of every child.

While children in some countries are limited by child labor and exploitation, or war and violence, children in the United States are often hampered by a hurried and pressured lifestyle that robs them of free play. Instead, the focus here is often on enrichment activities that hinge on parental fears that their children will be denied access to higher education opportunities. Children are also more and more engaged by electronics, a passive form of entertainment that can have harmful effects.

It's important to understand that brain development is cumulative. Early, simple connections and circuits form the foundation for more complex pathways and behaviors. Like muscles, connections and circuits that are used frequently become stronger and more efficient over time ("neurons that fire together, wire together"). But those con-nections and circuits that aren't utilized are pruned and eliminated ("if you don't use it, you lose it"). The bottom line is that creating the right conditions in early childhood is more effective and less costly than addressing problems later on in life.

| YOUR CONCERNS | POSSIBLE CAUSE | ACTION TO TAKE |
|---|---|---|
| *Your 2-month-old infant feels unusually stiff or floppy. His head falls backward if you pull him up while he's lying flat. At 6 months of age, he almost always reaches for objects with only one hand while keeping the other in a fist. At 10 months or older, he crawls lopsidedly; he pushes forward with his leg and arm on one side while dragging his other leg and arm. He moves about but doesn't crawl on all fours.* | Developmental delay Cerebral palsy (while sometimes caused by illness during pregnancy, may also follow a severe illness or injury during infancy) | Talk with your pediatrician, who will examine your infant and determine whether he should be seen by another health specialist. |
| *Your child seems more and more clumsy and has difficulty walking.* | Neurologic or muscular disorder | Talk with your pediatrician, who will examine your child and refer you to another health specialist, if necessary (see "Coordination Problems," page 56 ) |
| *Your "late talker" is also behind schedule in walking and other motor skills. He is older than 2 years and says fewer than 5 words. The words are unclear.* | Delayed development Hearing loss | Talk with your pediatrician, who will examine your child with special attention to hearing. Your child may need to be referred to another health specialist. |
| *Your child is having difficulty at school. He is having problems reading or with numbers. He has trouble keeping up with classmates in learning and social development.* | Delayed development Learning problems (See page 110.) Emotional stress | Talk with teachers to determine the extent of the problem. Your pediatrician will examine your child to rule out physical problems and recommend a treatment plan. |

## DEVELOPMENTAL MILESTONES

|  | DEVELOPMENTAL MILESTONES FOR THE FIRST 3 YEARS |
|---|---|
| 0 to 12 Weeks | • Eats and sleeps in first couple weeks of life<br>• Begins to motion toward mouth<br>• Opens and shuts fists<br>• Turns toward familiar voices<br>• Prefers human faces to other patterns |
| 3 Months<br>(Figure 2-8A) | • Makes gurgling, cooing, babbling, or other noises besides crying<br>• Usually keeps hands open<br>• Holds head up for a few seconds when held upright<br>• Responds to your voice |
| 6 Months<br>(Figure 2-8B) | • Plays with hands by touching them together<br>• Turns head to sounds coming from a different room<br>• Can roll over from stomach to back or from back to stomach<br>• When held under the arms, seems like he is trying to stand<br>• Reaches for you, when he sees you<br>• Produces a string of sounds |
| 9 Months | • Sits without support and without holding up her body with her hands<br>• Crawls and creeps on hands and knees<br>• Tries to drop or throw toys on purpose and likes to bang and shake toys<br>• Makes sounds that use vowels and consonants<br>• Holds own bottle |

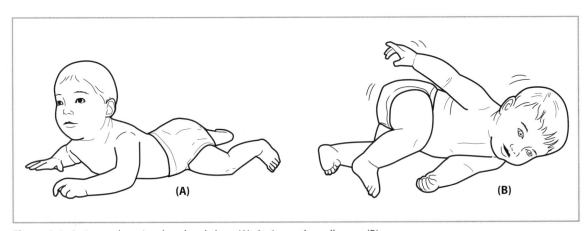

**Figure 2-8.** At 3 months, raises head and chest (A). At 6 months, rolls over (B).

## DEVELOPMENTAL MILESTONES

| | DEVELOPMENTAL MILESTONES FOR THE FIRST 3 YEARS |
|---|---|
| 12 Months | • Pulls up to a standing position<br>• Can walk holding on to furniture<br>• Likes to play peek-a-boo<br>• Says at least one word other than "ma-ma" or "da-da"<br>• Likes to explore objects and spaces<br>• Copies familiar behaviors such as using a cup or telephone |
| 18 Months | • Can use a cup without spilling<br>• Walks across large room without falling or wobbling from side to side<br>• Can feed self<br>• Says at least 4 to 10 words<br>• Can point to pictures that you name in a book<br>• Takes off own shoes |
| 24 Months | • Runs without falling<br>• Says 2-word sentences with total vocabulary of about 50 words<br>• Takes off own clothes and can point to at least one named body part<br>• Displays more and more independence<br>• Likes to play with or around other children |
| 36 Months | • Is easily understood by most adults and speaks in 3-word sentences most of the time<br>• Answers "what" questions about a story and can sit together for at least 5 minutes<br>• Can throw a ball overhand from a distance of 5 feet<br>• Can name at least one color |

## IN GENERAL

Autism spectrum disorders (ASDs) are a group of biologically based neurodevelopmental disorders that affect a child's behavior and abilities to interact and communicate with other people. Children with ASDs have ongoing struggles with social interactions. They often have trouble with give-and-take in normal conversations, difficulties making eye contact, a lack of facial expressions, and difficulties adjusting behavior to fit different social situations. They also engage in obsessive and repetitive patterns of behavior, interests, or activities.

Diagnosing a child with an ASD can be difficult. Unlike other health conditions, there are no blood tests, x-rays, or scans that can detect an ASD. Instead, diagnosis is made based on caregivers' descriptions of the child's development and by careful observations of characteristic behaviors by providers who have expertise with ASD. In some cases, the path to a diagnosis begins with a parent's hunch that something isn't quite right.

The severity of an ASD also varies widely among children. Every single case is different. Some children with ASDs have very mild forms, with only a few social difficulties and restrictive behaviors and the ability to function independently. Others have more severe forms of the disorder with noticeable disability and a lifelong dependence on others to meet their needs.

No one knows the exact cause of ASDs, although experts are fairly certain it's a combination of genetics and the environment. What we do know is that early diagnosis and treatment of an ASD is critical to how well a child and family lives with it. While most signs of ASDs are apparent by the time a child is 3 years of age, many children's ASDs are not diagnosed until they are much older.

Early diagnosis requires a working partnership between parents and pediatricians. Within this partnership, you, as the parent, should feel com-fortable discussing with your pediatrician any concerns you have about your child's behavior or development—the way she plays, learns, speaks, and acts. Your pediatrician will ask questions and probe for details, and he or she may even use a questionnaire that asks specific questions about your child's development. In order to know if something is a concern, it's important that you're able to spot the early signs of an ASD.

### Children with ASDs might

- Not point at objects to show interest in them (eg, not point at an airplane flying overhead)

- Not look at objects when others point at them

- Have trouble relating to others or might not have an interest in others at all

- Avoid eye contact and might want to be alone

- Have trouble understanding others' feelings or talking about their own feelings

- Prefer not to be held or cuddled or might cuddle only when they want to

- Appear to be unaware when people talk to them but might respond to other sounds

- Be very interested in people but might not know how to talk, play, or relate to them

- Repeat or echo words or phrases said to them or any words or phrases in place of normal language

- Have trouble expressing their needs using typical words or motions

- Not play "pretend" games (eg, not pretend to feed a doll)

- Repeat actions over and over again

- Have trouble adapting when a routine changes

- Have unusual reactions to the way things smell, taste, look, feel, or sound

- Lose skills they once had (eg, stop using words they previously used)

Adapted from Learn the signs. Act early. Autism spectrum disorders fact sheet. Centers for Disease Control and Prevention Web site. http://www.cdc.gov/ncbddd/actearly/pdf/parents_pdfs/autismfactsheet.pdf. Updated June 17, 2013. Accessed November 6, 2013

## Distinguishing a Child Who Has an Autism Spectrum Disorder

It isn't always easy for parents to know if their child has an autism spectrum disorder (ASD). Some of the symptoms of ASD may be seen in children with other types of developmental or behavioral problems or, to a lesser extent, in children with typical development. Also, not all of the symptoms are seen in all children. Some children may only display a few of the symptoms. This is what makes the process of diagnosing an ASD difficult. But here are some examples that may help you distinguish a child with an ASD from other children.

### At 12 Months

- A child with typical development will turn his head when he hears his name.
- A child with an ASD might not turn to look, even after his name is repeated several times, but he will respond to other sounds.

### At 18 Months

- A child with delayed speech skills will point, gesture, or use facial expressions to make up for her lack of talking.
- A child with an ASD might make no attempt to compensate for delayed speech or might limit speech to parroting what she heard on TV or what she just heard.

### At 24 Months

- A child without an ASD brings a picture to his mother and shares his joy over it with her.
- A child with an ASD might bring her a bottle of bubbles to open, but, when he does this, he doesn't look at her face or share in the pleasure of playing together.

## IN GENERAL

From time to time all children get bouts of diarrhea and pass frequent, watery stools. This symptom can signal a range of conditions, from a toddler's overconsumption of fruit juice to a mild viral infection, a bacterial or parasitic infection, or food poisoning. Diarrhea may also occur with vomiting (see page 168).

In most cases, sudden and severe diarrhea often goes away on its own as the underlying condition clears up. Until then, however, make sure your child has enough fluids to prevent dehydration. Also make sure your child returns to a normal diet as soon as possible. A short-lived loss of appetite isn't harmful in a well-nourished child. Usually your child will be ready to eat again once her symptoms clear up. If she has mild diarrhea and is vomiting, offer her an electrolyte solution in place of her normal diet.

Outbreaks of infectious diarrhea are common in children who attend child care centers, especially centers that care for children who aren't yet toilet trained. You should teach your child to wash his hands with soap and water every time he uses his potty-chair or the toilet. Chronic diarrhea, which lasts for longer than 2 weeks, should always be brought to your pediatrician's attention.

## Coping With Diarrhea

Water and salt lost in diarrhea must be replenished to prevent dehydration. For rehydration use only commercially available electrolyte solutions. Don't use sports drinks: their high sugar content can make your child's diarrhea worse. As your child begins to feel better, resume her normal diet.

If your child is vomiting, ask your pediatrician to recommend a commercially available electrolyte drink to keep up the body's normal water and salt levels until your child's vomiting has stopped. Give your child small amounts of the drink (no more than an ounce at a time) frequently, every 15 minutes or so, to have the best effect. If his vomiting persists or nothing is staying down, talk with your pediatrician. If your child's diarrhea isn't severe and her vomiting has stopped, let her eat a normal diet in moderation. You don't need to limit foods or drinks once she's feeling better.

### Call your pediatrician right away if your child has diarrhea with signs of dehydration such as

- Infrequent urination or no urination for 6 hours
- Dark urine
- Sunken eyes
- Refusal to drink
- Dry, sticky lips and mouth
- Lethargy (lack of energy) and decreased activity

### WARNING!

Over-the-counter antidiarrheal medications aren't recommended for children aged 2 years or younger. You should use them only if your pediatrician's says it's OK.

| YOUR CONCERNS | POSSIBLE CAUSE | ACTION TO TAKE |
|---|---|---|
| *Your child suddenly develops diarrhea with abdominal cramps, is vomiting, and has a mild fever.* | Infectious viral gastroenteritis with *Rotavirus* species or *Enterovirus* species | If your child is an infant, talk with your pediatrician at once. For an older child, follow the guidelines in "Coping With Diarrhea," page 70. Call your pediatrician if your child's diarrhea lasts more than 48 hours or her vomiting continues more than 12 hours. |
| *Your child has diarrhea with or without vomiting. He has blood in his stools and is feverish.* | Infectious bacterial diarrhea (eg, salmonella or shigella) | Talk with your pediatrician promptly. Follow the guidelines for rehydration (see "Coping With Diarrhea," page 70). |
| *Your toddler has had diarrhea for more than 2 days. He has several loose bowel movements every day but is otherwise healthy and gaining weight. He drinks a lot of juice, sweet drinks, and water.* | Nonspecific diarrhea (common in toddlers) Too much juice | Talk with your pediatrician, who will examine your toddler to rule out any serious health problems. He or she may suggest dietary changes, such as having your child consume smaller amounts of juices and sweet drinks, if any. |
| *Your child is vomiting. Others in your household have similar symptoms.* | Bacterial food poisoning | Call your pediatrician. Treatment will depend on the type and severity of food poisoning. |
| *Your toddler or young child has diarrhea with bloating or nausea. She is in a group child-care setting or school.* | Parasitic infection, such as giardiasis, especially if your toddler or young child attends group care | Call your pediatrician, who will examine your toddler or young child, order diagnostic tests as required, and recommend treatment. |
| *Your child has diarrhea during or just after antibiotic treatment.* | Medication side effect | Call your pediatrician. If your child needs an antibiotic, your pediatrician will prescribe an alternative and advise on diet. |
| *Your otherwise healthy school-aged child has alternating bouts of diarrhea and constipation that occur at times of stress. He has abdominal pain that starts and stops, nausea, bloating, or gas.* | Irritable bowel syndrome | Talk with your pediatrician, who will examine your child to rule out any serious disorders. If your pediatrician confirms irritable bowel syndrome, treatment of it may involve an increase in dietary fiber or medication that relieves cramps. This health problem is common but not serious. |
| *Your child's stools are bulky and foul smelling. Her symptoms are worse after eating certain foods. She is growing and gaining weight slowly.* | Malabsorption disorder | Talk with your pediatrician without delay, who will order diagnostic tests and recommend treatment, if required. |
| *Your child is passing bloody stools. She has pain in her abdomen and joints. She has lost her appetite and has nausea and fatigue.* | Infectious inflammatory bowel disease such as ulcerative colitis or Crohn disease | Talk with your pediatrician without delay; diagnostic tests and appropriate treatment are necessary. |

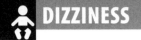

## IN GENERAL

When children say they feel dizzy, they usually mean they feel light-headed. This unsteady feeling sometimes accompanies a fever. Children with vertigo, on the other hand, sense that the room is spinning around or their body is veering out of control. It's somewhat common for healthy children, especially preteens and teens, to feel momentarily unsteady because of a minor change in blood flow when they stand abruptly after squatting or sitting. Unless your child actually faints, this feeling shouldn't concern you. The self-induced dizziness that results from spinning around or running in circles isn't a cause for concern either.

Some children get dizzy and nauseated when riding in a car; however, a child's dizziness rarely signals vertigo, which involves an unpleasant sensation of spinning and disorientation.

. . . . . . . . . . . . . . . . . . . . . . . . . . . . . . . . . . . . . . . . . .

### Talk with your pediatrician if

- Your normally coordinated child develops a staggering, "drunken" gait.
- Your child complains of dizziness and loses her balance or can't walk a straight line.
- Your child has dizziness and headaches that come and go and are worse when he lays down.

. . . . . . . . . . . . . . . . . . . . . . . . . . . . . . . . . . . . . . . . . .

### WARNING!

Vertigo is unusual in children. If your child has vertigo and ringing or buzzing in her ears, she should be seen by your pediatrician.

## Keeping a Sense of Balance

Our ability to remain upright depends on a delicate interplay between the nerves and muscles involved in hearing, sight, and touch. Through our sense of hearing we learn to place ourselves in relation to sounds. Our limbs and muscles are equipped with sense organs that help us gauge our position relative to our surroundings. A disturbance in any part of this balance mechanism may cause dizziness, vertigo, and nausea.

Dizziness usually goes away once the stimulus that caused it stops. Vertigo, on the other hand, is often an ongoing sensation caused by a problem with the inner ear. People with vertigo sometimes have tinnitus as well; this ringing or buzzing sound is caused by a related disturbance in the nerve we use to perceive sound.

| YOUR CONCERNS | POSSIBLE CAUSE | ACTION TO TAKE |
|---|---|---|
| *Your child is unwell and feverish with a temperature higher than 100°F (37.8°C).* | Lightheadedness due to illness<br>Fluid in the ear due to otitis media (inflammation of the middle ear) | Give your child acetaminophen or ibuprofen to reduce his discomfort. If his symptoms become worse or don't clear up in 1 to 2 days, talk with your pediatrician. If your child looks quite ill and lethargic (lacking energy), he may need an emergency evaluation for illnesses such as meningitis. |
| *Your child has had a moment of feeling dizzy or faint.* | Faintness due to heat, hunger, anxiety, or another stress | Have your child rest in a cool place. Offer her a drink that contains sugar, a light snack, and cold water. If she's still faint after 30 minutes, call your pediatrician (see page 188). |

| YOUR CONCERNS | POSSIBLE CAUSE | ACTION TO TAKE |
|---|---|---|
| *Your child is suddenly complaining that the room is spinning around. He is losing his balance and has tinnitus (ringing in his ears).* | Labyrinthitis (a viral infection of the inner ear) | Talk with your pediatrician, who will examine your child to confirm the diagnosis and rule out any other health problems. The viral infection usually clears up within a week without treatment; your pediatrician may prescribe medication to reduce your child's symptoms. |
| *Your child is unsteady after a recent viral illness, such as chickenpox.* | Post-viral cerebellar ataxia (weakness and loss of muscle coordination) | Talk with your pediatrician about a more thorough evaluation. |
| *Your child gets dizzy and nauseated while riding in a car, an elevator, or a boat.* | Motion sickness | Ask your pediatrician what measures you should take to prevent motion sickness in your child. |
| *Your child complains of dizziness after a fall or head injury.* | Head injury | Call your pediatrician without delay, who may order x-rays and other tests. If your child has lost consciousness or appears confused and disoriented, an emergency evaluation may be required. |
| *Your child complains of dizziness and disorientation. She has frequent, repeated, momentary lapses of attention.* | Absence seizure (an abrupt, transient loss or impairment of consciousness, not subsequently remembered, sometimes with light twitching or fluttering eyelids) | Talk with your pediatrician (see "Seizures," page 134). |
| *Your child has headaches that become worse when he lays down. He has trouble balancing or walking a straight line. He has nausea or is vomiting.* | Unusual health problem, such as a tumor, that requires diagnosis and treatment | Talk with your pediatrician. Although rare in children, these conditions can occur and require prompt treatment (see "Headache," page 96). |
| *Your toddler or young child topples over when sitting or standing still. She usually misses when she reaches for objects. She often misses when you ask her to touch her nose with her finger.* | In rare cases, ataxia (neuromuscular problem) | Talk with your pediatrician, who will examine your child and determine whether she should be seen by another specialist. |

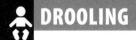
## IN GENERAL

Drooling and blowing bubbles is common in babies during the phase of development when getting what they need is centered on the mouth (Figure 2-9). This becomes especially apparent at 3 to 6 months of age. The increased flow of saliva that often signals the appearance of a new tooth seems to soothe tender gums; however, if your baby appears to be drooling excessively and looks ill, she may be having trouble swallowing, which requires medical attention.

### Role of Saliva

Drooling fulfills several important functions for your baby. His saliva softens and moistens food once solids are part of his diet, keeps his mouth moist and makes it easier for him to swallow, washes away food residues, and protects his teeth. Saliva also contains ptyalin, a digestive enzyme that changes starch into sugar. A natural antacid in saliva neutralizes stomach acid and aids digestion. Saliva also protects against tooth decay.

• Call 911 or your local emergency number, or take your baby to the nearest emergency department if he has a sore throat or cold symptoms and starts drooling, breathing hard and noisily, and gasping for breath with his mouth wide open, which may be epiglottitis, a now infrequent but serious medical emergency.

**WARNING!**

If your child is suddenly drooling, can't speak, and is having trouble breathing, she may be choking on food or a foreign object. Call 911 or your local emergency number, and while you're waiting for help, follow the first aid procedures related to choking (see pages 215–216).

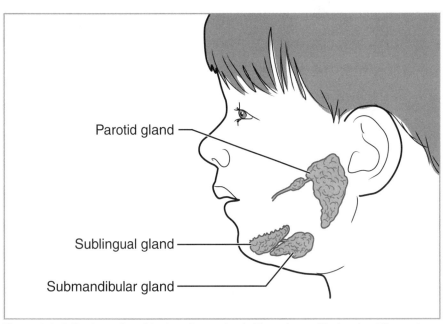

**Figure 2-9.** Saliva is produced in the salivary glands. The submandibular gland lies under the jaw, the sublingual gland is under the tongue, and the parotid is close to the ear.

| YOUR CONCERNS | POSSIBLE CAUSE | ACTION TO TAKE |
|---|---|---|
| Your infant is between 3 and 6 months of age. He is a little fussy, and he seems to want to chew and bite on firm objects, including your fingers. | Normal drooling | Comfort your baby, and give him a pacifier or a smooth teething ring to chew on (see "Dental Problems," page 62). |
| Your child has a fever of 101°F (38.3°C) or higher, a headache, and a sore throat. She has lost her appetite. She has pain on swallowing, and the glands in her neck are swollen. | Viral infection of the throat or mouth<br>Streptococcal throat infection<br>Tonsillitis (inflammation of the tonsils) | Call your pediatrician, who will examine your child and recommend treatment. If your pediatrician agrees, give your child acetaminophen or ibuprofen to reduce her fever. |
| Your child has spots or ulcerations inside of his mouth. He finds them painful. | Viral infection of the tongue or gums such as hand-foot-and-mouth disease<br>Herpes | Call your pediatrician, who will recommend treatment. |
| Your drooling child is straining and gasping for air with his mouth wide open. She has a severe sore throat. | Epiglottitis (inflammation of the flap of tissue that prevents food and liquids from entering the trachea [windpipe]) | Call 911 or your local emergency number, or take your child to the nearest hospital emergency department. This condition is serious and could cause your child to stop breathing. Once a grave threat, it has become less common since the introduction of the Hib vaccine for children. |
| Your child's face is turning blue. He is speechless; making short, loud noises; and trying to cough. | Choking | This is an emergency. Have someone else call 911 or your local emergency number while you start the Heimlich maneuver or chest compressions on your baby. If your child stops breathing and has no pulse, start CPR and keep it up until medical help arrives. For instructions on how to handle these emergencies, see page 215 or 216, depending on your child's age. |
| Your child has passed out. Her limbs and muscles are jerking and can't be controlled. | Seizure | During the seizure, make sure your child is safe from objects that could injure her (see page 222). Don't leave your child, but call your pediatrician as soon as possible, and follow his or her instructions. |

## IN GENERAL

Inflammation of the middle ear, called *otitis media,* is a common infection in young children. Most toddlers have had at least one episode by 2 years of age. Ear problems are common in children 2 years or younger because they are exposed to a host of germs before their immune systems are mature enough to resist infections. In addition, a young child's tiny eustachian tubes, which are canals that link the middle ear and pharynx, allow infectious material to remain in or travel up to the middle ear space. The impaired eustachian tube function also changes the pressure within the ear. This causes fluid to accumulate in the middle ear and bulging of the child's eardrum. Luckily children tend to outgrow these illnesses as their susceptibility to them decreases and their eustachian tubes mature.

When infants and young children who haven't yet learned to talk have an upper respiratory infection, it usually precedes the telltale signs of ear infection. These signs include nighttime crying and daytime irritability, fever (a temperature of 100.4°F [38°C] or higher), and loss of appetite. An infant with an ear infection will often cry in distress when feeding as his ear pressure changes with the sucking motion. A slightly older child may rub or pull at his ear. And once your child can talk, he will tell you if his ear hurts. Symptoms of ear pain, called *otalgia,* and a short-lived loss of hearing may appear rapidly in older children and teens. A middle ear infection may result in a sudden rupture of the eardrum with drainage of fluid from the ear canal.

If you suspect your child has an ear infection, call your pediatrician. Treatment will vary. In the past, antibiotics were routinely prescribed for all ear infections. This is no longer true. If an ear infection isn't severe, your pediatrician may recommend adopting a wait-and-see approach or giving your child acetaminophen or ibuprofen to relieve her pain. Other ear problems, however, may require antibiotics (Figure 2-10).

**Call your pediatrician if your child has earache along with**

- Discharge from his ear
- Swelling around his ear
- Headache
- Fever of 102.2°F (39°C) or higher
- Dizziness
- Hearing loss

**WARNING!**

Never leave your baby alone to finish a bottle while lying on her back. Formula or other liquid can sometimes travel up the eustachian tube and create ideal conditions for bacterial growth in her middle ear. Children who are exposed to secondhand tobacco smoke have an increased risk of developing upper respiratory infections; bronchiolitis, which is a lung infection; ear infections; and other health problems.

## Treating Ear Infection

Many pediatricians have raised concerns about whether or not the overuse of antibiotics directly relates to the rise in bacterial resistance. Their concerns have resulted in changes in the treatment of middle ear infections. The American Academy of Pediatrics (AAP) now recommends that pediatricians adopt a wait-and-see approach for children older than 2 years whose ear infection is mild and with symptoms that have developed within the last 48 hours.

If your child's ear infection is severe, however, your pediatrician will prescribe antibiotics. To warrant treatment with antibiotics, the severe pain must occur along with a fever of 102.2°F (39° C) or higher in a child who has been sick for at least 48 hours. Your pediatrician will also prescribe antibiotics if your child is between 6 and 23 months of age and has an ear infection in both ears, even if the infection has developed in fewer than 48 hours and the fever is less than 102.2°F (39°C). In addition, antibiotics may become necessary if your child's ear problem worsens or doesn't improve within 48 to 72 hours of the symptoms starting.

The goals of these new recommendations are to reserve antibiotics for serious conditions that demand powerful medication and to cut down on nonessential treatments that may promote the growth of resistant bacteria. If antibiotics are prescribed when they aren't needed, new strains of bacteria may develop. When this happens antibiotics may eventually stop working. The infections they're designed to treat will no longer be curable with them, and the bacteria they're treating will have become resistant.

Managing the pain of an ear infection, however, is still important. A warm pad over the ear and a dose of acetaminophen or ibuprofen may help ease your child's pain while her immune system fights off the infection.

Some children suffer ear infections that occur again and again. The AAP defines recurrent ear infection as one that occurs 3 different times in a 6-month period. Or it occurs 4 different times in 1-year, with one of the times occurring in the preceding 6 months. To treat recurrent ear infections that show signs of hearing loss, your pediatrician may recommend implanting tympanostomy tubes. These tubes are tiny cylinders surgically inserted into the eardrum to help prevent the buildup of fluid. The AAP doesn't recommend giving children with recurrent ear infection preventative antibiotics to reduce the frequency of ear infections, as this practice doesn't appear to be effective. Fortunately the tendency to develop recurrent ear infection becomes less likely as the child matures.

| YOUR CONCERNS | POSSIBLE CAUSE | ACTION TO TAKE |
|---|---|---|
| *Your child has a cold with a runny nose, cough, mild fever, or conjunctivitis (inflammation of the membrane that lines the eyelids). He appears to be having ear pain.* | Otitis media (middle ear infection) | Call your pediatrician, who will examine your child for an appropriate diagnosis. Depending on your child's situation, you may need to wait and carefully watch and listen to your child for more signs of infection. Your pediatrician may recommend treatment. |
| *Your child is complaining of pain, itching, or fullness in the ear. The pain is worse when she pulls on her earlobe, and a discharge is coming out of her ear. She has been swimming a lot or often dips her head under bathwater.* | Otitis externa, sometimes called *swimmer's ear* (an infection of the ear canal, the part of the ear that leads from the outer ear to the eardrum) | Talk with your pediatrician, who will examine your child and recommend treatment. Your child may need ear drops. Ask whether you need to take any other measures to prevent this ear problem from happening again. |
| *Your child's outer ear is red and swollen.* | Insect sting or bite Impetigo (a bacterial infection) | Check with your pediatrician. A cold compress will help relieve discomfort caused by an insect sting. If your child has impetigo, antibiotic treatment will be necessary. |
| *Your child is between about 18 months and 4 years of age and showing signs or complaining of ear pain. He doesn't have other symptoms such as runny nose or sore throat. He has been playing with small objects or paper. You see something stuck in his ear canal.* | Foreign object in the ear | Don't try to dig out the object; you may injure your child's ear. Call your pediatrician, who will examine your child's ear with a magnifying device and special lights. These tools make it easier to see and extract a foreign object. |
| *Your child has the feeling that something is moving around inside of her ear. She can hear buzzing, and she has pain.* | Insect in the ear | Most insects eventually find their way out; if not, talk with your pediatrician, who will confirm if there is an insect in your child's ear. If so, your pediatrician can remove it. |
| *Your child's ear has been injured in an accident. It is bleeding, cut, or bruised.* | Ear injury with cuts and bruising | Clean the outside of your child's ear gently with plain water, and lightly tape or bandage a sterile pad over his wound. Then call your pediatrician, who will want to examine your child. He or she will make sure that the internal tissues of your child's ear don't have an injury that needs attention. |
| *Your child's ear is sticking out at an angle. The area behind his ear is tender and painful.* | Mastoiditis (an infection of the bone of the skull that is near the ear) | Call your pediatrician at once to examine and treat your child. |

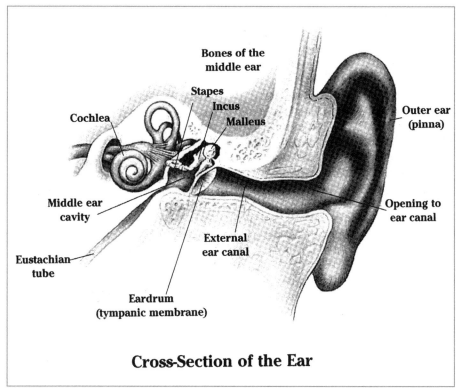

Bones of the
middle ear

Stapes
Incus
Malleus

Cochlea

Outer ear
(pinna)

Middle ear
cavity

Opening to
ear canal

Eustachian
tube

External
ear canal

Eardrum
(tympanic membrane)

## Cross-Section of the Ear

**Figure 2-10.** Often after the symptoms of acute otitis media clear up, fluid remains in the ear, creating another kind of ear problem called otitis media with effusion (middle ear fluid). This fluid may last several months and in most cases, disappears on its own. The child's hearing then returns to normal.

Swimmer's ear, also known as otitis externa, is a different illness than a middle ear infection. A swimmer's ear is an infection of the outer ear canal, the part of the ear that leads from the outer ear to the eardrum.

## IN GENERAL

When a child has a healthy attitude toward food, eating is a natural response to hunger, and meals are pleasant social occasions. The eating patterns we establish in our early years can influence our health and habits for a lifetime.

Sooner or later most children go through a phase of fussy eating (sec "Appetite Loss," page 28). During this often nerve-racking time, they refuse almost every food that's put in from of them and resist efforts to persuade them to eat. At the opposite extreme are children who appear to lack any appetite control. Luckily in most cases these minor feeding problems quickly pass; however, severe feeding problems can affect health.

Most feeding problems can be resolved if you provide your child with a variety of nutritious meals and snacks and let her have as much or as little as she wants.

Children need certain rules and boundaries in eating as in other aspects of their lives. Feeding done at different times that change often may make children worry that they're not going to be taken care of. In contrast, some parents use food as a pacifier, urging children to eat to ease any upsets. Constant snacking not only upsets normal appetite controls but can also lead to unwanted weight gain and poor eating habits.

### Talk with your pediatrician if your child is

- Losing or unable to gain weight
- Gaining too much weight

> ### WARNING!
> If your dinner table is turning into a battleground, or you're worried that feeding problems may interfere with your child's growth, it's time to seek professional help. Discuss your concerns with your pediatrician, who may advise you to consult other pediatric health specialists.

## A Common-Sense Approach to Feeding Your Child

Obesity has emerged as a major health problem that increases the risk for chronic illnesses. It is rapidly overtaking cigarette smoking as the leading preventable cause of disease in the United States. One of the key causes behind the obesity epidemic is overeating and inactivity. Often these habits are ingrained during childhood. As a parent, you can help make sure that your child will eat right if you practice the following guidelines:

- Serve a variety of foods in age-appropriate portions.
- Offer modest servings, with second helpings only if your child asks for more.
- Encourage your child to eat slowly.
- Time snacks so they don't interfere with meals.
- Don't use food as a bribe or reward.
- Learn to recognize when your child is asking for food but really wants your attention.
- Resist serving meals and snacks while children are watching television, listening to stories, or absorbed in play. This can lead to overeating from habit.
- Don't get upset when your child eats everything one day and almost nothing the next; appetites can vary. More important is considering what your child eats in the course of several days, not just at one meal or in a single day.
- Plan menus with attention to likes and dislikes, but don't be a short-order cook.
- Try to eat meals as a family.

| YOUR CONCERNS | POSSIBLE CAUSE | ACTION TO TAKE |
|---|---|---|
| Your baby is younger than 6 months. He is almost always restless and irritable. He is breastfed and unable to gain weight, even though he empties your breast. | Insufficient calorie intake | Talk with your pediatrician, who will examine your child and may recommend changes in his diet or your feeding method. If you're not sure you have enough breast milk to supply him, try pumping to check your milk production (also see "Feeding Problems in Babies," page 6). |
| Your baby vomits after most feedings. You persist in feeding her after she's turned away. You have been adding cereal to her bottle. Your baby is otherwise healthy. | Overfeeding | When your child avoids her bottle, she's telling you she has had enough. Babies take just as much as they need and may vomit if they're forced to drink more. (Vomiting is not the same as spitting up; see page 16). If vomiting continues even when your baby consumes less breast milk or formula, talk with your pediatrician. |
| Your baby refuses solid foods, even though your pediatrician says it's time your baby had the extra calories. He is about 4 to 6 months of age. | Normal transition to solid foods | Be patient, and continue breastfeeding or bottle-feeding. Stop solids if your attempts at solid feeding are upsetting your baby and you. When you try again, alternate breast milk or formula and solids so your baby associates a feeling of satisfaction with the sensation of spoon-feeding. |
| Your child aged 1 leaves most of the food on her plate. She is drinking less. She is otherwise happy and energetic. | Normal appetite decrease as the growth rate slows down | Give your child smaller portions, with second helpings only if she asks for them. This slowing down of the appetite is a normal stage in development, not a feeding problem. |
| Your school-aged child is still eating like a picky toddler. | Unsatisfactory eating habits | Keep your child on a regular (but not rigid) schedule for meals and sleep. He should avoid overstimulating games and entertainment around meals and bedtime. He should also avoid excessive snacking, especially in the 1 to 2 hours before meals. Try not to be a short-order cook and prepare meals "ordered" by your picky eater; instead of trying new foods, he will simply learn that refusing to eat what you prepare will result in a diet of only his preferred foods. |
| Your child is always eating. She hoards food. She is constantly snacking between meals. Her weight is noticeably more heavier than what it should be for her height and build. | Anxiety Stress Overeating Poor impulse control | Discuss your concerns with your pediatrician. Prepare regular meals and snacks with normal portions of foods that are average in calorie amount (but not diet foods). Encourage exercise and activities to take your child's mind off of food. |

## IN GENERAL

Common eye problems in childhood include infections, such as hordeolums (styes) and bacterial conjunctivitis (pink eye), and irritation caused by a foreign body or allergy. Babies' eyes are routinely treated at birth to prevent infections, which may be present in the birth canal. Eye infections that occur after the newborn period are seldom serious, as long as they're treated promptly by your pediatrician.

Injuries to the eye or eyelid should always be seen by a pediatrician, and a child with a potentially serious injury should be taken directly to the nearest emergency department. If you can't remove a foreign body from your child's eye or eyelid by washing it out with clean water, seek your pediatrician's help right away. For more information about eye problems, see "Cross-eye, Wandering Eye" on page 60 and "Vision Problems" on page 166.

### Talk with your pediatrician if your child has

- Redness, swelling, and eye discharge lasting for more than 24 hours
- Persistent (won't go away) eye pain
- Unusual sensitivity to light
- Excessive tearing
- Frequent blinking
- Decreased or blurred vision

### WARNING!

Some eye infections are highly contagious. Wash your hands before and after touching the area around your child's infected eye. Don't directly touch your child's eye or the discharge from it. Don't let the tip of an eye dropper or ointment tube touch the infected area. If your child has pink eye, consult a health professional for diagnosis and possible treatment. The role of antibiotics in preventing spread is unclear. Antibiotics shorten the course of illness a very small amount. Most children with pinkeye get better after 5 or 6 days without antibiotics. Launder his towel and washcloth after each use.

## Fireworks Injuries: Serious but Preventable

Fireworks are among the most common causes of serious, preventable eye injuries. Nearly half of all injuries occur in children younger than 15 years. Most injuries occur around Independence Day, with another surge during the New Year's period. Most often those injured are bystanders, including children. Fireworks injuries are usually permanent and can cause partial or complete blindness.

The sale of fireworks is completely banned in 4 states and restricted in others. Even where sale is legal, pediatricians who treat children injured by fireworks warn against consumer use of these products. Enjoy fireworks from a safe distance only at public displays conducted by professionals.

| YOUR CONCERNS | POSSIBLE CAUSE | ACTION TO TAKE |
|---|---|---|
| *Your baby's eye is always watering and has a frequent discharge. She may have a bulge under her eyelid near her nose.* | Blocked tear duct (common) | Your pediatrician will make sure your baby's eyes are not infected. Blocked tear ducts usually open on their own during the first few months of life, but your pediatrician may recommend that you gently massage the area or use eye drops. |
| *Your child feels pain when he blinks. He feels as if there's something in his eye.* | Foreign body in the eye | Wash out your child's eye with lukewarm water; if this doesn't help, call your pediatrician. |

| YOUR CONCERNS | POSSIBLE CAUSE | ACTION TO TAKE |
|---|---|---|
| The white of one of your child's eye has streaks or spots of blood on it. Her eyes are otherwise free of pain or irritation. | Subconjunctival hemorrhage (bleeding underneath the white of the eye) | These streaks or spots look alarming but aren't serious. They may follow coughing, sneezing, or a mild injury. If your child is a newborn, the streaks may be from the pressure of childbirth. If streaks increase or don't clear up within a week, call your pediatrician. |
| Your child's eyes are pinkish, irritated, and swollen. He may also have symptoms of an upper respiratory infection. | Conjunctivitis, possibly due to a viral infection such as the common cold | Talk with your pediatrician, who will determine if your child needs treatment. |
| Your child's eyes are red, tearing, and itchy. She has a runny nose and is sneezing. Allergies run in your family. | Allergic conjunctivitis (inflammation of the white front of the eye due to allergy) | Call your pediatrician, who may recommend treatment to relieve your child's symptoms and other measures to reduce your child's exposure to allergens (see "Allergic Reactions," page 26). |
| Your child's eyes are red. They have a discharge or are crusted shut in the morning. | Bacterial conjunctivitis | Your pediatrician will examine your child and determine if treatment is necessary. |
| Your child has a tender, red lump on his eyelid at the base of an eyelash. His eye is watery, and his eyelid is swollen. | Hordeolum (stye) | Your pediatrician will examine your child and advise applying warm compresses for 20 to 30 minutes 3 or 4 times a day. If your child's sty doesn't go away, your pediatrician may prescribe an antibiotic. |
| Your child has a non-tender or slightly tender swelling within her eyelid. | Chalazion (inflamed meibomian gland, which can dry out the eye's tear film) | Try applying a warm compress to your child's eyelids several times a day. If the swelling persists, talk with your pediatrician. |
| Your child's eyelids are red and scaly. They are crusted when he wakes up. He complains of burning or grittiness. | Blepharitis (inflammation of the oil glands in the eyelid margins) | Apply a warm compress to your child's eyelids several times a day. You can also try washing the affected area with baby shampoo. If it doesn't go away, call your pediatrician, who may prescribe treatment if the area is infected. |
| Your child's eye area is injured. It has bruising, bleeding, or swelling. | Eye injury | Call your pediatrician, or go directly to the nearest emergency department; any injury to the sensitive eye area should be examined. |
| One of your child's eyelids is swollen, red, warm, and tender. It is hard for her to open her eyes, and she's tearing. She has a fever and is generally unwell. | Periorbital cellulitis (a deep infection of the tissue around the eye) | Call your pediatrician at once. Left untreated, this infection may cause serious, long-lasting damage. Your child may need to be hospitalized for intensive treatment. |
| Your child's eye is unusually sensitive to light. He has had joint pain or a rash. His eye has been injured. | Iritis (deep inflammation, not infection) | Your pediatrician will examine your child and refer you to another health specialist, if necessary. |

## IN GENERAL

All children have fears and worries; indeed, well-defined fears mark different developmental stages. For example, an infant as young as 5 to 7 months of age may become anxious in the presence of a strange face. The vivid imagination of the preschooler may be expressed in fears of the dark or monsters. In typical school-aged children, imaginary threats are replaced by more realistic everyday fears, such as bodily harm during a thunderstorm due to a falling tree. In general healthy fears stop children from taking unnecessary risks but should not keep children from being able to live, learn, play, and interact with others in age- and developmentally appropriate ways. You should be concerned when your child's fear is persistent (won't go away), intense, and causes her to avoid appropriate interactions and experiences.

Certain fears may grow out of your child's experiences at home with your reactions, behaviors, and approaches to parenting after an event that impacts your family. For example, after a divorce or the death of a parent or other caregiver, a child may develop separation anxiety or depression. She may express these feelings with one or more fears or phobias. If you're overly worried or fearful yourself, it may foster shyness and make it hard for your child to attempts to try new things and stretch her abilities. Try to encourage healthy habits such as exercise, outdoor play, a balanced and consistent diet, proper sleep, avoidance of exposure to frightening or violent media, special time with parents, and open communication.

### Talk with your pediatrician if your child's fears

- Interfere with family activities
- Prevent her from making friends
- Create an excuse for her not to go to school
- Disrupt normal sleep habits
- Result in compulsive behavior (feeling the need to do something over and over again even though it has no true benefit or reward)

### WARNING!

Most childhood fears aren't a reason for concern, but some should alert you to look for a serious cause. This could include exposure to an adverse childhood experience such as neglect, physical or emotional abuse, witnessing trauma, or parental substance use. A sudden, intense fear of a once-trusted person may stem from exposure to one or more of these adverse experiences. Try not to dismiss intense fears as just another phase; instead, it may be a good idea for you to look for an experience or trigger that caused the fearful behavior.

| YOUR CONCERNS | POSSIBLE CAUSE | ACTION TO TAKE |
|---|---|---|
| *Your infant aged 5 or 6 months is less outgoing than before. He is fretful when he sees a strange face. He cries when you leave the room.* | Normal development Stranger anxiety | By now your infant is strongly attached to you and his other regular caregivers. Make a special effort to reassure him among new people or surroundings. Stranger anxiety peaks around the time your infant is 9 months of age, and most children outgrow it by the time they are about 2 years of age. |
| *Your infant or toddler often wakes up and calls for you at night. She is between about 10 and 18 months of age.* | Normal separation anxiety, which generally peaks in this age group | Quietly comfort your child and change her diaper if necessary. Put her back in her bed to stay until she's calm. Children usually settle down with reassurance. Nightly waking may continue for weeks or months. |
| *Your toddler screams, even when he recognizes a familiar babysitter. He sobs and tries to hold you back as you leave the house.* | Separation anxiety Seeking attention | Don't prolong your good-byes. Let your babysitter know in advance how he or she can settle your toddler down once you leave. Have the babysitter engage your toddler's attention with a book or game. Assure your toddler that you'll be back soon and then leave quickly. If your toddler's behavior persists, you may need to have him evaluated by his pediatrician. |

| YOUR CONCERNS | POSSIBLE CAUSE | ACTION TO TAKE |
|---|---|---|
| *Your toddler or preschooler is terrified by common events, such as thunder or noisy appliances.* | Normal fearfulness | The fears will fade with time. Take time to show your toddler how noisy appliances work, and let her have small doses of exposure to them over time. During storms hold her and talk calmly to show her you're not afraid. Have your child talk about how she feels so she can learn how to calm herself with your help. |
| *Your preschooler refuses to get into the bathtub or sit on the toilet.* | A still-developing sense of size and strength | If your child is afraid of being flushed down the drain, he may prefer showers or sponge baths. Let him use a child's toilet seat or a potty-chair until he's more confident. Spend time explaining to him how the bathtub and toilet works and how to be less afraid. |
| *Your child is especially fearful and withdrawn around people outside your family or in unfamiliar situations.* | Shyness | Prepare your child for new experiences by talking about them, but be careful not to make her more nervous by talking about these new situations too much. Let your child take her time in getting used to new situations. Ask her to talk about how she feels, and consider trying a role-play with her to practice the new situation. |
| *Your child adopts extreme delaying tactics or throws tantrums at bedtime.* | Fear of the dark Separation anxiety Fatigue Overstimulation | Follow the same bedtime routine every night. Avoid rough-housing and overstimulation. Place nightlights to orient him. Test out an earlier bedtime. If your child continues to have these behaviors, talk with your pediatrician. |
| *Your preschooler screams about an hour after falling asleep. She is unresponsive, although her eyes are open.* | Night terrors (Also see "Seizures," page 134.) | Quietly reassure your child, but try not to expect a response because she's not awake. The terror may last half an hour or more, but eventually your child will settle back to sleep. She will have no recall of the incident in the morning. |
| *Your preschooler wakes up in the night, afraid and crying.* | Nightmare | Your preschooler may not understand the difference between dreams and real life. Reassure your child that the dream wasn't real. Stay with her until she's calm. Ask her to talk about the dream and why it scared her. |
| *Your child is refusing to go to school. He complains of severe but vague symptoms (eg, headache, nausea, dizziness) to avoid school.* | School phobia (See page 84.) Separation anxiety Trauma or bullying, learning difficulties, or another school factor | Talk with your pediatrician, who will look for a physical problem or learning difficulty that may be causing the symptoms. After the evaluation, if no physical cause is found, your pediatrician may recommend counseling. Talk with your child's teachers to identify problems. Insist that your child attend school, but try to find solutions to specific problems. Also provide positive feedback and support to your child for his efforts. Be consistent about expectations at home and at school. Enlist the help of school staff in the process. |
| *Your child has developed fears or phobias after witnessing a violent event.* | Post-traumatic stress disorder | Talk with your pediatrician, who will evaluate your child's condition and may recommend counseling (also see "Anxiety," page 180). |

## IN GENERAL

Fever—an increase in body temperature—is one of our body's natural defenses against outside attacks, such as infections. Less commonly, fever may signal the presence of an internal threat, such as an autoimmune disorder. Normal temperature isn't a single number; it's a range of numbers: 97°F to 100.3°F (36°C–37.9°C). It also varies according to time of day and your child's age, general health, and physical activity. A mild illness may push up the temperature a notch, but pediatricians don't consider fever unless the temperature climbs to 100.4°F (38°C) or higher.

Most fevers are caused by illnesses that aren't dangerous, but fever in a child who is younger than 3 months (see page 8) or who has a medical condition (such as sickle cell anemia or immune suppression) should be promptly looked into. For most children, the fever itself isn't dangerous. In some children younger than 6 years, fever can cause a seizure (see page 134) that, while frightening for parents, doesn't usually result in serious problems; however, a pediatrician should always examine your child after the first febrile (fever-related) seizure to make sure the cause is not a more serious condition. If your child has a tendency to develop febrile seizures, he should be evaluated if there are 2 or more seizures in a 24 hour period, if he has additional symptoms, or if he doesn't return to his normal self within a couple hours after a seizure. Children generally outgrow febrile seizures by about 6 years of age.

Giving acetaminophen or ibuprofen to your child to reduce her temperature may make her more comfortable, help her rest comfortably, and prevent dehydration, but these medications don't alter the course of an illness.

### Call your pediatrician if your child

- Is 3 months or younger (see page 8)
- Appears ill and has unusual drowsiness or severe headaches, regardless of age
- Still appears ill after his temperature has been brought down
- Has delirium or hallucinations
- Refuses to drink
- Has an underlying disorder or treatment that affects his immune system
- Has traveled with your family outside of the country during the previous 8 weeks

> **WARNING!**
> Don't exceed the recommended dose of acetaminophen by giving your child a cold medication that also contains acetaminophen. Don't give acetaminophen or any other medications to a baby younger than 3 months without your pediatrician's advice. Unless advised by your pediatrician, don't give aspirin to your child to reduce her fever. The use of aspirin has been linked to an increased risk of Reye syndrome—a rare but serious disease affecting the brain and liver—following viral infections.

## Fever: A Symptom, Not an Illness

Many parents get very nervous when their child has a fever. In reality, a fever is a symptom, not an illness. Our body temperature is controlled by a part of the brain called the hypothalamus, which balances signals from heat- and cold-sensitive receptors throughout the nervous system. Among the factors that influence temperature are infections; medications; injury; inflammatory, autoimmune, and glandular disorders; and tumors. Temperature also rises with exercise or following prolonged exposure to heat. In general, if your child has a mild fever for a day or 2, is older than 3 months, seems well, and has no other symptoms, treatment isn't required. If your child is playful and drinking and sleeping well, you can hold off on giving him a fever-reducing medicine. But you should keep a close watch and be prepared to call your pediatrician in case new symptoms emerge or if the fever is above 101°F (38.3°C) for more than 48 hours.

Many doctors believe that fever may actually help shorten the course of infections by activating the immune system. Finding the cause of the fever is more important than getting rid of the fever itself.

| YOUR CONCERNS | POSSIBLE CAUSE | ACTION TO TAKE |
|---|---|---|
| Your child also has a cough, a runny nose, difficulty breathing, a sore throat, or muscle aches. | Common cold<br>Influenza<br>Another respiratory infection | Call your pediatrician, who will examine your child and will advise you on how to make him comfortable. |
| Your child also has a rash and a sore throat or swollen glands. | Another infectious illness such as strep throat, viral pharyngitis, mononucleosis, or hand-foot-and-mouth disease | Your pediatrician will diagnose the illness and recommend treatment. |
| Your child has pain in her ear. She also has a discharge from her ear. | Ear infection | Call your pediatrician. An ear infection may need to be treated (see page 76). |
| Your child also feels pain or a burning sensation during urination. She has abdominal pain. | Urinary tract infection | Your pediatrician will examine your child and, if necessary, prescribe antibiotic treatment. |
| Your child also has nausea or is vomiting with diarrhea and cramps. | Infectious gastroenteritis (viral or bacterial inflammation of the stomach and intestinal lining) | Give your child clear drinks but no food for a few hours. If his symptoms don't improve in 12 hours, call your pediatrician. |
| Your child has been feverish for 5 or more days. | Health condition that requires diagnosis and treatment | Call your pediatrician to arrange an examination. |
| Your child is irritable, lethargic (lacking energy), and feverish. She has a stomachache and swollen glands in her neck and a rash. Her lips and tongue are reddened. She also has conjunctivitis (inflammation of the membrane that lines the eyelids), and her hands and feet are swollen. | Kawasaki disease with fever and inflammation affecting the blood vessels | Call your pediatrician. The cause of this unusual disease is unknown, but your pediatrician will treat it to prevent any health complications caused by it. |
| Your child also has nonspecific symptoms such as fatigue and joint pains. He has a rash. | Lyme disease or another autoimmune disorder | Your pediatrician will examine your child and may order blood tests. Antibiotic treatment may be necessary. |
| Your baby recently had a high temperature for 3 to 5 days. She now has a spotty pink rash on her trunk (torso). The rash appeared when her temperature returned to normal. | Roseola infantum (a contagious viral illness) | Call your pediatrician, who will recommend ways to control the temperature. If your baby's condition doesn't improve, or the fever persists for more than 3 or 4 days, you'll need to talk with your pediatrician again. Keep your child away from other children. |

## IN GENERAL

Fractures—breaks in the normal structure of the bone—are common injuries among children younger than 12 years (Figure 2-11). They can be very serious, with the bone broken in several places or pushing through the skin (an open fracture). Less serious fractures, seen more often in children, involve a slight crack in the bone or a buckle (bulge) on the edge of the bone. Broken bones generally cause fewer problems in children than in adults because a child's bones are more flexible and better able to absorb shock. They also heal faster than an adult's bones.

A child's pliable bones often break in a greenstick fracture or a torus fracture. In a greenstick fracture, the bone bends like green wood but with a break only on one side. In a torus fracture, the bone buckles on one side but isn't separated.

Children are also vulnerable to growth plate fractures. These fractures may damage the growth plates at the ends of the bones and cause the bones to grow improperly or not at all. That is why your child, depending on her age and severity of the fracture, should have regular follow-up visits for at least 1 year after, especially for growth plate fractures.

Most childhood fractures need only to be kept free of movement long enough for the bone to grow back together. A molded cast of plaster or fiberglass is the usual treatment; surgical repair is seldom necessary. A little knot of bone, called a *callus,* forms over the fracture as a normal part of the healing process. Sometimes it can be felt beneath the skin. It requires no treatment and will eventually get smaller and disappear.

**Call your pediatrician or the orthopedic surgeon treating your child's fracture if you note any of the following symptoms:**

- Redness, swelling, and inflammation in the affected limb
- Temperature higher than 100.4°F (38°C)
- Toes (for a leg cast) or fingers (for an arm cast) turning blue or pale, becoming painful or numb, or swelling
- Increased pain in the fractured limb or the need for more and more pain medication
- Inability to wiggle the toes or fingers of the affected limb
- The cast breaking or loosening or the plaster getting wet or soggy

> **WARNING!**
> Don't try to move a child who has broken his leg or suffered another serious fracture. Call 911 or your local emergency number, and make your child as comfortable as possible while you're waiting.

## Preventing Childhood Fractures

Many broken bones in children can be prevented if parents follow these simple safety measures.

- Never leave your baby unattended on a changing table or bed.
- When driving, always place your child in well-secured car seat in the rear seat.
- Don't start the car until all seat belts are fastened.
- Make sure your children, when playing sports, wear protective gear (eg, wrist guards, helmets, knee pads, mouth guards) that meet US safety standards.
- Never allow your child to roller skate, ride a bicycle, or go in-line skating or skateboarding without a helmet. You should also be aware of the risks involved using trampolines, all-terrain vehicles, lawn mowers, and motorcycles.

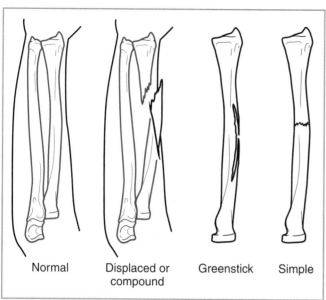

**Figure 2-11.** Types of fractures. In a displaced or compound fracture, the broken ends of the bone must be realigned; a segment of bone may penetrate through the soft tissue and skin. In a greenstick fracture, the break is on only one side of the bone. A simple fracture breaks through but doesn't displace the bone sections.

Normal    Displaced or compound    Greenstick    Simple

| YOUR CONCERNS | POSSIBLE CAUSE | ACTION TO TAKE |
|---|---|---|
| Your child had a severe blow to her head or face. Her nose is swollen, crooked, and painful to the touch. | Fracture of facial bones<br>Broken nose | Place a cold compress over her nose or the area around it to reduce pain and swelling. Call your pediatrician at once for further instructions. |
| Your child is having difficulty breathing following a fall or other accident. He has chest pain. | Broken rib | Call 911 or your local emergency number, or take your child to the nearest emergency department. |
| Your toddler is limping or refusing to walk. She is guarding a limb that's in pain. | Fracture<br>Sprain | Call your pediatrician without delay for an examination, x-rays, and treatment, if necessary. |
| Your active teen is limping. He has tenderness but no bruising in his shins. | Shin splints<br>Stress injury<br>Slipped capital femoral epiphysis (displacement of the head of the thigh bone) | Call your pediatrician, who will examine your child and prescribe appropriate treatment. Rest may be advisable. |
| Your child has swelling and pain at the site following injury to a bony part of her body, including fingers or toes. | Fracture | Call your pediatrician, who will examine your child, order x-rays if advisable, and recommend any treatment. |
| Your child has injured his head. There is blood or clear fluid leaking from his nose or ears. | Skull fracture | Call 911 or your local emergency number at once, or take your child to the nearest emergency department. |

## IN GENERAL

Gas is a common symptom of intestinal problems, but it's rarely a sign of a serious problem. Young babies who are eager to feed often gulp down air, which builds up as gas in their intestines. Many pediatricians believe that discomfort due to gas is one of the factors that can aggravate colic (see page 2).

A certain amount of gas is normally produced as food is digested; however, children as well as adults often have excess gas because their diet is too high in certain types of insoluble fiber, which ferments in the intestine. Many infants and toddlers also swallow air when crying or breathing through the mouth because of a stuffy nose. Older children gulp air when eating or chewing gum. Carbonated drinks may also be a factor. A few children who are older than 4 years have gas because they slowly over time lose the ability to digest the sugar in milk, called *lactose*.

### Call your pediatrician if your child has gas in his stomach or intestine with

- Severe abdominal pain
- Nausea and vomiting lasting for 12 or more hours
- Diarrhea that persists for more than 3 days
- Bulky, unusually foul-smelling stools

**WARNING!**
Don't treat your child's gas with over-the-counter indigestion remedies. If gas is troubling enough to be a concern, ask your pediatrician's for advice.

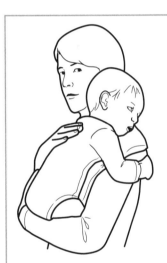 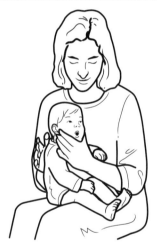 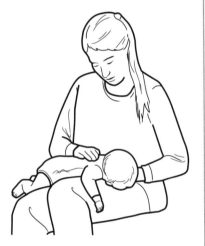

Option 1: Hold your baby upright with her head on your shoulder. Support her head and back while you gently but firmly pat her back.

Option 2: Support the baby on your lap in a sitting position with one hand and pat her back with your other hand.

Option 3: Lay the baby facedown on your lap. Use your knee to support her head a little higher than her chest, and gently rub her back.

**Figure 2-12.** Burping your baby. The best position for burping your baby is the one that makes her comfortable. Whatever position she prefers, protect your clothing with a towel or cloth diaper in case she spits up. Also, don't interrupt a feeding if it will upset your baby; instead, take advantage of natural pauses during a bottle feeding or when she switches breasts while breastfeeding.

| YOUR CONCERNS | POSSIBLE CAUSE | ACTION TO TAKE |
|---|---|---|
| *Your newborn or young infant passes a lot of gas during periods of colicky crying. She tends to gulp in her eagerness to feed.* | Aerophagia (swallowing air) during feeding | Give your baby more frequent burping breaks during each feeding and afterward (see Figure 2-12). Feed your bottle-fed baby with a slow-flow nipple appropriate to her age. |
| *Your preschooler or older child has gas along with frequent colds, sniffles, and a stuffed-up nose.* | Swallowing air during mouth breathing | Talk with your pediatrician, who will examine your child and recommend treatment, if necessary. |
| *Your school-aged child has a long history of gassiness with diarrhea that starts and stops, bloating, and discomfort.* | Intolerance to lactose or another food substance Celiac disease (gluten sensitivity) Another malabsorption problem Food allergy (rare) Irritable bowel syndrome | Talk with your pediatrician, who may recommend that you keep a food diary (see "Allergic Reactions," page 26) to track your child's daily food consumption and symptoms. Your pediatrician may also suggest an elimination diet to identify suspect foods. If your child thinks a certain food causes the discomfort, omit it from his diet for 1 or 2 weeks and bring it back to see if symptoms recur. |
| *Your child suddenly develops bloating, cramping, and diarrhea with excess gas.* | Infectious diarrhea Parasitic infection such as giardiasis | Talk with your pediatrician, who will examine your child and recommend treatment, depending on the cause of the diarrhea (see page 5). |
| *Your child has had gassiness and an upset stomach since taking an antibiotic or another medication.* | Medication side effect | Call your pediatrician, who may substitute another medication or recommend measures to keep side effects to a minimum, such as taking medication at meal times. |
| *Your child belches and passes gas noisily and often.* | High-fiber diet Carbonated beverages Attention-seeking behavior In general, your child's daily intake of fiber should equal her age plus 5 grams (eg, for a child aged 8 years, use $8 y + 5 g = 13 g$). | Reduce the amount of bran and other insoluble dietary fiber, and add more soluble fiber from fruits and vegetables. Eliminate carbonated beverages. Encourage moderate exercise, especially after meals. If passing gas is your child's way of seeking attention, let her know her behavior is unacceptable (but take care that your disapproval doesn't spur her on). |

## IN GENERAL

Genetics, nutrition, exercise, and general health determine how tall a child will grow. Most children who are either tall or short don't have a growth problem; they are simply growing the way they were genetically programmed to grow (by their family history). Parents often are surprised to learn that their baby's size at birth doesn't necessarily predict adult height. Adult height correlates better with height at 3 years of age.

At every physical examination, starting with your newborn visit, your pediatrician will measure your baby's length (height) and weight. Until your child turns 3 years of age, your pediatrician will also measure the size of her head to make sure she's growing at an appropriate rate. All of the measurements for weight, length (height), and head size should be plotted on growth curves, and your pediatrician should share this information with you. Whether your child is tall, short, or of average height isn't as important as your child's *rate* of growth. If your child is growing along one of the curves, it's likely that her growth is normal.

During the first 3 years of life, babies and toddlers often shift from one curve to another until they settle on their genetic curve, which pediatric specialists refer to as *shifting growth curves of infancy*. Because some babies are born long but have "short genes," or some babies are born short but have "long genes," shifting may be quite normal. Most children have found their genetic curve by the age of 2 or 3 years.

Nutrition is important to growth, and if a child takes in too few calories, growth may be slowed. Picky eaters, however, usually have a normal growth rate, even when they seem to eat very little, because they're consuming adequate calories within their limited food choices. Children who gain weight excessively are also at risk for future problems with obesity; overfeeding a child won't improve growth or health in the long run.

### Talk with your pediatrician if your child

- Either loses or is unable to gain weight
- Seems to be gaining too much weight

### WARNING!

Children grow best when they exercise regularly; discuss methods to increase your family's physical activity with your pediatrician.

## Addressing Growth Concerns

Some children who are small in stature have inadequate levels of the growth hormone. If a growth hormone deficiency is diagnosed, hormone treatment during the growing years can help a child reach an acceptable adult height. This treatment is reserved for children with proven glandular (hormonal) problems. Pediatricians don't advise treating a healthy, short child with growth hormone just to make him taller.

Other causes of a short stature include exposure to an infection, drugs, or alcohol while in the womb; chromosomal disorders; or extreme prematurity. In almost all cases, these problems are detected before birth or just afterward, and appropriate treatment is begun.

Sometimes children adopted from overseas may have decreased growth and delayed development because of malnutrition. They need special help and more calories than normal to catch up to a level appropriate for their age. Adoption agencies can put you in touch with support groups for parents in similar situations, and your pediatrician will help you with advice and recommendations.

| YOUR CONCERNS | POSSIBLE CAUSE | ACTION TO TAKE |
|---|---|---|
| Your infant or toddler is either losing or unable to gain weight. His growth rate is slow. | Failure to thrive | Talk with your pediatrician, who will measure and examine your child and review his diet, medical history, and other factors that may affect growth and weight gain. Your pediatrician will suggest an appropriate treatment plan. |
| Your child is healthy but somewhat shorter than most others her age. She is growing at a normal rate. | Normal short stature | Talk with your pediatrician. |
| Your preteen doesn't seem to be having the same growth spurt as his same-aged pubertal peers. | Constitutional growth delay | Talk with your pediatrician about your child's growth chart. Often there is a family history of a delayed pubertal growth spurt (a so-called "late bloomer"), and your child will eventually reach his likely, final adult height. |
| Your child is exceptionally small for her age. She is growing at a slow rate, and her weight is heavier than it should be. | Growth hormone deficiency Hypothyroidism (an underactive thyroid gland) | Talk with your pediatrician, who will examine your child and may refer her to an endocrinologist for further examination. |
| Your child is exceptionally tall for his age. He is normally proportioned, healthy, and growing consistently. | Tall stature | Make sure your child eats a healthy diet and exercises regularly. Discuss any concerns with your pediatrician. |
| Your child seems to be experiencing a growth spurt earlier than her same-aged peers. | Precocious (early) puberty | Discuss your concerns with your pediatrician, and consult your child's growth chart. |
| Your child has had a temporary slowdown in weight gain in the month of an illness. | Slowing of growth due to short-lived illness | Make sure your child has a selection of healthy foods and regular exercise. Talk with your pediatrician if your child's appetite and growth rate don't return a few weeks after recovery or starting treatment. |
| Your child is growing poorly and also has cramping, nausea, and diarrhea. | Inflammatory bowel disease such as Crohn disease or ulcerative colitis Celiac disease | Talk with your pediatrician about an evaluation and possible referral to a gastrointestinal specialist. Your pediatrician will also do tests to rule out any rare causes of short stature, such as kidney disease, liver disease, and electrolyte disturbances. |

## IN GENERAL

Almost all newborns lose some or all of their hair. This is normal and to be expected. The baby hair falls out before the mature hair comes in. Hair loss in the first 6 months of life isn't a cause for concern.

Babies also lose their hair from rubbing their scalp against the mattress or because of a head-banging habit. When the rubbing or banging behavior stops, this type of hair loss will correct itself.

Around 4 months of age, many babies also lose hair on the back of their scalp as the hair grows in at varying times and rates. In very rare cases babies may be born with alopecia (hair loss), which can occur by itself or in association with certain abnormalities of the nails and the teeth. Later in childhood, hair loss may be due to medications, a scalp injury, or a medical or nutritional problem.

An older child may also lose her hair if it's braided too tightly or pulled too hard when combing or brushing. Hot combs may also contribute to hair breakage. Some children (younger than 3 years) twirl their hair as a comforting habit and innocently break it off or pull it out. This behavior usually stops by the age of 4. Other children (usually older ones) may pull their hair out on purpose but deny doing so. Others are simply unaware that they're doing it, which is a sign of emotional stress and something you should discuss with your pediatrician.

Some children may experience hair loss because of an autoimmune condition called *alopecia areata*.

In this disorder, children lose hair in a circular area, causing a bald spot. In general, when it's limited to a few patches, the outlook for complete recovery is good. But when the condition persists or worsens, steroid creams and even steroid injections and other forms of therapy at the site of the hair loss may be used. Unfortunately if the hair loss is extensive, it may be difficult to renew its growth.

### Talk with your pediatrician if your child has hair loss that can't be explained along with

- Fatigue
- A red rash across the bridge of his nose
- Fever or other symptoms of illness
- Loss of lashes and eyebrows

### WARNING!
Use a soft brush of natural or nylon bristles; hard bristles can break your child's hair and irritate her scalp.

## Coping With Hair Loss

Sometimes an otherwise healthy child suddenly loses hair in patches. The hair loss may be because of an autoimmune condition called *alopecia areata*. Although the cause is unknown, it often affects other family members. No predictable, safe, and effective treatment has been developed, but in most cases the hair grows back within 6 to 12 months. Your pediatrician may refer you to a pediatric dermatologist for treatments such as topical corticosteroids or other medications. The condition may recur.

| YOUR CONCERNS | POSSIBLE CAUSE | ACTION TO TAKE |
|---|---|---|
| *Your baby is only a few weeks or months of age, and his hair is falling out.* | Telogen effluvium (normal loss of baby hair) | Baby hair is gradually replaced by mature hair. Wash your baby's scalp frequently, and use a soft hairbrush daily. If there's no sign of hair by 12 months, talk with your pediatrician. |
| *Your baby has a bald spot at the back or side of her scalp.* | Loss of baby hair caused by rubbing or lying in one position | New hair will cover the spot as your baby becomes mobile. Changing your baby's position frequently can help. If several bald patches appear or your baby's scalp is irritated, talk with your pediatrician. |

| YOUR CONCERNS | POSSIBLE CAUSE | ACTION TO TAKE |
|---|---|---|
| Your baby has greasy, crusty patches on his scalp. | Seborrheic dermatitis (cradle cap) | Wash your baby's scalp frequently with a mild shampoo and gently towel-dry It. Rub it with baby oil or petroleum jelly before washing it to help lift the crusts. If the crusts are extensive, your pediatrician may prescribe a cream. |
| Your toddler or school-aged child is losing hair in round, scaly patches. His scalp is itchy. | Tinea capitis (ringworm) | Call your pediatrician, who will examine your child and prescribe an oral antifungal medication if appropriate. |
| Your child's hair loss is especially noticeable around her hairline. She wears braids or a ponytail. She uses a curling iron or hair straightener, or she has a permanent wave. | Traction (damage due to overstyling or chemicals) | Vary your child's hairstyle daily to prevent damage from tight pulling. Avoid using chemical treatments such as dyes, straighteners, and perms. Use a mild shampoo, and don't use a hair dryer. |
| Your child lost a lot of hair following an illness with fever. | Telogen effluvium (an interruption of the hair growth cycle) | The hair usually grows back within 6 months, but bring the hair loss to your pediatrician's attention (see "Coping With Hair Loss," page 94). |
| Your preschooler or school-aged child has dandruff. Members of the family have psoriasis or seborrheic dermatitis. | Psoriasis (red, itchy, scaly patches) Seborrheic dermatitis (greasy scales on the skin) | Talk with your pediatrician, who will examine your child and refer him to a pediatric dermatologist (skin specialist) if necessary. |
| Your child pulls or twists her hair. She twists her hair while she sucks her thumb. | Trichotillomania (hair pulling) sometimes related to stress or an emotional problem | Ask your pediatrician how to manage this problem. Try to identify and remove sources of stress. |
| Your child has an autoimmune disorder such as lupus. | Hair loss due to a chronic disorder | Talk with your pediatrician to make sure your child's condition is being appropriately treated. Discuss ways to help your child deal with his hair loss. |
| Your physically maturing teen is losing his hair. Family members on either side of the family are bald. | Hereditary male or female pattern baldness | There is no proven treatment for baldness; medication is only partly effective. Help your child accept his hair loss. Talk with your pediatrician about ways to develop cosmetic solutions. |
| Your older child or teen is losing clumps of hair. | Alopecia areata (an autoimmune condition) | Talk with your pediatrician. In most cases the hair eventually grows back. There is no proven, universal cure, although corticosteroid treatment is sometimes used. |
| Your child is being treated with irradiation or chemotherapy for a serious illness. | Toxic alopecia or anagen effluvium caused by the effects of treatment | The hair will grow back within 2 to 3 months of stopping the treatment. In the meantime provide head coverings such as baseball caps or bandanas. A particularly sensitive child might prefer a wig. |

## IN GENERAL

Headaches are among the 3 most common recurring pain symptoms that pediatricians often see; stomachaches and earaches are the other ones. Headaches may be classified as *primary*, meaning they're not triggered by an underlying disease (eg, tension-type headaches and migraine headaches), or *secondary*, meaning there's an underlying trigger (eg, benign causes, such as a viral illness and caffeine withdrawal, to more serious but rare diseases such as brain tumor). In more than 90% of cases a pediatrician can classify the headache with a physical examination and a review of a child's medical history. Extensive tests are seldom needed, and only in rare cases does headache signal a serious condition. Most headaches disappear with rest, proper hydration, food if the child is hungry, and the end of a viral illness. Nonprescription medications such as acetaminophen and ibuprofen often relieve headaches.

### Call your pediatrician if your child has a headache and any of the following symptoms:

- Unusual drowsiness or confusion
- Reluctance to bend her neck forward
- Repeated awakening with a headache but without other signs of illness
- Irritability
- Refusal to drink
- Temperature higher than 102°F (39°C)
- Vomiting but no diarrhea
- Muscular weakness or loss of coordination

### WARNING!

If your child has frequent headaches, wakes up with a headache, has a sudden severe headache, or has vomiting as well, bring it to the attention of your pediatrician. Most recurrent headaches are benign; however, your pediatrician may want to rule out any underlying disorder.

## Migraine Headaches in Children

Your child may have the health problem migraine if she experiences recurrent headaches with symptom-free gaps between them and has some or all of the following symptoms: throbbing head pain, often on one side of the head; nausea or vomiting; abdominal pain; a visual or sensory sensation, such as blurring or flashes of light or numbness of the hands and feet); relief of headache following sleep; and a family medical history of migraine.

Most migraine attacks in children aren't severe and can be managed at home. Talk with your pediatrician about the best methods to avoid triggers and treat migraines. Attacks may be triggered by hormonal changes, certain foods, stress, and other factors. If your child has symptoms suggestive of migraine, your pediatrician will recommend a treatment plan. Keeping a headache diary can help a child identify and avoid migraine triggers. A typical headache diary will include notations of the date, time, duration, location, and severity of the headache, as well as environmental factors such as foods eaten before the onset of headache, stressful situations, and other possible triggers. At the first sign of an attack, your child should rest in a quiet, darkened room. Non-prescription medications such as acetaminophen and ibuprofen are often effective for mild migraine headaches. In many cases children with migraine have fewer, less severe headaches once they've been examined by a doctor and reassured that they don't have a serious health problem.

| YOUR CONCERNS | POSSIBLE CAUSE | ACTION TO TAKE |
|---|---|---|
| Your toddler had a bump or fall but didn't lose consciousness. | Mild trauma (Serious injury is very rare with typical toddler falls and collisions.) | Comfort your toddler and encourage him to nap; try a dose of acetaminophen or ibuprofen. If sleep doesn't relieve the pain and upset, and the headache lasts for several hours or gets worse, call your pediatrician. |
| Your child is feverish and unwell. She has a sore throat, runny nose, or other symptoms. | Common cold Streptococcal throat infection (strep throat) Another respiratory infection | Headache often adds to the general sense of feeling unwell during infectious illness. Talk with your pediatrician, who will perform diagnostic tests and prescribe treatment. |
| Your child also has pain in the face and jaw. His nose is runny, and he's tired and irritable. | Sinusitis (an inflammation of the sinuses, airspaces within the bones of the face) Dental problem | You may need to see your child's dentist if a tooth is causing the pain (see "Dental Problems," page 62). You may need to see your pediatrician, who may prescribe treatment for sinusitis (see "Treating Sinusitis," page 132). |
| Your child complains of a dull, non-throbbing headache that feels like a tight band around her head. | Tension headache possibly linked to emotional stress | Give acetaminophen or ibuprofen for occasional headaches, but if they occur frequently, talk with your pediatrician. Try to uncover and remove sources of emotional stress. |
| Your child complains of head pain when she has ice cream, chilled drinks, or other cold foods. | Cold-foods headache caused by a sensitive nerve Tooth sensitivity | Some people get head pain when cold food touches their soft palate. This sensitivity problem is harmless and wears off without treatment. If it bothers your child, help her avoid cold foods. |
| Your child gets headaches when reading or doing close-up work. She blinks or squints a lot. She has neck and shoulder pain when working at a desk. | Eyestrain, change in vision, and possible need for glasses Furniture needing adjustment Poorly positioned computer screen | Talk with your pediatrician, who will examine your child's vision and recommend a consultation with an eye specialist, if necessary. Adjustments to your child's regular workstation may also be required. |
| Your child has a temperature higher than 102°F (39°C). He is sleepy and irritable. His neck is stiff and sore. The light hurts his eyes. | Meningitis or another infection requiring urgent treatment | Call your pediatrician at once. Bacterial meningitis is much less common now that Hib, meningococcal, and pneumococcal vaccines are available, but viruses, unusual bacteria, and other organisms may also causes meningitis. Your pediatrician will want to examine your child. |
| Your child is having severe and more and more frequent headaches. They are worse when she lies down or on waking. She is clumsy or walking oddly. She is vomiting. The headache awakens her. | Tumor | Call your pediatrician without delay. Tests and referral to a pediatric neurologist or neurosurgeon may be needed to identify the cause of the headache. |
| Your teen is feeling sluggish, fatigued, drowsy, or tired. He experiences headaches on the weekend. | Caffeine withdrawal | A teen who abruptly stops or cuts back on caffeine use after a steady intake may develop a headache due to caffeine withdrawal. This headache occurs 1 or 2 days after cutting back. Some teens may experience weekend headaches if their caffeine intake drops regularly on weekends. Once the caffeine habit is broken, caffeine-withdrawal headaches should disappear within 1 or 2 weeks. |

The Big Book of Symptoms

## IN GENERAL

Before you bring your newborn home from the hospital, he needs to have a hearing screening.

Although most babies have normal hearing, 1 to 3 of every 1,000 babies is born with some degree of hearing loss. Without newborn hearing screening, it's difficult to detect hearing loss in a baby during the first months and years of life. About half of the children with hearing loss have no risk factors for it.

Newborn hearing screening can detect possible hearing loss in a baby's first days of life. If a possible hearing loss is found, further tests will be done to confirm the results. When hearing loss is confirmed, treatment and early intervention should start as soon as possible. Early intervention refers to programs and services available to babies and their families that help with hearing loss and learning important communication skills.

Even if your newborn passes the newborn hearing screening test, remember that this is just a screening test and doesn't guarantee that your baby's hearing is normal. If you suspect a hearing problem in your child at any age, you should notify your pediatrician and consider having an audiologist formally assess your child's hearing.

A pronounced loss of hearing, or deafness, raises a barrier to communication that interferes with every aspect of a child's development. There are 2 main types of hearing loss. In the first, called *conductive deafness,* structural problems in the outer or middle ear block the transmission of sound. Common causes of conductive hearing loss include infections, injury, and wax buildup. Many children with this type of hearing loss can be helped by treatment for infection, surgery, or other measures to remove a blockage.

The second type, *sensorineural hearing loss,* may be inborn or caused by illness. In about two-thirds of the cases of childhood sensorineural hearing loss, the cause is genetic, although hearing loss that runs in the family may not show up until later in life. Children are sometimes born deaf because their mothers had a viral infection (eg, German measles, or rubella) or took certain medications (eg, the antibiotic streptomycin) during pregnancy. Most people with sensorineural deafness benefit to some degree from hearing aids.

Hearing aids won't restore hearing completely to those with significant sensorineural hearing loss, but they will help your child develop spoken or oral language if the hearing impairment is mild or moderate. Should your child have severe or profound hearing impairment in both ears and receive no benefit from hearing aids, she will become a candidate for a cochlear implant. Since 1990 cochlear implants have been approved by the government for children older than 1 year. There is now enough experience with them to say that cochlear implants work well for the most children who have normal brain function.

### Talk with your pediatrician if your child

- Responds to your speech only when he can see your face
- Is not speaking or making sounds appropriate to his age level
- Does not seem to hear certain sounds
- Cannot understand what's said on television or radio unless the volume is very high

### WARNING!

Always call your pediatrician if your child complains of ear pain. Left untreated, infections of the ears can cause permanent hearing loss.

### Preventing Injury From Headphones

If your child is exposed to an MP3 player, an iPod, or another portable device, it's important to carefully regulate the volume. Kept at a volume similar to normal speech, headphones may do no harm. But if children turn up the volume to block out external noise, they subject their ears to an assault that can cause permanent hearing loss. If others in the room can hear sound while the child is wearing headphones, the volume is at an unsafe level and should be turned down. Some experts believe there's no safe way to use headphones. They contend that one of the best ways to protect the hearing is not to use headphones at all. One practical measure is not to allow your child to turn up the volume beyond 60% either on a digital readout or using a volume wheel. This assures that the sound is within safe limits.

Never allow your child to wear a portable headset while walking, skating, or cycling. It blocks out warning noises, and the risk is all the greater because your child will concentrate on the music and not be alert to traffic and other potentially dangerous situations.

| YOUR CONCERNS | POSSIBLE CAUSE | ACTION TO TAKE |
|---|---|---|
| Your baby doesn't turn her head when you call. She doesn't respond when you clap, even when she's not looking at you. | Hearing impairment | Call your pediatrician without delay. After testing your baby's hearing, your pediatrician may recommend consultation with another health specialist, if necessary. |
| Your infant of 6 or 7 months doesn't babble and imitate the tone of your voice. He doesn't respond to the sounds around him. | Partial or complete hearing loss | Call your pediatrician promptly. He or she will test your infant's hearing and provide referral to another specialist, if needed. |
| Your child has been less responsive since having an ear infection. | Fluid buildup following otitis media with effusion (middle ear infection) | Talk with your pediatrician, who will examine your child and provide appropriate treatment. If the problem persists, your pediatrician may refer your child to a pediatric otolaryngologist. |
| Your child has gradually become hard of hearing. | Blockage of outer ear canal by foreign body or wax buildup | Talk with your pediatrician, who will examine your child's ear using a lighted instrument called an otoscope. He or she will also remove the blockage. Don't try to remove wax or other material yourself; you may force it farther into the ear and injure the ear. |
| Your child has had an injury to the ear. | Trauma Perforated ear drum | Call your pediatrician, who will examine your child's ear and treat your child appropriately. |
| Your child has been hard of hearing since recently riding a plane or a rollercoaster ride. | Barotrauma (injury due to change in ear/air pressure) | Hearing loss due to pressure change usually clears up by itself. If there's no improvement in 2 or 3 days, call your pediatrician. |
| Your child gets severely dizzy and loses her balance. She has attacks of nausea and vomiting. She complains of ringing in her ears, called tinnitus. | Neurologic disorder | Talk with your pediatrician, who will examine your child to determine whether she needs treatment. |

# HEADBEAT IRREGULARITIES

## IN GENERAL

The human heart is divided into 4 chambers: the left and right atria at the top and the left and right ventricles on the bottom. These chambers are separated by valves that keep the blood moving through the heart in the proper direction. Their muscular walls contract in rhythm to keep the heart efficiently pumping blood. The muscle contractions are triggered by electrical impulses from a group of cells in the right atrium, called the *sinoatrial node* (or *sinus node*). Each electrical impulse that powers a heartbeat arises in the sinus node, flows through the left and right atrial walls, and is relayed through a second group of pacemaker cells—the atrioventricular node—to the ventricles. An error at any stage of the conduction system may result in a disturbance of the normal heartbeat pattern known as the *sinus rhythm*.

At birth, a baby's heart beats as often as 120 to 140 times a minute, increasing to more than 170 with crying and slowing to between 70 and 90 during sleep. The very rapid newborn rate slows over time, but the normal childhood range of heartbeats remains quite wide from 70 to 100 beats per minute. The rate speeds up during exercise and slows at rest. Preteens and teens in advanced athletic training may have a resting heart rate of only 40 to 50 beats per minute. A fever can also quicken the heart rate.

Minor variations in children's heart rate and rhythm, called *arrhythmias* or *dysrhythmias,* occur for many reasons. Occasional palpitations (strongly-felt heartbeats) or flutters are common and usually harmless. In most cases a slight irregularity in the basic sinus rhythm is of no consequence; certain irregularities and patterns, however, may signal a health problem and must be looked into. A change in rhythm is dangerous only when it's so pronounced and prolonged that it interferes with the heart's ability to pump blood efficiently. In the rare cases where treatment is necessary, the heartbeat can be regulated by medication or the use of an electronic pacemaker. Some children with serious changes in rhythm may be treated with a special catheter inserted into the heart through a large vein and, rarely, some may need surgery.

**Call your pediatrician right away if your child has a change in heart rhythm with any of the following symptoms:**

- Breathing difficulty
- Chest pain
- Dizziness, light-headedness, or paleness
- Confusion
- Loss of consciousness

> **WARNING!**
> If your child's heartbeat is unusually slow or remains fast over a prolonged period, the change may be serious and should be brought to your pediatrician's attention.

## Prolonged QT Interval Syndrome

A rare inherited condition may cause a child, preteen, or teen to faint and have severe heartbeat irregularities during exercise or an emotionally stressful experience. This heart problem is known as *prolonged QT interval syndrome* because of the characteristic pattern—an abnormal lengthening of the QT interval—seen when an electrocardiogram is performed during carefully monitored exercise. Sometimes the condition isn't inbo0rn but occurs with another form of heart disease. When inherited, it may also be associated with deafness. If one member of your family is diagnosed as having prolonged QT interval syndrome, tell your pediatrician. Other family members should also be tested. This heart problem can be controlled by medication or, rarely, a defibrillator implanted in the body. Your child should also be extra careful while participating in strenuous activities such as unsupervised swimming or climbing that could put her at risk.

| YOUR CONCERNS | POSSIBLE CAUSE | ACTION TO TAKE |
|---|---|---|
| Your child's heartbeat seems irregular. It speeds up when she breathes in and slows down when she breathes out. She is otherwise well and active. | Sinus arrhythmia (a normal variation in heart rate) | If the irregularity is worrying you, bring it to your pediatrician's attention. A simple examination will show whether further testing, such as an electrocardiogram, is needed. |
| Your newborn's pulse seems unusually slow (less than 70 beats per minute). | Dysrhythmia Bradycardia (an abnormally slow heartbeat) | Talk with your pediatrician, who will examine your baby's heart and determine whether further consultation is required. |
| Your child's heartbeat has felt uneven since he had an illness with fever. | Uneven beats (common during recovery from an illness with fever) | In most cases this health problem resolves itself over time without treatment. If it persists or gets worse, discuss your concerns with your pediatrician. |
| Your child complains that she can feel her heart beating faster while at rest. She drinks caffeinated soda or energy drinks. | Excessive caffeine or energy drink consumption, which leads to fast and irregular heartbeats Dysrhythmia | Caffeine can cause the heart to race or miss a beat. Help your child cut out chocolate and replace colas and other caffeine-containing drinks with juices, milk, and water. If there's no change in 1 or 2 days, talk with your pediatrician. |
| Your child noticed a thumping or racing sensation in his chest while taking medication, such as an antihistamine for allergies or a cold medication. | Side effect of the medication | Call your pediatrician, who will either withdraw the medication or prescribe a substitute. |
| Your child has previously been diagnosed and treated for a heart condition. | Inborn or acquired heart condition | Inborn heart disorders are usually associated with disturbances in heart rhythm. If new irregularities appear or become more noticeable, bring them to your pediatrician's attention. |
| Your child is having night terrors. She is unusually tired and taking many naps, is irritable, and faints sometimes. Her mother has an autoimmune disease such as lupus. | Atrioventricular block (an abnormality in the heart's electrical system) | Talk with your pediatrician, who will examine your child and refer him to a pediatric heart specialist for evaluation, if necessary. This condition can usually be well controlled with use of medication or a pacemaker. |
| Your child feels extra or missed heartbeats and recently had streptococcal throat infection (strep throat). | Ectopic beats (a complication of strep throat which may be associated with various conditions, including rheumatic fever) | Talk with your pediatrician, who will examine your child to determine whether further tests and treatment are necessary. |
| Your child is suddenly pale and tired. He is sweating while at rest and has had several fainting episodes. Other young members of the family have had repeated fainting or a history of heart disease. | Arrhythmia that leads to inefficient heart pumping Anemia Prolonged QT interval syndrome (See page 100 for a definition.) | Talk with your pediatrician, who will examine your child, order tests if appropriate, and possibly refer your child to another specialist. |

## IN GENERAL

An attack of indigestion can cause tremendous discomfort, such as gas, a feeling of being overly full, and heartburn. Heartburn is a burning sensation caused by stomach acid flowing back into the esophagus and irritating its lining. This backward flow, or *gastroesophageal reflux,* also causes the sour taste that sometimes occurs after a heavy or fatty meal. Infants may be affected by reflux (see "Feeding Problems in Babies," page 6).

Makers of over-the-counter remedies claim that indigestion is caused by too much acid, but it's actually caused by acid in the wrong place. The trigger is sometimes too much food. A sphincter at the end of the esophagus relaxes to let food pass and closes tight to keep it in the stomach. Various triggers, however, can cause the sphincter to open at the wrong time. Pressure due to an overfull stomach, obesity, or lying down after eating may force it open. A meal heavy in fats slows down stomach emptying and contributes to overloading. Foods that can make the sphincter muscle relax include tomato-based products, chocolate, caffeine, and peppermint. Certain medications, such as some used to treat asthma, may also have this effect.

As long as your infant is growing at a normal rate, it's unlikely that he has a serious gastrointestinal problem.

**Talk with your pediatrician if your infant has**

- Persistent (won't go away) vomiting
- Poor weight gain

### WARNING!

Don't treat your child's indigestion with over-the-counter antacids, acid-suppressing remedies, or homemade concoctions of baking soda. Regular use of antacids and certain pain medications can injure the stomach lining. Use these and all medications only on the advice of your pediatrician.

## Coping With Gastroesophageal Reflux

Time the evening meal so your child has 1 or 2 hours of quiet relaxation but nothing more to eat or drink before bedtime. After meals she should sit up in a straight chair while reading, doing homework, or another calm activity to give the digestive process time to work. Lying down soon after eating encourages the reflux of stomach contents into the esophagus. She may sleep more comfortably if you raise the head of her bed with bricks or a wedge, which are available in pharmacies. Sleeping with the upper part of the body elevated uses gravity to discourage reflux.

If your child is troubled by indigestion or other symptoms related to gastroesophageal reflux disease, your pediatrician may also prescribe a medication to reduce stomach acid or suppress the acid flowing into the esophagus.

| YOUR CONCERNS | POSSIBLE CAUSE | ACTION TO TAKE |
|---|---|---|
| *Your newborn between 2 and 6 weeks of age vomits at every feeding. The vomiting is projectile or forceful. She is unable to gain or even lose weight.* | Pyloric stenosis (See "Feeding Problems in Babies," page 6.) | Call your pediatrician at once. |
| *Your newborn older than 6 weeks is vomiting after each feeding (but not forceful, projectile vomiting).* | Gastroesophageal reflux disease (spitting up due to relaxation of the sphincter between the esophagus and stomach) | Talk with your pediatrician. Some vomiting or spitting up is normal; most infants outgrow the problem by about 1 year of age (see "Feeding Problems in Babies," page 6). |
| *Your child is vomiting after every meal and has a serious developmental delay.* | Gastroesophageal reflux disease due to developmental problem | Talk with your pediatrician; your child may need further evaluation or medical or surgical therapy. |
| *Your child is complaining of a stomachache and an occasional sour, burning taste in her throat.* | Gastritis (inflammation of the stomach) Peptic ulcer (possibly linked to *Helicobacter pylori* infection) | Talk with your pediatrician. He or she may refer you to a pediatric GI specialist. |
| *Your child has burning in his chest, hoarseness, chronic cough, or wheezing. He has had pneumonia. He is gaining weight only slowly.* | Respiratory effects of gastroesophageal reflux | Your pediatrician will examine your child and may review your child's diet with you. Your child may benefit from medical treatment as well as cutting down on fatty foods, tomato-based products, and colas. |
| *Your child has a burning pain in her chest. She rushes when she eats her food or sometimes eats too much. She has gassiness or bloating.* | Aerophagia (swallowed air) Overeating Esophagitis (inflammation of the esophagus) Eating too fast | Pace meals so that your whole family eats in a more relaxed fashion. Your pediatrician will examine your child to determine whether your child's health problem requires treatment. |
| *Your school-aged child or teen has frequent gassiness, bloating, cramps, and diarrhea after meals. He is growing slowly.* | Malabsorption problem such as lactose intolerance Celiac disease (The small intestine is hypersensitive to gluten.) Irritable bowel syndrome Chronic inflammation of the intestinal tract (eg, Crohn disease or ulcerative colitis) | Talk with your pediatrician, who will examine your child and may provide a referral to a specialist in pediatric gastroenterology, if necessary. Dietary changes may be advised. |

## IN GENERAL

Each child is born with a temperament—a personality and disposition—that emphasizes certain characteristics over others. Parents are often astonished to find that their newborn already seems adventurous or hesitant, impatient or accepting, outgoing or shy. Some children are more prone to a negative mood, are less adaptable, or are more sensitive and reactive, with the result being that they're more easily made irritable. Although a child's basic nature is inborn, her temperament and outlook are influenced by her experiences, interactions with parents and others, and sense of self-worth.

Like grown-ups, most children feel irritable, agitated, or short-tempered at times. If your child can't tell you why, it may be because he either can't pinpoint the trouble or can't yet express himself in words. In general, a sudden and severe physical or psychological cause for irritability leads a child to act very differently from his everyday behavior. If a child often seems irritable, there may be an underlying health problem or stressful factors in his family or school environment. It's important to recognize the difference between a passing mood and the fretful crying that signals that your child needs your attention to deal with fever, pain, cold, heat, hunger, or other physical reasons for irritability. An occasional irritable mood may not be serious, but a child who is almost always irritable may need medical, developmental, or psychological attention. Many babies from about 2 weeks of age up to 6 months have daily bouts of irritable crying and colic (see page 2). Although upsetting to the parents while it lasts, this irritability isn't a symptom of illness and usually disappears on its own by the time the baby is 6 months or younger. A child between the ages of 18 months and 3 years may find himself frustrated as he's learning better ways to communicate with those around him, resulting in irritability. This phase passes as the child becomes more independent. It's not unusual for a preteen or teen to be irritable during the mood swings associated with adolescence, hormonal changes, academic pressures, and possibly depressed mood (see page 182).

**Call your pediatrician if your child is unusually irritable and has**

- A fever higher than 100.4°F (38°C)
- Pain, including a sore throat, stiff neck, or headache
- Unusual drowsiness
- Vomiting without diarrhea
- Severe temper tantrums where she can't be soothed
- Decrease in school performance
- Increase in aggression
- Mania symptoms

### WARNING!

Don't ignore irritability and hope it will go away by itself. If the cause is physical, the irritability should be addressed. If stress is altering your child's mood, the cause should be identified and, if possible, eliminated.

## Coping With Irritability

Although your child has her own unique disposition, she also copies the examples she sees. If she usually gets an irritable, impatient response to her questions, sooner or later she may mimic this behavior and treat others the same way. If your child often seems grouchy and irritable but has no health problem that could be causing discomfort, take a look at potential triggers in her environment, changes in peer relations, psychosocial changes and stressors, and other possible causes of this change in mood. Avoid placing your child in difficult situations, let her express her opinions, and don't ask if she wants to do something when you really mean you want her to do it.

| YOUR CONCERNS | POSSIBLE CAUSE | ACTION TO TAKE |
| --- | --- | --- |
| Your infant is older than 3 months, and his temperature is higher than 100.4°F (38°C). He is fretful. | A viral or bacterial infection | Call your pediatrician, who may want to examine your baby and will prescribe any necessary treatments. |
| Your infant or older child has sniffles and a runny nose. She is coughing. | Common cold<br>Another upper respiratory tract infection | Call your pediatrician for advice (see "Cough," page 58; "Breathing Difficulty/Breathlessness," page 50; "Runny/Stuffy Nose," page 132). |
| Your toddler is limping or guarding one of his limbs. There is swelling, redness, or warmth. | Fracture, infection, or injury to the leg or hip | Call your pediatrician for an examination and x-rays, if necessary (see "Fractures/Broken Bones," page 88). |
| Your child wakes up irritable every morning. She often breathes through her mouth because of a stuffed-up nose. She is always tired. | Allergy<br>Interrupted sleep due to enlarged tonsils or adenoids and upper airway blockage<br>Sleep apnea | Talk with your pediatrician, who will examine your child for signs of a chronic allergy (see "Allergic Reactions," page 26), tonsil or adenoid enlargement, and upper airway blockage (see "Breathing Difficulty/Breathlessness," page 50), and prescribe any necessary treatment. |
| Your child's stools are hard pellets. He has been unable to move his bowels for several days. He complains of a stomachache. | Constipation | Make sure your family's diet includes plenty of fresh vegetables, fruits, and other sources of fiber; encourage your child to drink several glasses of water or diluted juices each day (see "Constipation," page 54). |
| Your school-aged child is constantly irritable and fatigued. She goes to bed late. She is involved in many after-school activities. | Not enough sleep<br>Health problem requiring treatment | Your child's schedule may include more than she can manage. Where possible, provide for more rest and make sure she's getting enough exercise. If these measures don't help, or if your child has other symptoms, call your pediatrician to arrange an evaluation. |
| Your school-aged child is irritable, anxious, or easily distracted. | Emotional stress due to academic or social problems at school<br>Tension in the family | If your family is under stress, explain the situation without overburdening your child; try to keep the daily impact to a minimum. Questioning may give you an idea of what's bothering your child at school. Speak with teachers to identify problems. |
| Your child is just grumpy without any symptoms of illness. | Shows signs of frustration | Discuss coping techniques with your pediatrician. Let your child make his own choices when there is room for reasonable compromise. |

## IN GENERAL

When a child gets an itchy rash, he may have been exposed to an irritant or allergen. Or he contracted a viral infection. Children who develop allergic reactions to medications may also develop intense itching.

Itching without a rash occurs for many reasons, especially in children with dry skin or atopic dermatitis (eczema) and when central heating and winter air dry out the skin. Fungal and yeast infections can be itchy, too, though apart from ringworm or diaper rash due to yeasts, they're not often seen before adolescence.

Some children scratch from habit, which irritates the skin and prompts further scratching. Those with eczema are especially vulnerable to the itch-scratch-itch cycle. In some children the skin gets cracked and sore and may become infected.

Itchy skin without a rash is linked to a few systemic conditions, but these are rare in children. Girls may be embarrassed by itching due to vulvovaginitis (see page 164), and teenaged boys are prone to the itchy fungal infections known as *jock itch* (in the groin area) and athlete's foot. Your pediatrician may recommend over-the-counter products to treat these latter 2 conditions, and you should encourage your child to dry himself thoroughly after showering or bathing.

### Call your pediatrician if your child

- Has itching along with swelling of her lips or face
- Develops an itchy rash after starting a new oral medication
- Has a patch of eczema that is showing signs of infection, such as swelling, warmth, and pus
- Has a nervous habit of scratching that is causing skin problems or social difficulties

### WARNING!

If your child has itchy skin, use mild soap for laundry, and avoid detergents that contain dyes and perfumes. Rinse clothes thoroughly, and put them through a second plain water cycle, if necessary, to remove soap residue.

## Managing Eczema

Eczema, also known as *atopic dermatitis,* is a very common skin condition that causes reddened, itchy skin. Sometimes the skin is covered with juicy red bumps that weep and crust over. In chronic eczema, which may last for many months or years, the skin thickens, becoming scaly, cracked, fissured, and darkly pigmented.

Eczema typically occurs in children whose families have a tendency to develop eczema and allergies, although in most children the rash isn't caused by allergy. It may appear at any age but in most cases it develops by 5 years of age. In babies between 2 and 6 months of age, eczema appears as itching, redness, and bumps on the face and scalp, perhaps spreading to the arms and trunk. In about half the cases the rash disappears by 2 or 3 years of age. Many children outgrow it by about 6 years of age, others by puberty. In others it may recur from time to time even in adolescence and adult life.

If you suspect certain foods are causing the rash, avoid them. Apply moisturizers while your child's skin is damp. Use a pH-neutral soap that's perfume free. Daily bathing, if brief, not too hot, and followed right away with hydration either with an over-the-counter emollient (softening agent) or prescription, can help keep your child's skin hydrated. Sedating antihistamines may be recommended by your pediatrician to help get your child to sleep when itching is most intense at bedtime. In children with eczema and environmental allergies, oral non-sedating antihistamines may also be useful. A topical (applied to the skin) steroid may be needed for short periods when a child has severe eczema. It should not be used long-term. But a relatively new group of non-steroidal topical medications called *topical calcineurin inhibitors* may be prescribed for sensitive areas such as the face and genital area in children older than 2 years of age.

| YOUR CONCERNS | POSSIBLE CAUSE | ACTION TO TAKE |
|---|---|---|
| Your baby has patches of red, rough skin. Other family members have eczema and allergies. | Atopic dermatitis (eczema; see "Skin Problems," page 207) | Your pediatrician will examine your baby and recommend treatment for this common condition. Don't dress your baby in itchy clothing. |
| Your child has red, flaky patches or a moist rash. The affected areas come into contact with allergens such as dyes in clothing or nickel in jewelry. You recently switched brands of soap or detergent. | Allergic contact dermatitis (See "Skin Problems," page 207.) | Use cold compresses to soothe the irritation. Try to identify and avoid the source of irritation. If the rash is severe, talk with your pediatrician who will examine your child and recommend treatment. |
| Your child has broken out in an itchy rash after a cough, fever, and upper respiratory symptoms. | Rash due to virus | Call your pediatrician, who will examine your child and prescribe any necessary treatments. |
| Your child developed a blistering rash after being outdoors. The rash looks like a series of lines. | Poison ivy, oak, or sumac  Nettles or other stinging plants | Wash the area with soap and water, and rinse it for 10 minutes. Wash your child's clothes. Apply cool compresses. If the rash is severe, call your pediatrician. |
| Your child has an itchy rash in an exposed area. There are bumps with red spots in the centers. | Bites of insects, such as chiggers, mosquitoes, or fleas | Apply cool compresses (also see "Bites and Stings," page 40). If the rash persists or bites show signs of infection, talk with your pediatrician. |
| Your child develops a widespread, itchy, red, bumpy rash within a week of starting a new medication. | Allergic reaction to the medication | Stop the medication and talk with your pediatrician as soon as possible. |
| Your child is constantly scratching. You see either nits (egg cases) in his hair or reddish tracks on his skin. | Skin parasites such as head lice (on the scalp) or scabies (on the body) | Call your pediatrician, who will recommend treatment and measures to eradicate the parasites from your home. Notify your child's school or child care center. |
| Your child has itchy ring-shaped patches on the skin and bald patches on her scalp. | Ringworm | Call your pediatrician, who will prescribe treatment and advise how to stop the infection from spreading. |
| Your child has developed a rash while taking a medication, such as an antibiotic. | Medication side effect | Call your pediatrician, who will examine your child and prescribe a different antibiotic, if necessary, as well as treat the skin problem. |
| Your child has itching around the anus that's more intense at night. | Pinworms (See "Rectal Pain/ Itching," page 128.) | Your pediatrician will examine your child and prescribe appropriate treatment. Ask your pediatrician how to prevent the spread of infection. |
| Your teenaged son is complaining of itching around his genital area. | Jock itch (fungal infection)  Intertrigo (dermatitis in the skin folds) | Your pediatrician will recommend treatment. Encourage your son to soap thoroughly during showers and baths and to dry thoroughly before dressing. |
| Your teenaged daughter is troubled by itching in her vaginal area. She is also experiencing a discharge and unusual odor. | Vulvovaginitis (See page 164.) | Talk with your pediatrician, who will prescribe appropriate treatment. |

## IN GENERAL

Pains resulting from a minor injury to the arm or leg are usually short-lived. But children may also have persistent (won't go away) pain in the joints because of infection or arthritis. If your child has joint pain that lasts longer than 1 or 2 days, and she seems reluctant to move her affected limb, call or make an appointment to see your pediatrician (also see Fractures/Broken Bones," page 88; "Knee Pain," page 194).

**Call your pediatrician if your child has joint pain along with**

- Fever
- A rash
- Warmth, swelling, or tenderness
- Difficulty using an arm or leg

**WARNING!**
Don't ignore complaints of joint pain. Joint pain in children isn't normal and should be evaluated by your pediatrician.

## Preventing Lyme Disease

Lyme disease is an infection caused by bacteria transmitted through the bites of deer ticks in certain regions of the United States. Ticks are about the size of a poppy seed, and they live in grassy, wooded, and marshy regions. They can be found year-round but are most plentiful in spring, summer, and fall.

The most distinctive symptom of Lyme disease is an enlarging circular rash, sometimes with the appearance of a bull's-eye (page 40), which usually appears 3 to 10 days after the tick bite. The rash doesn't always follow a bite, however, and for some people Lyme disease is signaled only by influenza-like symptoms such as headache, fever, fatigue, and aches in the muscles and joints. Antibiotic treatment is usually effective if given within a month of the bite. Left untreated, Lyme disease may cause severe symptoms, including visual disturbance, facial paralysis, and joint pain and arthritis. The infection is harder to treat in the later stages.

Dress your child protectively when he ventures into wooded areas. He should wear long-sleeved shirts and tuck the legs of his pants into his socks. A hat can help keep ticks away from favored spots along the hairline and behind the ears. Encourage your child to stay on cleared trails. You can also use an insect repellent that contains no more than 30% DEET on any exposed areas. Just make sure to always wash off the repellent with soap and water.

Check your child for ticks every evening when he's been playing outdoors. By removing a tick as soon as you see it, you lower the chance of your child getting Lyme disease. A tick needs to be attached to the skin for about 48 hours in order to transmit the infection.

| YOUR CONCERNS | POSSIBLE CAUSE | ACTION TO TAKE |
|---|---|---|
| *Your child has joint pain following an injury caused by a fall or a sudden movement. But he can move his limb.* | Bruise Muscle or ligament strain | Apply an ice pack to your child's sore joint; use a cold compress but no ice if your child is younger than 2 years. If the pain doesn't get better after 24 hours, call your pediatrician. |
| *Your child is suddenly limping. She has pain in one hip. She is between 2 and 10 years of age. She recently had a mild respiratory illness.* | Toxic or transient synovitis (inflammation of the hip joint), probably caused by a viral infection | Call your pediatrician. If viral synovitis is suspected, your pediatrician may recommend rest and acetaminophen or ibuprofen. This acute hip pain usually clears up with no aftereffects. The condition could also be an early bacterial infection, so if pain with movement or fever develops, contact your pediatrician. |

| YOUR CONCERNS | POSSIBLE CAUSE | ACTION TO TAKE |
|---|---|---|
| Your toddler or preschooler is holding his arm close to his side. His elbow is very tender. He resists if you gently try to straighten his arm. He was recently pulled or swung by his arms. | Pulled elbow, also called *nursemaid's elbow,* caused when soft tissue becomes trapped in the joint | Call your pediatrician right away for an examination. Fold a scarf or soft towel into an arm sling, but don't try to treat the injury yourself. Your pediatrician may manipulate your child's elbow to release the trapped tissue. He or she may also discuss with you how to help your child avoid such injuries. |
| Your child has severe pain and some swelling in the joint at the tip of a finger. She is an active ball player. | Mallet finger, also called *baseball finger* | Apply an ice pack to this minor injury, which occurs when a ball bends a fingertip back. If your child's finger is still painful and swollen after a couple of days, talk with your pediatrician. |
| Your child has soreness and stiffness in his hands, wrists, knees, and ankles. He recently had symptoms suggesting a viral infection. | Post-viral joint pain | Joint pains following a viral infection usually go away within 1 to 2 weeks. If your child has a fever, develops redness or swelling of his bone or joint, or isn't better after a week, call your pediatrician. |
| Your child has pain, redness, and warmth in one or more joints. Her temperature is higher than 100.4°F (38°C). She is having trouble moving her limbs. She recently had an infection or a tick bite. | Inflammation or infection Septic arthritis Juvenile idiopathic arthritis Lyme disease (See "Preventing Lyme Disease," page 108.) Rheumatic fever Lupus | Contact your pediatrician. He or she will examine your child and order blood tests to clarify the diagnosis. Long-term treatment may be required. Your pediatrician may also refer your child to a specialist in joint disorders. |
| Your son limps because of pain in his hip, thigh, or knee. He is generally free of symptoms other than leg pain. He is between about 4 and 9 years of age. | Legg-Calvé-Perthes disease (hip disorder initiated by a disruption of blood flow to the head of the thigh bone, usually in boys) or another condition requiring diagnosis and treatment | Talk with your pediatrician, who will examine your son and determine whether he needs further tests and treatment. |
| Your child also has a purple rash on his legs, feet, or buttocks. He has pain in his abdomen. | Henoch-Schonlein purpura (an autoimmune condition) | Call your pediatrician, who will examine your child, order appropriate diagnostic tests, and prescribe necessary treatment. |
| Your preteen or teen (aged 10 to 13) has hip and knee pain. She is having trouble walking. She is overweight. | Slipped capital femoral epiphysis (displacement of the head of the thigh bone) | Talk with your pediatrician, who will examine your child and determine whether treatment is required. |

## IN GENERAL

If your child is having trouble at school, it may mean he has a learning problem. This doesn't mean your child is less intelligent than other children; it's just harder for him to learn. Failure in school can cause frustration and disappointment for your child as well as your family. Sometimes a learning problem is at the root of an apparent behavioral problem (see "Attention-Deficit/Hyperactivity Disorder," page 30, "Behavioral Concerns," page 38, or "Temper Tantrums," page 156). When the learning problem is identified and addressed, a child's behavior generally improves. The cause of a child's learning problem varies. Learning problems tend to run in families. In many cases no definite cause is ever identified. In rare cases learning difficulties follow a head injury or brain infection.

Some children have problems with basic skills such as reading, writing, spelling, and numbers. Others have trouble with language skills, including listening, understanding, remembering, and speech. Still others have difficulties with balance, writing, and coordination—skills that require the child to integrate messages from the motor (muscle) and sensory systems. Poor social skills often hamper children with learning problems. They misunderstand and respond inappropriately to friends, teachers, and parents. Like social and emotional problems, learning problems need to be dealt with as soon as possible. Problems may be obvious before a child enters preschool or show up only when she can't keep up in the later grades.

Your child's teachers can refer you to resources available in your local district. They will also work out classroom strategies and suggest steps you can take at home. Psychological counseling may be advised. If your pediatrician diagnoses serious attention problems, behavior therapy and medication may be prescribed to improve your child's concentration.

**Talk with your pediatrician as well as your child's teachers if your child**

- Has trouble reading words or numbers
- Is not achieving grade level
- Has temper tantrums or behavior problems
- Seems depressed
- Tries to avoid going to school

### WARNING!

Despite claims and publicity, treatments such as megavitamins, patterning exercises, eye exercises, and additive-free diets haven't been found to benefit children with learning problems. Seek the advice of your pediatrician before starting any treatments.

## Gifted Children Need Help Too

Children who have high abilities in reading, language, mathematical reasoning, science, performing or fine arts, or sports are often considered gifted. These children usually have lots of interests, read more—and read more difficult—books than others the same age. They are often able to work on their own at an early age. Their outstanding talents give them a great potential for achieving personal satisfaction as well as for making a contribution to society.

Just as children with learning problems need help, gifted children also deserve special programs to develop their talents. Without such programs, some gifted children don't meet their potential in the classroom. When unable to get emotional rewards from their achievements in school, they lose faith in themselves and feel more and more unsuccessful and isolated from their peers. They may become bored and disruptive.

Providing programs for gifted children isn't always easy. Without special training, teachers may find it difficult to deal with the advanced thinking of a gifted student. School budgets often can't afford teachers who are trained to work with gifted children. Most gifted children benefit from an approach that combines independent study, advanced special classes, and use of outside resources, where appropriate. A student with outstanding ability in one field, such as music or performing arts, may be considered for application to a specialized school.

| YOUR CONCERNS | POSSIBLE CAUSE | ACTION TO TAKE |
|---|---|---|
| *Your child's speech is hard to follow. He has trouble finding words or organizing his thoughts. He often misunderstands you. He has trouble with recall.* | Slow development<br>Language/speech disability<br>Attention or memory problems | Talk with your pediatrician, who will evaluate your child and advise whether treatment is necessary. |
| *Your school-aged child speaks well but has trouble writing. She puts off assignments or doesn't complete written projects. She asks others to write for her.* | Dysgraphia<br>   (writing difficulty)<br>Fine motor problems | Ask your child's teacher for an evaluation by the educational psychologist. Request a meeting to discuss the specific problem and possible solutions. The school's learning center may provide help with organization and writing mechanics, or outside tutoring may be recommended. |
| *Your child finds it hard to understand what he reads, but he can follow what is read to him. He has trouble remembering printed information.* | Learning difficulty<br>Dyslexia<br>Poor vocabulary<br>Difficulty with concepts<br>Attention problems | Ask your child's teachers and the school psychologist to evaluate the problem. Find out if the school learning center can provide appropriate help or whether tutoring is advisable. |
| *Your child has problems memorizing. It is hard for her to retell a story in the right sequence. She has trouble with math facts.* | Memory/thinking difficulty<br>Attention problems<br>Few memory strategies | If these problems are causing difficulties at school, ask for an evaluation and possibly a referral to the school learning center. Get advice on improving your child's memory, organizational skills, and concentration. |
| *Your child's behavior is causing concern. He is aggressive toward other students or teachers. He is defiant at home. He is unable to keep up.* | Learning problem<br>Behavioral problem<br>   (See page 38.)<br>Hyperactivity<br>   (See page 30.)<br>Depression<br>   (See page 182.) | Ask your child's teachers to identify areas of concern and seek their recommendations for management. Talk with your pediatrician, who can advise as to whether psychological counseling is needed. |

## IN GENERAL

Temporary pain in a child's arms or legs is usually because of minor falls, collisions, or muscle strains. A visit to the pediatrician is usually unnecessary, and a cold compress and pain medication (eg, acetaminophen or ibuprofen) is the only treatment that's needed. On the other hand, pain due to an obvious, more serious injury, such as a fracture, requires medical care at once. And even when there's no sign of injury, your child should be seen by a pediatrician if her limb or leg pain lasts for more than 1 or 2 days or grows more intense.

### Talk with your pediatrician if your child's limb pain is severe or occurs along with

- Limping
- A lump in a bruised muscle that doesn't go away within 1 or 2 weeks
- Difficulty in moving the affected limb
- Swelling or pain that continues to increase after 24 hours

### WARNING!

Don't ignore limb pains and muscle aches. Your pediatrician may identify a physical cause that can be treated. Stress, too, can cause nonspecific symptoms such as pain.

## Avoiding Overuse Injuries

Exercise that's too much for your child's developmental stage or physical condition may result in overuse injuries such as sprains, strains, stress fractures, shin splints, and tendinitis. Pain in legs and limbs often results from injuries to bones, soft tissues, and the growth cartilage that's found only in children. Children are especially vulnerable to overuse injuries because their bone length grows at a faster rate than their muscle mass. The difference in growth rate places uneven stresses on the musculoskeletal system.

Unless carefully managed, overuse injuries may cause adverse long-term effects. To help your child avoid overuse injuries, encourage him to stick to the following guidelines:

- Begin and end every sports or exercise session with warm-up exercises, such as walking, slow jogging, or riding a bicycle, followed by gentle stretching exercises.
- Gradually work up to new levels in the frequency, duration, and intensity of exercise.
- Don't over-train.
- Follow your coach's instructions when learning an activity.
- Check your shoe size at least every 3 months, and buy athletic shoes at a shop where the salespeople are trained in fitting sports shoes for children.

| YOUR CONCERNS | POSSIBLE CAUSE | ACTION TO TAKE |
| --- | --- | --- |
| The pain came on suddenly with movement. There is swelling or stiffening at the site of the pain. | Muscle strain or sprain | Apply a cold compresses to relieve soreness and swelling, and have your child elevate and rest the affected area. If pain persists, call your pediatrician, who may want to examine your child. |
| Your child complains of cramping pain in the muscles of his thigh, his calf, or the arch of his foot. The pain usually comes on at night after an active day. | Muscle spasms from overuse | Gently but firmly rub the affected area to relieve your child's discomfort. |

| YOUR CONCERNS | POSSIBLE CAUSE | ACTION TO TAKE |
|---|---|---|
| *Your active teen is limping. He has tenderness but no bruising in the shins.* | Shin splints<br>Stress injury<br>Slipped capital femoral epiphysis (displacement of the head of the thigh bone) | Call your pediatrician, who will examine your child and prescribe appropriate treatment. Rest may be advisable. |
| *Your school-aged child (5 to 10 years) has pain in her legs almost every night. She is otherwise well and without symptoms.* | Growing pains (nonspecific pains of unknown cause) | If the pains are worrying your child, discuss your concerns with your pediatrician. Your pediatrician may want to examine your child to rule out any serious causes of pain and will discuss ways to manage stress at school and home. |
| *Your child has a temperature higher than 101°F (38.3°C). He also has a runny nose, sore throat, and watery eyes.* | Viral infection | Make your child comfortable; give him cold drinks or chicken soup to soothe the sore throat and acetaminophen or ibuprofen to reduce fever and ease discomfort. If symptoms persist or get worse over the next 48 hours, or the temperature rises above 101°F (38.3°C), call your pediatrician. |
| *Your preteen or teen is limping since taking part in a highly active exercise or sports program. One or both of her shins are painful. You can feel a slight swelling over the tender area.* | Shin splints | Apply a cold compress to reduce pain and swelling; rest the limb until the pain is gone. Have your child resume exercise slowly over time and prevent further problems by conditioning. Begin and end exercise sessions with warm-ups and stretching. Acetaminophen or ibuprofen may be given for pain relief. |
| *Your child has pain and swelling in his joints. He also has fever or a rash.* | Infection that requires diagnosis and treatment<br>Juvenile idiopathic arthritis<br>Juvenile polyarthritis<br>Rheumatic fever<br>Lyme disease | Call your pediatrician, who will do an examination and laboratory tests for diagnosis and treatment (also see "Joint Pain, Joint Swelling," page 108). |
| *Your child has severe pain in one area. The surrounding skin is swollen, warm, and tender.* | Infection of bone (osteomyelitis), skin, or joint | Call your pediatrician, who will examine your child and perform diagnostic tests, including x-rays. If a bone infection is present, your pediatrician will advise consultation with another health specialist. |
| *Your child is complaining of frequent, severe leg pain. She is unusually pale and tired. She has swollen glands. She has an unusual number of bruises.* | In rare cases, a tumor, blood disorder, or other condition that requires diagnosis and treatment | Call your pediatrician, who will examine your child, perform appropriate diagnostic tests, and recommend any necessary treatment. |

## IN GENERAL

As babies discover the different parts of their bodies, they learn to associate particularly pleasurable feelings with touching their genitals. This isn't sexual activity; it's just a comforting sensation. Parents should neither discourage or call needless attention to a baby's normal curiosity. There will be time to teach your child about privacy and modesty later on.

Masturbation—stimulation of the genitals—is normal and, up to about 6 years of age, common among both boys and girls. From that age until puberty, self-stimulation may decline as children develop a greater social awareness and sense of modesty; nevertheless, masturbation remains a normal activity and usually continues in private. As hormones and sexual tensions surge during puberty, healthy preteens and teens may accept self-stimulation as an expression of their emerging sexuality.

Some parents find it difficult to accept the notion of masturbation, possibly because it implies an acknowledgment that children are sexual beings. Those who cling to now-dispelled myths may react with embarrassment and outrage. Parents who are aware of their child's masturbation should accept it as part of normal development. They may even recognize it as an opportunity for teaching their children about sexuality and the differences between public and private behavior.

### Talk with your pediatrician if your child

- Engages in compulsive masturbation every day, whether in private or in public
- Persists in public masturbation even after you've told him that such activity is acceptable only in private
- Masturbates and shows symptoms of emotional disturbance, such as bedwetting or fecal soiling, aggressiveness, destructive behavior, or social withdrawal
- Exhibits sexual activity or talk that's inappropriate f or his age

### WARNING!

At times excessive masturbation or a public display may be a sign that your child is under emotional strain, is overly preoccupied with sex, or isn't receiving the emotional comfort she needs. It may also signal that a child is being sexually abused. If you have any concerns, discuss them with your pediatrician.

### Signs of Inappropriate Stimulation

Children who are enlisted into sexual activity frequently become preoccupied with sexual matters. Their unusual behavior may be a cry for help, which is especially urgent when a sexual predator has sworn the child to secrecy. Television and the Internet are also sources of explicit sexual material. Although you may not allow such material in your own home, your child may have access to it at the homes of friends and schoolmates.

If you suspect sexual abuse, or you have concerns about certain people in your child's life, talk with your pediatrician. He or she will examine your child for signs of abuse and may be able to elicit information that your child is shy about discussing with those closer to him. If abuse has occurred, your pediatrician has a responsibility to report the abuse to the appropriate authorities.

| YOUR CONCERNS | POSSIBLE CAUSE | ACTION TO TAKE |
|---|---|---|
| *Your baby boy frequently has penile erections when you remove his diaper or when he's asleep.* | Normal response to pleasurable sensation<br>Full bladder | This is quite normal in a healthy little boy. |
| *Your baby or toddler reaches for her genitals when you change her diaper.* | Normal exploration and familiarization with her body | Young children find it comforting to feel their bodies. This activity will gradually grow less frequent as more independence enables your child to explore the world outside of her body. |
| *Your toddler or preschooler covers or rubs his crotch or exposes his genitals when he needs to urinate.* | Confusion about physical sensations and urges | Some young children are confused by the sensations they feel when their bladders are full or they need to defecate. Teach your child to tell you when he feels the urge so you can help him get to the potty-chair or bathroom in time. |
| *Your preschooler or school-aged child often rubs her genitals when others are around.* | Emotional tension | Try to eliminate the source of tension and reassure your child. Ask your pediatrician to examine your child to rule out any physical causes. When your child stimulates herself in public, suggest that she might be more comfortable on her own but can rejoin the family when she feels ready. |

## IN GENERAL

Not long ago, media meant television, movies, newspapers, magazines, and books. These days the term *media* refers to all of these forms of communication as well as computers, tablets, cell phones, DVDs, and, of course, everything on the Internet, from Web sites to social media to blogs. No doubt, media serve a useful purpose in communicating information and ideas, but too much time spent engaged in media—at the expense of physical, academic, and social pursuits—can affect your child's health.

The excessive use of media can impact your child's physical health because more often than not, media use doesn't involve physical activity and is instead a sedentary activity. Children who spend too much time on media are more likely to be overweight and to consume unhealthy foods that are often featured in advertisements. Overuse of media can also impact your child's emotional and mental well-being because of the exposure to violence and inappropriate images and videos. And because so many children now are using social media to connect, social media can affect your child's self-esteem and confidence if peers are using social media sites to bully your child, a form of torment aptly named *cyberbullying*. Media usage can also interfere with a good night's sleep.

The safe use of all media has become a major public health concern. Because media can influence how children think, feel, and behave, the American Academy of Pediatrics (AAP) encourages parents to help their children form healthy media use habits early on. Here is what the AAP recommends.

- Create a family media use plan. Limit screen time—texting, games, movies, and cell phones—to no more than 2 hours a day. Turn off the television when your child is doing homework. Turn off all media at bedtime, and keep TVs and Internet access outside of your child's bedroom. Carefully choose the movies and programs your child watches. If your child is younger than 2 years, it's best to discourage TV. Studies show that early exposure to TV may negatively affect development, including speech delay and higher risk for attention problems.

- Watch and use media with your child. Use it as a time to bond with your child, and look for teachable moments. Help your young child distinguish advertisements from TV shows. Make use of the TV Parental Ratings guidelines to help you determine which shows are appropriate for your child. Recognize that some reality shows, news programs, and movies are not suitable for children.

- Encourage your child to participate in other activities. Help your child cultivate hobbies such as art, music, and imaginative play. Get your child outdoors and involved in sports or activities that involve movement. Spend time reading with your child to encourage her love of reading and learning.

- Watch your own media habits. Be vigilant about how you use media in front of your child. Children learn from watching their parents, so make sure you're limiting your own screen time and engaged in other activities.

## Positive Ways to Use Technology

Using media appropriately, sparingly, and wisely is possible. The key is using media in ways that are appropriate and helpful, without allowing it to overtake your life. Watching movies and programs that you enjoy as a family is one way to enjoy family time. Many forms of media are also helpful for staying in touch when schedules get hectic. As your child gets older for instance, technology can be useful for checking in on the day's plans. It's also an easy way to communicate quick, simple messages (eg, "Can you pick me up at 5?"). Children are known for asking lots of good questions; you and your child can perform some online research on a topic together to learn more about a subject your child is interested in.

Never use technology to engage in an argument or to make an accusation. Save confrontations for in-person discussions.

| YOUR CONCERNS | POSSIBLE CAUSE | ACTION TO TAKE |
|---|---|---|
| Your child is more and more upset and withdrawn. He spends a lot of time on his cell phone texting. He may tell you that classmates are making fun of him on a social media site. | Cyberbullying or sexting | Ask to look at your child's cell phone, social media, and e-mail. Save all messages, texts, and postings. Talk with other parents about what's going on. Contact your school for guidance. If your child's safety is at risk, call the police. Talk with your pediatrician if your child starts experiencing other symptoms such as insomnia (see page 142), loss of appetite (see page 28), or depression (see page 182). |
| Your child acts out a lot of violence and seems to have more aggression than usual. She is having trouble sleeping and has frequent nightmares. | Overexposure to violent media | Set limits on your child's use of media. Remove televisions, computers, and gaming devices from her bedroom. Talk with your child about what concerns you in violent movies and games. Use the V-chip in your TV to block programs you find objectionable. |
| Your child is gaining weight. When he exercises, he's prone to injury. | Too much time on media | Limit the amount of time your child spends in front of a screen. Encourage him to get involved in physical activities. |

## IN GENERAL

Pain in the mouth is most often caused by infections, allergies, canker sores, or injury. Pain arising from the throat is often confused with mouth pain.

### Call your pediatrician if your child

- Is refusing to drink because of mouth pain
- Complains of mouth pain along with swelling of the lips or breathing difficulty
- Has a mouth ulcer that lasts longer than 1 week
- Has swelling on the gums, roof of the mouth, or lips

### WARNING!

If a child's mouth is sore he may be reluctant to drink. Encourage your child to drink enough to keep his tissues properly hydrated.

## Geographic Tongue

The normal tongue is a healthy pink, its upper surface covered with papillae—hair-like projections of tissue—encircled by taste buds. Sometimes parents are concerned to see that their child's tongue is covered with bright red patches with white borders forming a map-like pattern. These painless patches tend to fade and reappear in new sites on the tongue. This condition, known as *geographic tongue* or *benign migratory glossitis,* isn't serious. It doesn't require treatment. The exact cause is unknown, although the tendency seems to run in families.

| YOUR CONCERNS | POSSIBLE CAUSE | ACTION TO TAKE |
|---|---|---|
| *Your breastfed baby has developed small, ulcerated patches on the roof of her mouth.* | Sucking blisters | These minor, superficial ulcers aren't painful; they're caused by nipple pressure during breastfeeding and disappear after weaning. If they look inflamed, or your baby is refusing to nurse, talk with your pediatrician. |
| *Your baby is drooling a lot and keeping his fist in his mouth most of the time. He is between about 4 and 8 months of age.* | Normal behavior that occurs with teething | Give your baby a smooth teething ring or a pacifier, if he finds it comforting (see "Dental Problems," page 62). |
| *Your baby is hungry but unwilling to feed. She has whitish patches on her tongue and inside her cheeks. She has been taking an antibiotic.* | Oral thrush (yeast infection) | Call your pediatrician, who will examine your child to determine the cause of her discomfort and prescribe appropriate treatment. Yeast infections are fairly common in babies; in older children they may occur when antibiotic therapy upsets the normal flora of the mouth. |
| *Your school-age child is complaining of pain on swallowing due to a sore throat.* | Viral or streptococcal infection of the throat (strep throat) | Talk with your pediatrician, who will examine your child and prescribe appropriate treatment. |
| *Your child has painful ulcers on the inside of his lower lips, his cheeks, or his tongue.* | Aphthous ulcers (canker sores) | If these ulcers don't disappear in a week or recur repeatedly, talk with your pediatrician. The exact cause is unknown. |

| YOUR CONCERNS | POSSIBLE CAUSE | ACTION TO TAKE |
|---|---|---|
| *Your child has painful, yellowish spots in her mouth. The glands in her neck are swollen. She has a fever. There is a red, crusted fever blister or cold sore on your child's lip. Her gums are reddened, swollen, or painful. There are blisters on her tongue.* | Mouth infection caused by virus such as herpes or coxsackie | Talk with your pediatrician who will evaluate your child's general health and recommend methods to reduce discomfort, including a soothing mouthwash or a pain medication to apply to the sore area. Cold liquids may be comforting. |
| *Your child has dry, reddened lips. They are scaling and cracked in the corners of his mouth.* | Cheilitis (chapped lips) possibly caused by sensitivity to foods and worsened by alternate wetting and drying | Apply a bland lip salve or petroleum jelly, especially during cold weather. Don't apply lanolin-based salves, which may cause further problems with sensitivity. |
| *Your child has a sore on the end or side of her tongue or one sore spot on the inside of her cheek.* | Sore caused by chipped tooth Self-injury caused by biting (nervous habit) | If the sore is caused by a rough spot on a tooth or filling, talk with your child's dentist, who will examine your child's teeth and file off any sharp points. Ask your child if she's biting the insides of her cheek, and encourage her to stop the habit. |
| *Your child has sore patches on his tongue or inside his mouth. He is taking a prescription drug such as an anticonvulsant or an antibiotic.* | Medication side effect | Call your pediatrician, who will examine your child and adjust his medication if necessary. |

## IN GENERAL

The most frequent causes of muscle pain in children are the minor injuries incurred during sports and play. Children often have temporary aches and pains when they increase their athletic activity, begin a new sport that requires new movements, or play an old sport at a higher level. Children also experience growing pains during periods of normal growth (see "Limb/Leg Pain," page 112).

Some viral illnesses, especially influenza, can cause achy muscles and usually occur with fever, fatigue, and a feeling of being generally unwell. Emotional tension and anxiety may also take the form of muscle pain in the neck and shoulders, particularly in teenaged girls. A child who has tight, painful muscles due to stress must learn to unwind. Exercise is among the best ways to relieve muscle pain because it promotes the release of endorphins, our body's natural painkillers and mood elevators. Children who are physically active may have a few bumps and scrapes, but they're much less likely to have nagging stress-related pain than their more sedentary friends.

Even children with chronic illnesses can keep fit and have fun with physical activity. A child with a disability should be encouraged to become as active as possible without taking unnecessary risks. Your pediatrician can advise you about suitable sports.

In rarer cases muscle aches can be a first sign of muscle inflammation, called *myositis;* bone infection, called *osteomyelitis;* or a joint infection, called *septic arthritis.* If your child's symptoms persist and worsen, see your pediatrician as soon as possible.

**Talk with your pediatrician if your child's muscle pain occurs along with**

- An inability to move the affected area
- A persistent (won't go away) swelling or lump

**WARNING!**

Use ice—never heat—to treat new muscle injuries. Heat increases the blood flow to the injured area, in turn increasing hemorrhage and worsening inflammation.

## RICE Treatment for Muscle Injuries

If your child strains a muscle or injures a limb, apply the following RICE treatment to minimize swelling (Figures 2-13 and 2-14). Don't use any other treatment, including pain relievers, until a doctor has examined your child and diagnosed the injury. If your child is injured while playing a sport, keep him from putting weight on the injured limb as you help him off the playing field.

1. **R**est: Stop the activity and rest the injured part.
2. **I**ce: Place an ice bag (a package of frozen vegetables from the freezer will do) wrapped in a towel over the injured area. If your child is younger than 2 years, use a cloth wrung out in cold water; excessive cold can damage delicate tissues in young children. Don't apply ice directly to the skin and don't leave the wrapped ice bag on the skin for longer than 20 minutes or apply it more often than every 2 hours; excessive exposure to cold can damage tissues.
3. **C**ompression: Remove clothing from the injured spot. An elastic bandage may be helpful to prevent swelling and promote healing; however, it's very important to make sure the bandage isn't too tight. An overly tight bandage can cut off circulation.
4. **E**levation: Raise the injured arm or leg higher than the level of the child's heart, and keep it elevated until the pain and swelling begin to go down.

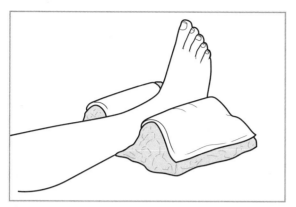

**Figure 2-13.** Rest and ice. Place an ice bag over the injured area. Protect the child's skin with a towel.

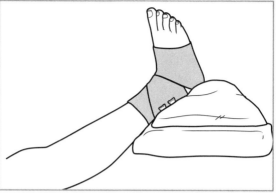

**Figure 2-14.** Compression and elevation. Keep the injured limb elevated until the pain and swelling begin to go down.

| YOUR CONCERNS | POSSIBLE CAUSE | ACTION TO TAKE |
|---|---|---|
| *Your child is complaining of sharp, cramping pain in her calf or thigh. The muscle feels hard and tense. She either had an unusually active day or was confined in one position (such as in a car) for a long period.* | Muscle cramp due to fatigue or reduced circulation | Rub the area to increase circulation. If the pain doesn't improve after an hour, or your child has frequent muscle cramps, talk with your pediatrician. |
| *The pain began suddenly during sports or strenuous activity. The area is slightly swollen.* | Muscle strain | Have your child rest, and apply the RICE treatment (see page 120). If the pain and swelling get worse, call your pediatrician. Encourage your child to begin and end activity sessions with warm-up exercises and stretching to help prevent strains. |
| *Your child had severe pain following an injury, such as twisting an ankle or falling on a wrist. The area is rapidly swelling.* | Sprain (torn ligament) Fracture | Call your pediatrician. |
| *In addition to aching muscles, your child has a fever, runny nose, sore throat, or cough.* | Influenza or another viral infection | If your child's temperature is 101°F (38.3°C) or higher, call your pediatrician; otherwise, encourage your child to rest and give him acetaminophen or ibuprofen to relieve muscle aches and reduce fever. Make sure drinks are available to replace lost fluids. |
| *Your child is complaining of pain and stiffness in her shoulders, upper arms, and neck. She is otherwise healthy. She could be under unusual stress because of events at home or school.* | Emotional tension Functional pain | Try to identify sources of stress and deal with them. Encourage your child to exercise regularly. If pain and tensions persist, discuss your concerns with your pediatrician. |
| *Your child has a persistent (won't go away) lump in a muscle.* | Tumor (rare) | Talk with your pediatrician, who will examine your child and perform diagnostic tests. |

## IN GENERAL

Even slight damage to the delicate mucous membrane lining of the nose can rupture tiny blood vessels and cause bleeding. Babies rarely have nosebleeds, but toddlers and school-aged children often do. Fortunately, most children outgrow this common but rarely serious event by the time they are teens. A tendency for nosebleeds often runs in the family. Many children have nosebleeds for no apparent reason.

A nosebleed usually comes on suddenly, with blood flowing freely from one nostril. A child who has nosebleeds at night may swallow the blood in his sleep. He will vomit it up or pass it in his stools later. Most nosebleeds stop by themselves within a few minutes. For persistent (won't go away) bleeding, see "Stopping a Nosebleed."

Nosebleeds are unlikely to signal serious illness, although bleeding can result from injury. Children may cause bleeding by picking their noses; toddlers often injure the nasal membranes by forcing objects into their nostrils. Children are especially prone to nosebleeds during colds and in the winter months when the mucous membranes become dry, cracked, and crusted or when a chronic condition such as allergic rhinitis damages the membrane.

A child with a chronic illness that causes forceful coughing, such as cystic fibrosis, may have frequent nosebleeds. And parents of children with clotting disorders such as hemophilia or von Willebrand disease, should be vigilant about harmful habits such as nose-picking. If your child's nosebleeds last for longer than 8 to 10 minutes routinely, your pediatrician may wish to test for a blood clotting disorder.

### Call your pediatrician right away if

- Your child is pale, sweaty, or not responding to you.
- You believe your child has lost a lot of blood.
- Your child is bleeding from the mouth or vomiting blood or brown material that looks like coffee grounds.
- Your child's nose is bleeding after a blow or injury to any part of the head.

### WARNING!

Consult your pediatrician before giving your child medicated nose drops or nasal sprays to treat problems that affect the nose and respiratory passages. Although sold over-the-counter for the relief of congestion, some medications may actually increase congestion after a few days' use. This increased congestion is known as the *rebound effect,* and can be even more uncomfortable and difficult to treat than the original problem. For a natural nose spray, try using a saline, salt water spray.

## Stopping a Nosebleed

- Stay calm; the nosebleed is probably not serious, and you should try not to upset your child. Your child will pick up on your emotional cues.
- Keep your child sitting or standing and leaning slightly forward. Don't let him lie down or lean back because this will allow blood to flow down his throat and might make him vomit.
- Don't stuff tissues or another material into the nose to stop the bleeding.
- Firmly pinch the soft part of your child's nose—using a cold compress if you have one, otherwise your fingers—and keep the pressure on for a full 10 minutes. Don't look to see if your child's nose is bleeding during this time; you may start the flow again.
- If bleeding hasn't stopped after 10 minutes, repeat the pressure. If bleeding persists after your second try, call your pediatrician or take your child to the nearest emergency department.
- While most nosebleeds are benign and self-limited, a child with severe or recurrent bleeding or bleeding from both nostrils should be evaluated by a pediatrician. If necessary, your child will be referred to an ear-nose-throat specialist.

| YOUR CONCERNS | POSSIBLE CAUSE | ACTION TO TAKE |
|---|---|---|
| Your child has a runny nose due to a cold or allergic rhinitis (hay fever). She has allergies. | Swelling and irritation of the nasal tissue | To stop bleeding, pinch the soft part of your child's nose. Use of a cool mist humidifier in your child's bedroom at night may help relieve stuffiness and keep the membranes moist. Don't add medications or aromatic preparations to the humidifier. If your child has not been evaluated for allergies, talk with your pediatrician. |
| You live in a very dry climate. Your house is overheated. The winter air is very dry. | Drying of nasal mucous membranes | Try a cool mist humidifier in your child's room at night. Saline nose drops may help keep tissues moist. If bleeding is severe or recurrent, talk with your pediatrician. |
| Your child had a fall or a bump on the nose. He picks his nose. He blows his nose very hard. | Trauma (injury) to the nose | Follow the steps in "Stopping a Nosebleed," page 122. If bleeding doesn't stop after two 10-minute attempts, or if your child had a severe blow to the head, call your pediatrician at once. |
| Your child has frequent, fairly severe nosebleeds for no apparent reason. | Abnormal formation of blood vessels in the nose. Polyps or another growth in the nose. Bleeding problem (See "Bleeding and Bruising," page 42.) | Talk with your pediatrician, who will examine your child and provide a referral, if advisable, to an ear-nose-throat specialist. |
| Your child is taking medication, whether a doctor's prescription or an over-the-counter product such as medicated nose drops or nasal spray. | Side effect of the medication | Stop any over-the-counter medication. Call your pediatrician, who will prescribe an alternative treatment, if necessary. |
| Your child was once diagnosed with a blood-clotting disorder. | Abnormal blood clotting. Bleeding following self-injury such as nose-picking or scab-picking. | Explain how self-injury is causing nosebleeds, and urge your child to stop. Seek your pediatrician's advice about different approaches. |
| Your child has a chronic illness that causes forceful coughing. She needs medications or extra oxygen for a chronic illness. | Pressure injury due to forceful coughing. Effect of medications on nasal mucous membrane | Talk with your pediatrician, who will recommend measures to keep the nasal tissues moist and prevent nosebleeds. |

## IN GENERAL

A naturally fair child may look paler during the winter months when there are few opportunities to play outdoors. Some children will look paler if they have fatigue or dark blotches under the eyes because of allergies, called *allergic shiners*.

If your child looks unusually pale, your pediatrician will examine her nail beds, her lips, the creases of her palms, and inside her lower eyelids. As long as these areas are rosy pink and there's no weakness or unusual fatigue, your child is probably quite healthy.

> ## WARNING!
> A child with mild anemia usually has pale-to-normal skin color and few symptoms. When anemia is advanced, the child is pale, irritable, and lacking in energy. The symptoms may develop so slowly over time, however, that parents have difficulty recognizing them.

### Talk with your pediatrician if your child looks unusually pale and also

- Has bruising in places that don't usually get injured
- Has swellings in his neck or abdomen
- Feels weak and extremely tired all the time
- Has prolonged bleeding, including nosebleeds lasting more than 10 minutes or menstrual periods lasting more than 7 days

## Managing Anemia

Blood contains several different types of cells. The most numerous are red blood cells, which absorb oxygen in the lungs and distribute it throughout the body. These cells contain hemoglobin, a red pigment that carries oxygen to the tissues and carries away carbon dioxide, which is the waste material. When the amount of hemoglobin is decreased, you'll experience a condition called *anemia*. People who have anemia can't get oxygen to their body cells. Anemia may occur when the production of red blood cells slows, too many red blood cells are destroyed, there isn't enough hemoglobin within the red blood cells, or red blood cells are lost from the body.

Children are most likely to become anemic because they fail to get enough iron in their diet. Iron is a mineral essential to the production of hemoglobin. Young babies get iron-deficiency anemia if they start on cow's milk too early without taking an iron supplement. Cow's milk contains very little iron, and the small amount is poorly absorbed through the intestines into the body. In infants younger than 12 months, the cow's milk can irritate the bowel and cause a decrease in red blood cells.

Children can also develop anemia from blood loss. In rare cases it may be due a clotting problem, especially in young babies who lack vitamin K. Sometimes the red cells are prone to being destroyed, a condition called *hemolytic anemia*, which results from disturbances on the surface of the red cells or other abnormalities. Some children develop anemia from inherited conditions such as sickle cell anemia or thalassemias, or an enzyme deficiency.

Because there are so many kinds of anemia, it's important to first identify the cause of your child's anemia. If it's due to a lack of iron, your child will be given a medication that contains iron. Don't give the medication with milk because milk blocks iron absorption. Follow the medication with a glass of orange juice, which contains vitamin C, a vitamin that helps iron absorption. Be sure to brush your child's teeth after every dose because liquid iron can turn the teeth a grayish black color. Know that iron can also turn the stools black, which is normal. To prevent iron deficiency, make sure you give your breastfed baby an iron supplement, and feed him iron-fortified foods when you introduce solid foods. If your baby is formula-fed or partially breastfed, give him formula with added iron (4-12 mg of iron per liter), beginning at birth and through age 12 months. Make sure your older child eats foods that contain iron such as fortified grains and cereals, egg yolks, green and yellow vegetables, yellow fruits, red meat, potatoes, tomatoes, and raisins.

| YOUR CONCERNS | POSSIBLE CAUSE | ACTION TO TAKE |
|---|---|---|
| *Your child is pale but active and healthy. She is eating and sleeping well.* | Normal fair complexion | Your child is naturally fair. Pay special attention to sun protection when she plays outdoors. |
| *Your child between 8 months and 2 years is pale, fretful, and lethargic (lacking energy).* | Anemia of infancy iron-deficiency anemia | Your pediatrician will examine your child and may order blood tests. If your child is anemic, your pediatrician will review your child's diet and, if necessary, prescribe extra iron. |
| *Your child has dark blotches under his lower eyelids. He has had several late nights or unusual activity. He is otherwise healthy.* | Tiredness Allergies | If your child is overtired, make sure he gets enough rest to make up for daytime activities. If he also has a stuffy nose or other symptoms of allergies (see "Allergic Reactions," page 26), ask your pediatrician for advice. |
| *Your child recently had a viral infection. She has been taking a prescribed medication, such as an antibiotic.* | Temporary, normal decrease in red blood cell production following acute (sudden and severe) illness | Your pediatrician will examine your child, order blood tests, and—if the diagnosis is confirmed—provide a treatment plan. |
| *Your child has been diagnosed with an autoimmune disease or other chronic illness. She has digestive problems.* | Autoimmune hemolytic anemia Anemia secondary to a chronic illness | Talk with your pediatrician, who may order blood tests and, if necessary, prescribe treatment, including iron supplements. |
| *Your child has unexplained bruising. He is sometimes feverish.* | Leukemia (a type of blood cancer) Tumor | Your pediatrician will examine your child and order necessary diagnostic tests. |
| *Your infant is about 6 months of age. Her hands or abdomen are swollen. She seems fretful and in pain. Her family heritage is from Africa.* | Sickle cell anemia | Call your pediatrician, who will examine your infant, perform blood tests, and, if appropriate, prescribe treatment. |
| *Your infant is between 6 and 12 months of age. He is fretful and is losing or unable to gain weight. Your infant's family has ancestors in Asia, Africa, the Middle East, Greece, or Italy.* | Thalassemia (an inherited blood condition that mainly affects people from the Mediterranean) | Call your pediatrician, who will examine your infant, order blood tests, and prescribe any necessary treatment. |
| *Your toddler or preschooler often eats nonfood items such as paint chips. She seems less advanced than other children her age. She often has stomachaches and vomiting.* | Lead poisoning | Talk with your pediatrician promptly for treatment as well as advice on getting rid of lead in your home and environment. |

## IN GENERAL

As a developing baby approaches delivery, his spine begins to straighten out from its original C-curve in preparation for the changes in posture and movement that will highlight the first few years of life. After birth, the neck (cervical spine) curves forward, readying itself to support the head. At the same time, the chest (thoracic spine) curves backward, and there is a corresponding inward curve of the lower spine. This graceful curvature protects the spine from undue stress. Changes in posture can alter the natural curve and place stress on the vertebrae (the interlocking bones of the spine).

To find the balance needed for walking, a toddler curves his lower back inwards while, at the same time, pushing his belly and buttocks out in the typical, potbellied, 2-year-old stance. As the body matures, posture becomes more erect until, at maturity in the late teens, the spine is properly curved and a young adult is standing tall. At regular checkups, your pediatrician evaluates your child's spine, shoulders, and hips, along with his gait and stance, for symmetry and balance and makes careful note of any abnormal curves. If your pediatrician detects any abnormalities, she will determine the cause and provide any necessary treatment.

**Talk with your pediatrician if your child has a change in posture together with**

- Persistent or increasing back pain
- Fever, weight loss, and feeling generally unwell
- Weakness in the legs or limping
- Persistent vomiting
- Evidence of a curved spine, such as one shoulder or hip consistently higher than the other
- Torticollis, or tilted head, of infancy

## WARNING!

Conditions that interfere with good posture should always be brought to the attention of your pediatrician. While some require treatment, others eventually correct themselves. When your pediatrician recognizes that a disorder will clear up without treatment, the best course is careful observation with no intervention. In the meantime, parents and child must be patient.

## Good Posture Now May Prevent Back Problems Later

Habits of poor posture in children become exaggerated in self-conscious preteens and teens: slouching, slumping, head down, and shoulders rounded. Boys may slouch because they don't want to stand out from the crowd, and girls stoop because they are afraid of appearing taller than their friends, especially boys. Poor posture starts around the time of breast development in many girls; some are embarrassed because their breasts are growing, others because they're not.

Encourage your child to practice good posture. Whether sitting, standing, or exercising, the body should be straight but relaxed, with head level, shoulders down and back, and abdomen and buttocks tucked in.

| YOUR CONCERNS | POSSIBLE CAUSE | ACTION TO TAKE |
|---|---|---|
| Your child usually slouches, keeping his shoulders rounded and his chest sunken. He is otherwise healthy with no complaints of pain. | Postural kyphosis (round back) caused by habitual poor posture | Encourage your school-aged child to correct his posture to avoid problems later on. If kyphosis persists, talk with your pediatrician, who will examine your child to rule out serious problems. |
| Your child keeps her shoulders hunched. She has back pain. She is unable to straighten up. | Idiopathic kyphosis Scheuermann disease | Talk with your pediatrician, who will examine your child and provide a referral to another specialist. Treatment usually involves exercises and braces; surgery is rarely required for this relatively common condition. |
| Your toddler seems to be slow in walking. His legs seem weak. He is unusually clumsy. His belly is particularly prominent, while his spine curves backward. | Neuromuscular condition Metabolic disorder Bone disease requiring investigation and treatment | Talk with your pediatrician, who will evaluate your toddler and determine the appropriate management. |
| Your baby is holding his head to one side with his chin up. When lying on his stomach, he always sleeps with the same side of his face toward the mattress. His head movement is limited. He recently had an upper respiratory infection. | Wryneck (torticollis); in older children, possibly linked to a viral illness such as an upper respiratory infection or sore throat | Talk with your pediatrician, who will examine your baby and order x-rays. Your pediatrician may recommend special exercises, position changes, or, rarely, surgery. |
| Your child seems to be holding one shoulder higher than the other. His hips are uneven. His spine appears curved when he bends over. | Curvature of the spine (scoliosis) Asymmetry Unequal leg length | Talk with your pediatrician, who may refer your child to a pediatric orthopedist. (Also see "Back Pain," page 34.) |
| Your child is walking with difficulty. She has pain or stiffness in her lower back and hips. Her joints are painful. | Inflammatory disorder such as juvenile idiopathic arthritis or other condition requiring diagnosis and treatment | Call your pediatrician, who will examine your child and determine whether referral to another specialist is advisable. |

## IN GENERAL

Frequent causes of rectal discomfort in children include constipation, poor hygiene, and pinworms. Pain associated with bowel movements may lead to constipation and an anal fissure, a painful tear in the mucous membranes lining the anus, which often leads to more constipation because of stool holding and pain. To many children, itching caused by pinworms, which is usually most intense at night, is just as distressing as the pain associated with constipation or anal fissure. Scratching the itch site further irritates the skin and increases the risk of infection. Streptococcal infection can cause dermatitis with redness and intense discomfort around the anus.

Serious causes of rectal pain are uncommon in children, as are hemorrhoids. Though they are common, uncomfortable, and less serious in adults, hemorrhoids may be a symptom of a more serious disease in children.

Be sure to watch for to any bruising near the anus. It raises the disturbing possibility that your child has been sexually abused, especially if your child is reluctant to give a reason for the bruising and discomfort.

### Talk with your pediatrician if your child has

- Rectal pain and bleeding
- Severe constipation and rectal discomfort
- Hemorrhoids
- Itching that is more intense at night
- A sore, red rash around the anus
- Bruising near the anus

### WARNING!

An anal fissure won't heal unless measures are taken to soften hard stools that can tear the anus. The healing process may take weeks. It may require help from your pediatrician to retrain your child so that she stops withholding stool and learns to respond to the urge to defecate.

## Managing Pinworms

Pinworms are found everywhere, at every age and economic level. Especially common in children, they are easily transmitted from one child to another in child care and schools. The infection is annoying but harmless, although pinworms may carry fecal bacteria to the female genital tract and cause vulvovaginitis (see page 164).

Children ingest pinworm eggs carried under fingernails, on clothing or bedding, or in house dust. The eggs hatch in the stomach and the larvae migrate to the intestine, where they mature into white worms about 1 centimeter long. At night, female worms deposit eggs near the child's anus. The child scratches the itching this causes and traps more eggs under her fingernails—only to ingest them again or shed them where they will find their way to new hosts.

If your child has itching, is unusually fidgety, or has trouble getting to sleep, press adhesive tape to the skin around the anus in the morning, then remove it. Show the tape to your pediatrician; adhering eggs and worms will confirm the diagnosis.

Pinworms can be eradicated with a short course of medication. Because reinfestation is common, the treatment may need to be repeated at intervals. Wash bedding and clothing in hot water to get rid of eggs and prevent pinworms from spreading.

| YOUR CONCERNS | POSSIBLE CAUSE | ACTION TO TAKE |
|---|---|---|
| Your child has pain when he moves his bowels and for several minutes afterward. There is fresh blood on the toilet paper, on the stool, or in the toilet bowl. | Anal fissure | Talk with your pediatrician, who can diagnose an anal fissure by examining the anus. Most anal fissures occur during passage of hard stools (see "Constipation," page 54). Treatment may involve stool softeners to break the cycle of hardened stools, laceration, and stool withholding, and local cream to protect the skin. |
| Your infant or preschooler has a sore, red rash around the anus. | Perianal dermatitis caused by streptococcal infection | Call your pediatrician, who will examine your child and, if necessary, prescribe an antibiotic. Clean the child's anus with plain water after bowel movements and apply petroleum jelly, zinc oxide ointment, or a similar barrier cream to protect the skin. |
| Your child uses wet wipes after using the toilet and has irritation of the skin around the anus. | Overuse of wet wipes | Even wipes labeled "for sensitive skin" can cause irritation. Minimize the use of wet wipes and encourage plain water baths on a regular basis to help promote good skin hygiene and health. |
| Your child fidgets and scratches her anus. The itching is worse at night. There are white, threadlike worms less than an inch long moving in her stools. | Pinworms (See "Managing pinworms," page 128.) | Talk with your pediatrician, who will examine your child to confirm the diagnosis and prescribe appropriate treatment. Ask whether other family members should also be treated to prevent the spread of infection. |
| Your child is having painless bleeding from the anus. She seems healthy and active otherwise. | Inflammatory polyps Meckel diverticulum, a saclike pouch in the small intestine (ileum) | Talk with your pediatrician, who will examine your child to determine whether the bleeding is due to polyps and should be referred to another specialist. |
| Your child's rectum protrudes through the anus and stays outside after a bowel movement. He was straining on the toilet. He has previously been diagnosed with a chronic condition such as cystic fibrosis. | Rectal prolapse (procidentia) | If your child isn't in pain, cover your finger with toilet tissue and push the rectum back into its proper position. (Pieces of toilet tissue that stick will pass out with a bowel movement.) If your child finds it hard not to strain, suggest that he keep his feet on a low footstool while seated on the toilet. Stool softeners might help. Talk with your pediatrician if you can't replace the rectum, if it happens frequently, or if it's tender or bleeding. |
| Your toddler or preschooler is walking oddly and showing signs of rectal pain. She resists suggestions that she use the potty or bathroom. You see something in the rectum. | Foreign object in rectum (your child's natural curiosity) | Call your pediatrician, who will examine your child and identify the foreign object. A small object can sometimes be left to pass on its own; if it's large, sharp, or otherwise dangerous, your pediatrician will refer you to another specialist right away. |
| Your child has pain and a sore, red swelling or "pimple" near the anus. | Perianal abscess or fistula Crohn disease | Talk with your pediatrician, who will examine your child to determine whether treatment is necessary. |

## IN GENERAL

Head banging and rocking are quite common among normal children and are also seen in those with developmental problems. In normal children, repetitive head banging and rocking, while alarming to parents, are harmless and gradually stop over a period of months. If they continue, your child should be evaluated by your pediatrician. Head banging can occur during a temper tantrum (see page 156) as well.

Some experts theorize that the actions begin as normal behavior and are part of an infant's efforts to master movement as he gradually gains control of his body. Thus, an infant who starts head rocking as early as 4 or 5 months may be rocking his whole body at 6 to 10 months as he develops more skills.

Nobody knows why children bang their heads and rock, but it's interesting that these rhythmic habits—body rocking, head banging, and head rolling—all stimulate the vestibular system of the inner ear, which controls balance. They aren't usually associated with developmental delay, although children who have certain types of disabilities often repeat movements, as do children with autism spectrum disorders and others with oversensitive nervous systems.

Children usually outgrow rocking, rolling, and head banging between 18 months and 2 years of age, but repetitive actions are sometimes still seen in older children, preteens, and teens.

**Talk with your pediatrician if your child is frequently nodding or shaking her head and**

- Doesn't interact with you
- Has developmental delays

**WARNING!**
Children are rarely, if ever, harmed by this behavior, but if you're concerned that your child may injure himself or the behavior isn't diminishing over months, talk with your pediatrician.

## Coping With Head Banging

Rhythmic, repetitive motions at bedtime are a common early childhood behavior that seems to calm babies and toddlers even as it mystifies their parents. It's hard to understand how an infant or young child could derive comfort from rocking back and forth, knocking his head into the railings of his crib, or banging his head into the mattress. Nevertheless, a small percentage of infants and young children sooth themselves this way for 15 minutes or longer while preparing for sleep. Children usually outgrow rocking, rolling, and head banging between 18 months and 3 years of age. While distressing for parents, it's generally harmless, though your child may experience a minor bump, bruise, or callus. If the activity continues, becomes more intense, or occurs in the daytime, ask your pediatrician for an evaluation.

Pull the crib away from the wall and place it on a thick rug. Fit rubber or plastic carpet protectors on the legs of the crib to lessen noise and make it harder for your baby to move the crib as he rocks. Some pediatricians suggest using a metronome or playing music with a strong beat to regulate the head banging.

Place a mobile over the crib to divert your baby with different shapes and bright colors. A mobile with a built-in music box that plays a repetitive tune can be soothing for a baby trying to fall asleep. Watch your baby's reaction to mobiles; however, some babies find them frightening and cry until they are removed. In any case, mobiles must be removed when babies are making serious attempts to sit, get up on all fours, or pull themselves to a standing position. Music playing softly in the room may put your baby in the mood for sleep.

| YOUR CONCERNS | POSSIBLE CAUSE | ACTION TO TAKE |
|---|---|---|
| Your baby of about 6 months rocks vigorously in his crib for up to 15 minutes at a time, or even longer. This activity often occurs when he's left alone to fall asleep or listen to music. Your baby rocks when he's tired. | Body rocking as part of a baby's normal development | Body rocking is harmless and seems to comfort your infant. It will gradually stop as your baby becomes more mobile and is usually gone by the age of 2 or 3 years, although some form of body movement may last through adolescence. |
| Your child bangs his head hard and often—as many as 60 to 80 times a minute—against solid objects such as his crib. The head banging follows a head-rolling or body-rocking phase. Your child also sucks his thumb or rubs a blanket as he bangs his head. | Head banging | This inexplicable behavior seems to comfort the child. Your child is getting comfort from this activity, even it distresses you. In fact, it probably doesn't seem to worry your baby (most often a boy), who often looks relaxed and happy while banging his head. It usually starts at about 6 months and stops around 2 years of age. |
| Your baby has made a bald spot on her head with her constant head rolling or shaking. She is otherwise active and happy. Her eyes move normally. | Head rolling or rubbing | This harmless habit may also appear in a child who can sit up. It may start as early as 6 months and usually disappears before the child reaches 2 years of age. |
| Your child, who is developmentally disabled, bangs her head or performs other rhythmic actions. You're concerned that she may injure herself. | Developmental disorder or behavior typical of an autism spectrum disorder | Talk with your pediatrician, who may prescribe a short-term medication to calm your child and recommend a helmet to protect her head. |

## IN GENERAL

A runny or stuffy nose usually clears up in a few days without any treatment. The most common cause is an upper respiratory viral infection such as a common cold (rhinovirus) or, in winter, flu (influenza). When a runny nose is accompanied or followed by other symptoms, your child may have a more serious problem. In such cases, you should talk with your pediatrician.

## Treating Sinusitis

The sinuses are air spaces in the bones above and adjacent to the nose (Figure 2-15). Each of the 8 sinuses is lined with mucous membranes that drain into the nose.

An acute sinus infection is usually set off by a cold, influenza, or hay fever. If the sinus membranes become inflamed, swollen, and possibly infected, your child may complain of a headache, stuffy nose, and perhaps tenderness around the eyes or other parts of the face. Nasal discharge is likely to become unusually thick and tinged with green or yellow. Your child also may have a fever and will probably act sicker than he does when he has an ordinary cold.

Treatment depends on the underlying cause. Antibiotics may be prescribed to clear up a bacterial sinus infection. Taking a steamy shower, placing a misting humidifier in your child's bedroom, or using a saline nasal spray may help to drain blocked sinuses. Ask your pediatrician for advice on the best approach for your child.

**Call your pediatrician if your child's runny or stuffy nose is accompanied by**

- Unusual sleepiness or lethargy
- Difficulty breathing
- A temperature above 100.4°F (38°C) in an infant younger than 3 months and above 101°F (38.3°C) in an infant older than 3 months
- Neck pain or stiffness
- An earache or sore throat
- Swollen glands
- Eye redness or swelling
- A rash

### WARNING!

Don't treat your child's stuffy nose with nonprescription nasal sprays unless your pediatrician gives the go-ahead. These medications may provide temporary relief, but there is sometimes a rebound effect that can worsen the problem. A better option is over-the-counter nasal saline rinse or spray.

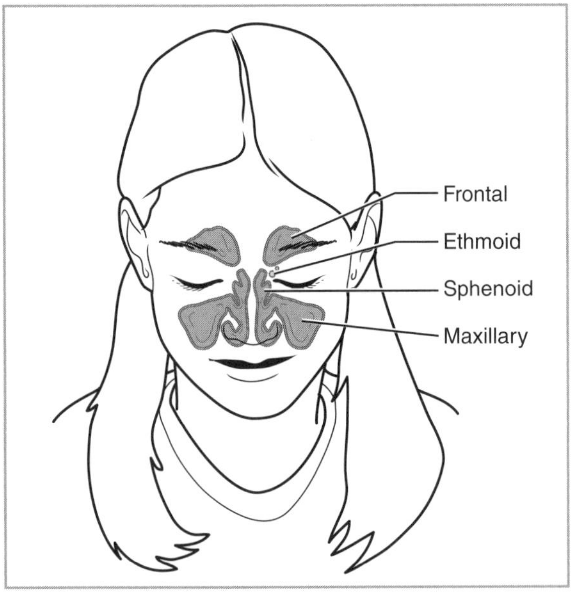

Frontal

Ethmoid

Sphenoid

Maxillary

**Figure 2-15.** The size and shape of sinuses vary from one person to another, but this illustration shows a typical conformation. The frontal sinuses, which develop at about age 8, are situated in the forehead and are a frequent cause of sinus headaches. The maxillary (upper jaw) sinuses, located to the side of the nostril, are the largest. The sphenoid sinuses are more toward the center of the head; the ethmoid sinuses are made up of many air pockets on each side of the nose.

| YOUR CONCERNS | POSSIBLE CAUSE | ACTION TO TAKE |
|---|---|---|
| Your child's main symptom is a clear, watery discharge. Your child is active as usual with little or no fever. | Common cold | You may want to keep your child at home for a day or two, but no special action or medication is needed. A cold will run its course in about a week. |
| Your child also has an earache. She is fussy and irritable. | An ear infection | Ask your pediatrician to examine your child and confirm the diagnosis. If it persists, an antibiotic may be needed. (See "Earache, Ear Infection," page 76.) |
| Your child also has a sore throat. The throat symptoms are severe. | Most likely a cold, but other infections such as strep throat should be ruled out. | See your pediatrician, who will examine your child and may order a throat culture. If strep throat is diagnosed, an antibiotic will be prescribed. (See "Sore Throat," page 144.) |
| Your child is feverish and unusually sleepy or lethargic. | Complications of an upper respiratory infection | Talk with your pediatrician, who will examine your child and recommend treatment. |
| Your child's neck and glands are swollen and tender. | An infection, which may be viral or bacterial | See your pediatrician, who will want to examine your child and may recommend treatment. |
| Your child's nose has been runny for more than a week, or it recurs periodically. Her nose is itchy and her eyes are red, itchy, or watery. | Hay fever (allergic rhinitis) or another allergic response | Talk with your pediatrician, who may want to test for specific allergies. (See "Allergic Reactions," page 26.) |
| Your child's nose has a discharge that has lasted more than 10 days. It has gotten thicker or changed in color. He has a headache. | Sinus infection | See your pediatrician to confirm the diagnosis. Your pediatrician will prescribe appropriate treatment (see "Treating Sinusitis," page 132). |
| Your child's nose has a foul-smelling discharge coming from one nostril. | Foreign object in the nostril | Talk with your pediatrician, who will examine your child and, if necessary, remove the object. |
| Your child has trouble breathing. She snores and wakes up frequently. | Enlarged tonsils and adenoid | Ask your pediatrician to examine your child and, if necessary, perform diagnostic tests. |
| Your child had a recent fall or facial injury. | Nose injury (eg, deviated septum) or other structural problem | Call your pediatrician for tests and x-rays, if necessary. |

## IN GENERAL

A convulsion or seizure is an episode of abnormal electric discharges in the brain. A few children have convulsions when their temperature rises rapidly. Most outgrow these benign febrile seizures and suffer no long-term effects; indeed, most who have one febrile seizure never have another. Because serious infections may also cause seizures, however, call your pediatrician when a feverish child has a seizure.

Recurrent seizures are known as epilepsy. The cause isn't always clear and children must be evaluated. Epilepsy can generally be controlled with medication, and there are certain epileptic syndromes (eg, simple absences, petit mal) that children outgrow.

### Call your pediatrician right away if a convulsing child

- Remains unconscious for more than 2 minutes
- Has difficulty breathing

### WARNING!

If your child has epilepsy, explain first aid measures to teachers and caregivers. Ask your pediatrician about precautions for potentially dangerous activities. A child with epilepsy should not be left unsupervised in a bath or swimming pool, no matter how old he is.

## Conditions That Resemble Seizures

Several conditions may be mistaken for convulsions because they involve jerking movements and alterations in consciousness. They include night terrors (see "Fears," page 84) and breath-holding spells (see "Bluish Skin," page 44). Children with asthma sometimes have paroxysmal coughing that causes fainting spells resembling seizures. Your pediatrician will differentiate these conditions from seizures.

| YOUR CONCERNS | POSSIBLE CAUSE | ACTION TO TAKE |
|---|---|---|
| *Your child is twitching, unconscious, and feverish. He is irritable and unwell.* | Febrile convulsion associated with an infectious disease | Your pediatrician will want to diagnose and treat the cause of the fever. It is also important to make sure that a more serious condition such as meningitis isn't responsible. |
| *Your child "switches off"—stops speaking or hearing—for several seconds at a time. She is unaware of the incident.* | Absence seizures (petit mal) | Your pediatrician will perform tests and may refer your child to a neurologist. Petit mal seizures can often be controlled with medication, and children will often outgrow the milder forms of this epilepsy. |
| *Your child loses consciousness for a minute or longer. She twitches. She loses control of her bladder, bites her tongue, or vomits.* | Generalized seizure (grand mal epilepsy) Some partial (focal) seizures | Your pediatrician will examine your child, order diagnostic tests, and provide a referral to a neurologist if advisable. Many but not all cases of epilepsy can be controlled reasonably well with medication. |
| *Your infant of 6 months or older has repeated symmetric flexion contractions of the neck, trunk, and limbs when drowsy.* | Infantile spasms | Talk with your pediatrician, who will examine your baby and may refer him for a neurologic evaluation or testing. |
| *Your child has a seizure while on anticonvulsant medication.* | Need to adjust dosage | Your pediatrician will order tests and possibly change the medication. |

## IN GENERAL

Despite its rigid, rocklike appearance, bone is in a state of constant change, renewing and remodeling based on the nutrients available and the load it bears. This process of renewal and remodeling continues throughout life.

Between birth and age 4 years, your child's skeleton doubles in size from an average length of 20" to about 40". Bone growth continues at a steady but somewhat slower rate until puberty, when a gain of 4" in a single year isn't unusual. The rate of growth is influenced by growth and sex hormones. Malnutrition, lack of vitamin D, and chronic illness slow bone growth and may interfere with proper bone formation. Long-term treatment with certain medications (eg, prednisone, other steroid drugs) can also impair bone development.

Glandular disorders, such as thyroid problems, sometimes interfere with skeletal development, causing short stature and disproportionately short limbs that can resemble dwarfism in severe cases. Pituitary disorders and a few other very rare conditions may cause a child to grow abnormally tall, with disproportionately large hands and feet, bony deformities, and developmental problems.

### Talk with your pediatrician if

- Your toddler walks with a limp.
- Your child's spine appears crooked or her limbs are asymmetric.
- Your child seems to be growing slowly, her head appears unusually large, and her arms and legs look bowed.
- Your child seems to be growing abnormally fast and her hands and feet look disproportionately large.

### WARNING

At birth, many babies have what appear to be leg or foot deformities that reflect the effects of a confining position in the womb. In most cases, the bones straighten out without treatment during the first year of life.

## Chest Wall Deformities

A frequently seen chest wall abnormality is funnel chest (pectus excavatum or hollowed chest), in which the breastbone (sternum) is sunken and the chest cavity correspondingly narrowed. Funnel chest is usually just an isolated congenital abnormality and may, in fact, run in the family. Occasionally it may signal the presence of an unusual connective tissue disorder such as Marfan syndrome (see "Growth Problems," page 92) or the nutritional disorder, rickets. Children with chronic obstructive disease of the airways may develop a funnel chest deformity, which becomes less noticeable or even disappears when the underlying condition is successfully treated. Funnel chest is rarely a cause for concern, and surgery is not usually necessary.

An unusually prominent sternum causes the shape known as pigeon breast (pectus carinatum, meaning keel-shaped chest). In an otherwise healthy child, this is of no consequence.

| YOUR CONCERNS | POSSIBLE CAUSE | ACTION TO TAKE |
|---|---|---|
| *Your newborn's head looks misshapen. It has become flattened on one side in the weeks since his birth.* | Normal molding of skull | Your baby's skull is subject to great pressure during birth; this causes no harm and the head will gradually resume a normal shape. If flattening has occurred since birth, it's simply the result of pressure and will disappear as your baby is able to change his position. |
| *Your toddler recently started to walk unaided. She is limping.* | Disorder of the hip, such as developmental dysplasia of the hip, or other condition requiring treatment | Talk with your pediatrician. Although usually diagnosed at birth, this condition may not be apparent until your child starts to walk. Your pediatrician will refer your child to a pediatric orthopedist. |
| *One of your child's shoulders is higher than the other. Her hips look uneven. Her spine is curved.* | Scoliosis, or curvature of the spine | Talk with your pediatrician, who will determine whether your child should be seen by a pediatric orthopedist. Treatment may be required. (See "Back Pain," page 34.) |
| *When lying on his stomach, your baby always sleeps with the same side of his face toward the mattress. His head movement is limited. He recently had an upper respiratory infection.* | Wryneck (torticollis) In older children, possibly linked to a viral illness such as an upper respiratory infection or sore throat | Talk with your pediatrician, who will examine your baby and order x-rays. Your pediatrician may recommend special exercises, position changes, or, rarely, surgery. (Also see "Posture Defects," page 126.) |
| *Your preteen is worried because one side of his rib cage looks much smaller than the other.* | Thoracic (rib cage) asymmetry | This common phenomenon is normal. It is always present from birth but may not be noticeable until ages 9 to 13 years or when growth speeds up at puberty. It has no medical significance and no treatment is needed. |

## IN GENERAL

Children's skin problems are often caused by allergic reactions (see page 26) or infections. But many of the skin disorders that plague adults are also seen in children. Skin disorders can usually be identified by a simple inspection backed by detailed questioning and a physical examination. In some cases, however, diagnostic tests may be necessary, especially if the problem is confused by injury, infection, or attempts at treatment.

In general, skin that is inflamed or oozing need to be dried out, while chronic, dry conditions should be moisturized. A condition should be diagnosed before treatment is started. If the skin problem is an allergic reaction, it will recur unless your child avoids contact with the offending substance. When your child develops hives from certain foods, these foods should be removed from his diet.

Soaps containing perfumes and deodorants may be too harsh for children with sensitive skin. Many pediatricians recommend non-soap cleansing lotions for babies and neutral, full-fat soaps for toddlers and older children. Laundry soap or detergent residue on clothing and bedding can also irritate sensitive skin. Use a laundry product that is free of dyes and perfumes, and double rinse to eliminate irritating chemicals. Soaps and lotions containing lanolin may be irritating to those with atopic dermatitis. Children who can't tolerate woolen clothing next to the skin are likely to be hypersensitive to lanolin-based products. If you're in doubt about any product, use plain warm water to wash your child. When a moisturizer is needed, it should be applied to damp skin immediately after a bath or shower.

Some synthetic fabrics and the dyes and other chemicals used in manufacturing also can he irritating to sensitive skins. Washing new clothes before wearing may help. If not, wear undyed cotton clothing next to the skin.

**Talk with your pediatrician if your child has**
- Ring-shaped red or scaly patches on the body or scalp
- Spreading blisters that turn crusty and scaly
- A rash while taking a prescribed medication
- Many small, itchy, red lumps and track marks in the skin

**WARNING!**
Pediatricians warn against the use of all-purpose over-the-counter skin medications, which may contain substances that can sensitize a child's skin and worsen irritation. Talk with your pediatrician before applying a fluorinated steroid cream to your child's face. How quickly a child's skin absorbs creams can vary widely.

## Pigmentation Disorders

Apart from common pigmented birthmarks, freckles, and moles, disorders of skin pigmentation are more often because of a lack of pigment, rather than excess pigment. Albinism, an inborn lack of pigment in the skin, eyes, and hair, is noted at birth with areas of depigmentation (sometimes with areas of dark pigmentation in the white patches) that vary from a few patches to total body involvement. Albinos with total body involvement are extremely vulnerable to the sun's effects; they should not go outside unless well protected with clothing, sunglasses, and sunblock.

Vitiligo, in which pigment loss occurs after birth and may be progressive, turns the skin white in patches that often appear in a symmetric pattern. Patches frequently occur around the mouth and eyes and over prominent bones. Vitiligo may be linked to autoimmune disorders (eg, diabetes mellitus, thyroid disease), although the cause is still unknown. In some cases, pigment gradually returns, although the skin may remain lighter. Patches burn easily and should be protected with a sunscreen with a high sun protection factor (SPF).

Patches of darker pigmentation frequently appear on the skin following inflammation, such as in children with eczema or contact dermatitis. These are best left alone because they generally fade with time.

| YOUR CONCERNS | POSSIBLE CAUSE | ACTION TO TAKE |
|---|---|---|
| Your baby has developed a raised, spotty rash a day or two after getting over a fever. He had only mild, vague symptoms while his temperature was elevated. | Roseola infantum (exanthem subitum), an infection usually caused by human herpesvirus 6 | Call your pediatrician; if roseola seems the likely diagnosis, you may be advised to lower your baby's fever with acetaminophen or ibuprofen. You should also keep your baby away from other children. |
| Your child has bright red, warm, raised patches suddenly appear on her cheeks. She also has mild symptoms such as slight fever and a rash that is spreading. | Fifth disease (erythema infectiosum), a viral infection | Call your pediatrician, who may examine your child to make sure the rash is due to fifth disease. This mild parvovirus infection usually clears up within 10 days, but the rash may recur. |
| Your child has developed small red bumps that hurt and are warm to the touch. They appear to be oozing pus. | Cellulitis caused by methicillin-resistant *Staphylococcus aureus* (MRSA) or other bacteria | You can start warm wet compresses with tap water and a washcloth. Talk with your pediatrician immediately if your child appears ill or develops a fever or if the infection doesn't improve or spreads. An oral antibiotic may be required. |
| Your child has itchy, red patches with small blisters and scaling or crusting. Her skin was exposed to a possible allergen, such as soap, jewelry, or new clothing. | Contact dermatitis | If you can trace the patches to a particular irritant, remove it and see if the rash improves (see "Allergic Reactions," page 26). If you can't, or if the patches don't disappear, talk with your pediatrician, who may prescribe treatment. |
| Your child has a cold sore or fever blister near her mouth. | Herpes virus infection (See "Mouth Pain," page 118.) | Talk with your pediatrician, who may recommend measures to make your child comfortable until the sore heals. |
| Your child has hardened, red patches in areas that itch or started as eczema. | Lichen simplex Chronic eczema or contact dermatitis | This roughening of the skin occurs when a child repeatedly scratches an area of eczema or contact dermatitis. It will gradually disappear if the contact allergen or irritant is removed or the eczema is treated. |
| Your toddler or older child has developed a dusting of brown spots on parts of the body exposed to sunlight. | Freckles (ephelides) | Freckles are common and run in families. They are typically darker in summer, paler in winter, and not dangerous but signal sun damage. Protect your child's skin with sunscreen, a T-shirt, and a hat. |
| Your child has occasional small brown spots appearing on her face and body. | Moles (nevi) | Most people get moles in childhood and adolescence. A mole doesn't require attention unless it's disfiguring or could become irritated (eg, on the shaving area of a teenaged boy's face). But if you see a change in the size, color, or shape of a mole, talk with your pediatrician, who may refer you to a dermatologist. |
| Your child has 6 or more noticeable spots about the color of milky coffee (café au lait) on his body. | Condition requiring diagnosis and treatment (eg, neurofibromatosis) | Talk with your pediatrician, who will examine your child and refer you, if necessary, to another specialist. |
| Your child has spreading, shallow, red blisters that are forming crusty scabs. | Impetigo (streptococcal or staphylococcal infection) | Call your pediatrician; if your child has impetigo, antibiotic treatment will be required. |

| YOUR CONCERNS | POSSIBLE CAUSE | ACTION TO TAKE |
|---|---|---|
| Your child has one or more painful, red, warm lumps under the skin. A lighter area is visible at the top of each swelling. | Boils (infected hair follicles) | Apply hot compresses to relieve pain and swelling. Don't squeeze the boil. Cover it with an adhesive bandage if it's open or exposed. If it fails to heal or more boils appear, call your pediatrician, who may prescribe an antibiotic and other treatments. |
| Your child has several painless, rough-surfaced lumps on her hands, elbows, or feet. | Warts | Warts are caused by a virus and eventually disappear without treatment. If the warts make it difficult for your child to use her hand or foot or are disfiguring, your pediatrician may advise removal or topical treatments. |
| Your child has a lump on the sole of his foot. There is a small opening in the swelling. It is slightly painful. | Plantar (sole of the foot) wart, also called *verruca* Callus | Talk with your pediatrician, who will prescribe treatment or advise on foot care to remove the callus. |
| Your child's facial skin looks oily. She is developing whiteheads and pimples in the oily areas. | Acne | Skin changes are normal as children near puberty. Make sure your child cleans her face each night and morning. If she develops pustules or a rash, talk with your pediatrician, who may recommend more specific acne treatment. |
| Your child has numerous small, itchy bumps. You see nits (egg cases) on her hair. There are red or grayish lines near the itchy bumps, and you may see live crawlers in the scalp. | Infestation with parasites such as lice or scabies | Consider treating everyone with an over-the-counter lice medication now and repeat in a week. Notify your child's school or child care facility. But continue sending your child to school. If you still find live lice in your child's scalp after the second treatment, talk with your pediatrician about new, more effective treatment options. |
| Your child has red, scaly rings that are pale in the center on his body. He has patchy hair loss on his scalp. | Ringworm (tinea corporis on body; tinea capitis on scalp) | Talk with your pediatrician, who will prescribe appropriate treatment. |
| Your child complains of itching between his toes or on the soles of his feet. The skin is scaling or peeling in these areas. His fingernails or toenails are yellowish. | Athlete's foot (tinea pedis) | Talk with your pediatrician, who will prescribe an antifungal cream or ointment. If the infection is severe, oral medication may be needed. If weather permits, your child should wear open sandals to help clear up the infection. |
| Your school-aged child or teen has a rash with oval, coppery patches of scaly skin. The rash is on his trunk and started with a single, "herald" patch. | Pityriasis rosea | Talk with your pediatrician to make sure of the correct diagnosis. If pityriasis rosea is confirmed, the rash will disappear on its own in 8 to 12 weeks. Your pediatrician may recommend a cream to ease itching. Baths and showers should be tepid; heat may make the itching worse. |

| YOUR CONCERNS | POSSIBLE CAUSE | ACTION TO TAKE |
|---|---|---|
| Your school-aged child has developed thick, red, scaly patches on his face and body. They are particularly noticeable on his elbows and knees. He also has dandruff. | Psoriasis (Attacks may be associated with strep throat or viral infections as well as winter, when your child has less sun exposure.) | Talk with your pediatrician, who will examine your child. If the lesions appear to be psoriasis, referral to a dermatologist may be advised. |
| Your child has a hard knot of skin over a recently healed skin injury. He has a skin tag forming on an area that was intentionally pierced, such as an earlobe. | Keloid | Talk with your pediatrician. These skin over-growths aren't harmful, but they can grow to unsightly proportions. They are more common in people who are dark skinned, especially those of African descent. |
| Your toddler or older child is looking yellowish. Her stools are pale and her urine is dark. She has lost her appetite. She is nauseated or vomiting and generally unwell. She has a stomachache. | Hepatitis (probably viral) | Call your pediatrician, who will examine your child and prescribe appropriate treatment. Ask your pediatrician when your child may return to child care or school. |
| Your child has developed several blister-like spots surrounded by red halos on her face and body. She is feverish and irritable. | Chickenpox (varicella) | Chickenpox is rare these days, thanks to the effectiveness of the varicella vaccine. Call your pediatrician to confirm the diagnosis. Acetaminophen or ibuprofen may relieve discomfort. Adding powdered oatmeal or baking soda to bathwater helps soothe the itching; your pediatrician may also prescribe a medication. If any spots get very red, warm, and tender, they may be infected, in which case antibiotic treatment may be required. |
| Your child's skin turned yellow, although the whites of his eyes still look white. | Carotenemia, possibly from frequent consumption of yellow, orange, and red (carotene-containing) vegetables | Talk with your pediatrician, who will examine your child to rule out a serious disorder. This condition usually appears in children who are eating large amounts of carrots or tomatoes and is harmless. |

## IN GENERAL

Proper sleep, including overnight sleep and day-time naps, helps children grow properly, boosts the immune system, and aids family harmony with well-rested parents. But sleep can be a challenge in children of all ages.

Older infants, children of all ages, and adults experience multiple sleep cycles during a full night of sleep. Some older infants may experience awaking during a lighter phase of sleep. If your baby is waking up more than once a night at 6 months, you can modify your infant's sleeping environment to encourage a better night's rest. If she's still sleeping in your room, she may sense your presence and should be moved to another room nearby. If her bed is very small, she may be ready to move to a full-sized crib. If her room is dark, leaving a night-light on may reassure her that she's in familiar surroundings. White noise, such as from the hum of a running fan, can help muffle outside noises.

By about 1 year of age, your increasingly active child may find it hard to wind down at bedtime. This is when a regular evening routine of story, songs, and a quiet game is essential. Don't expect your baby to fall asleep during the routine; instead, settle her into her crib while she's still awake so she learns to fall asleep on her own. Tuck her in, say your good nights, and leave the room. She may cry for a moment but will soon calm down and fall asleep. If she's still crying after about 5 minutes, go in and comfort her, let her know you're nearby, but don't stay longer than a minute or two. Repeat this sequence several times if necessary, each time waiting a little longer to go in and check on her. Be consistent but flexible.

Toddlers can be notoriously difficult about going to bed. You can help the process with a consistent nightly routine that allows her to settle down and provides comfort. It may include a book, a bath, and some snuggling. Letting your toddler take a beloved object to bed and making sure she's comfortable can help the process along. Even older children will benefit from the comfort that comes with a regular, calming routine.

As children get older and more active, they are usually sufficiently fatigued by the time they hit their pillows. But some children may have fears, separation anxiety, and school worries that keep them awake. Some kids also have trouble sleeping when they are excited about an upcoming event such as a holiday or birthday. An occasional bad night makes for a grumpy mood the next day but is usually harmless. To help your child sleep well, try and keep her on a consistent sleep schedule.

. . . . . . . . . . . . . . . . . . . . . . . . . . . . . . . . . . . . . . . . . . .

### Call your child's pediatrician if she

- Awakens every day with a headache
- Has severe allergy symptoms that disrupt sleep
- Is experiencing increasing fears that are occurring during the day too
- Has sleep disturbance related to a temperature above 101°F (38.3°C) or other signs of illness (Also see "Fever in Babies and Children," page 86.)

. . . . . . . . . . . . . . . . . . . . . . . . . . . . . . . . . . . . . . . . . . .

**WARNING!**
Placing a television or computer in your child's bedroom can be disruptive to sound sleep. The American Academy of Pediatrics recommends not allowing televisions or computers in your child's room. Technology stimulates the brain and makes it more difficult for a child to achieve a restful state.

## Medications and Sleep

Certain drugs can make it hard for your child to sleep. Children who have attention-deficit/hyperactivity disorder, for instance, may require medications that improve concentration but cause sleeplessness. Drugs given for seizures may disrupt nighttime sleep too. For some parents, it might be tempting to give your child a medication to help him sleep. Some people use diphenhydramine (eg, Benadryl) or melatonin, a naturally occurring hormone associated with sleep, to induce sleepiness. If you do want to try a medication, discuss it with your pediatrician first. Most of these remedies should be used as short-term solutions. It's more important to use behavioral interventions (eg, regular sleep schedule, soothing routine, avoidance of television and caffeine) to help create good sleep habits.

| YOUR CONCERNS | POSSIBLE CAUSE | ACTION TO TAKE |
|---|---|---|
| Your toddler cries every night before sleep. | Your child is learning to fall asleep by himself | Look in on your toddler every 5 to 10 minutes and quietly repeat your usual sign-off, such as, "Good night." Be consistent to help your toddler learn to fall asleep on his own. |
| Your child throws a tantrum every night before bed. | Normal developmental phase | Avoid letting your child become overtired, overstimulated, or unnecessarily frustrated. Make sure your child isn't going to bed hungry or thirsty. Stay calm and reassuring, but leave the room soon after you respond. |
| Your child is fearful about going to bed. | Anxieties about events (real or imagined) that get worse at night | Reassure your child that she's safe and her parents are looking out for her. Discuss her fears during the day. Stay in her room while calming her, but keep discussions to a minimum. Talk with your pediatrician if fears aren't resolved. |
| Your child awakens in the middle of the night and can't fall back to sleep. | Associating sleep with something that is absent when he awakens | Eliminate unwanted sound or light, and make changes with what he associates with sleep. No child should fall asleep with a television on. Ensure that your child falls asleep under environmental conditions that are similar to the conditions that will be present overnight. |
| Your child awakens and appears confused. She sometimes says things that make no sense. She has no memory of the event the next day. | Confusional arousal | These events are common in young children and will resolve on their own. Avoid trying to comfort your child when she gets up because that may upset her. There is no need to do anything, and these events usually stop after age 5 years. |

## IN GENERAL

Parents who have been through a winter or two with young children won't be surprised to learn that a sore throat is one of the most common complaints in school-aged children. Often, it's the first symptom of a common cold. But while sore throats and colds are more common in the winter, sore throats caused by viruses also occur during the summer months, especially among toddlers and preschoolers.

Antibiotics can cure strep throat and other bacterial infections. But if a sore throat is caused by a virus, the only treatment is rest and the passage of time. You can make your child more comfortable by reducing his temperature with acetaminophen or ibuprofen and giving cool drinks and soft foods that are easy to swallow. Viral throat infections usually clear up by themselves in 3 to 5 days, but bacterial sore throats may lead to complications if left untreated.

Some children wake up almost every morning with throats that are sore and dry from breathing through their mouth. One reason may be a blocked nose due to allergies, large adenoid, or other conditions. The discomfort usually disappears once a child has had a drink to remoisten the back of the throat. If a recurring sore throat is caused by allergies, your pediatrician will recommend treatment for the allergies. A cool-mist humidifier in the bedroom may also help. Occasionally, you may notice white spots on your child's tonsils when she doesn't have a sore throat. The spots are food particles in the tonsil pits. If the child is otherwise well, no attention is required.

### Call your pediatrician if your child has a sore throat along with

- A temperature of 102°F (39°C) or higher
- Ear pain
- A rapid onset of new symptoms such as nausea, swollen glands, rash, severe headache, breathing difficulty, or red, tender joints
- Dark urine up to 3 or 4 weeks after the sore throat
- A rash
- Pus (light-colored flecks) on the tonsils

### WARNING!

If your pediatrician diagnoses a bacterial (strep) infection, an antibiotic will be prescribed. Make sure your child takes all the medication for the whole prescribed time, even though the sore throat may feel better after a day or two. Stopping the medication before all the germs are eradicated may allow the sore throat to return.

## Tonsils: In or Out?

Before antibiotics were used to treat throat infections and prevent complications, tonsils were routinely removed in children who had frequent sore throats (Figure 2-16). Pediatricians still recommend removal of the tonsils and adenoid when the tonsils swell so much that they interfere with swallowing or breathing or cause sleep problems or snoring, or when a child has recurrent, severe abscesses around the tonsils. This procedure is also advised when a child has had at least 6 to 7 strep throats in one year.

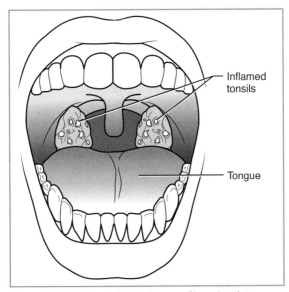

**Figure 2-16.** The tonsils are clumps of lymphoid tissue located in the rear of the throat.

Inflamed tonsils

Tongue

| YOUR CONCERNS | POSSIBLE CAUSE | ACTION TO TAKE |
|---|---|---|
| Your child has developed a sore throat over a few days. He also has a runny nose or cough. | Common cold or other viral infection of the upper respiratory tract | Keep your child comfortable, with plenty of drinks to replace lost fluids (see "Runny/Stuffy Nose," page 132). You can give acetaminophen or ibuprofen to reduce fever. In children older than 5 years, sucking a hard candy or throat lozenge may give some relief; for those 8 years or older, gargling with salt water (half a teaspoon of salt in 8 ounces of warm water) may soothe the pain. Consult your pediatrician if the cold doesn't improve after a week or other symptoms develop. |
| Your child's throat is red and inflamed. You can see pale flecks on her tonsils. She has swollen glands in her neck or a stomachache. Her temperature is 101°F (38.3°C) or higher. | Strep throat Infectious mononucleosis Another throat infection | Call your pediatrician, who will diagnose your child and advise on treatment, which may include an antibiotic. Your child may go back to school or other activities 24 hours after the start of treatment, provided her temperature is 100.4°F (38°C) or lower. |
| Your child is complaining of a sore throat during the summer months. You can see blisters on his throat. | Infection by coxsackie or another virus | Call your pediatrician, who will examine your child and advise appropriate treatment. (See "Mouth Pain," page 118.) |
| Your baby refuses to drink or take solid food. She is irritable. You can see white patches on her tongue and gums. | Thrush | Call your pediatrician, who will examine your baby. If she has this common yeast infection, treatment will be prescribed. (See "Mouth Pain," page 118.) |
| Your child is in a lot of pain, feverish, and drooling. She is having difficulty breathing. | Serious cause of throat pain such as epiglottitis, abscess, tonsillar infection, or foreign body | Take your child to the nearest emergency department or call 911 or your local emergency number. (See "Breathing Difficulty/Breathlessness," page 50.) |
| Your child is having severe pain, especially when drinking or eating. He is drooling. His gums and tongue hurt. He has a fever, and his neck glands are swollen. | Herpes infection of the mouth (herpetic gingivostomatitis) | Call your pediatrician promptly for an examination and treatment recommendations. |

## IN GENERAL

Many children can say several words clearly by the time they're 1 year old. During the second year, most toddlers increase their expressive, verbal vocabulary, and after the second birthday, they bubble over with increasingly complex sentences, ideas, and questions. Many factors influence speech development, including genetics, birth order, and interactions with parents. For some children, a period of stammering occurs when the ability to speak can't keep up with the flow of thoughts. It's not usually a sign of future speech problems and will pass with time.

When you're evaluating how well your child speaks, it's important to distinguish between speech and language. Speech is the production of understandable sounds, whereas language is the underlying mental function around communication that includes expressive (speaking) and receptive (understanding) speech. Common causes of speech problems are hearing loss (see page 98), developmental delay (see page 64), and lack of verbal stimulation. Early detection can help prevent a speech problem from interfering with learning. If your pediatrician believes your child may have a speech or language problem, your pediatrician will examine her, test her hearing, and, if necessary, refer her for more evaluation and treatment. Most schools also monitor children's speech and recommend treatment for those with potential problems.

**Talk with your pediatrician if, at about 2½ years,**

- Your child's speech is very hard to understand.
- Your child doesn't use 2-word sentences.
- Your child doesn't follow simple verbal instructions.

> **WARNING!**
> Some parents are so eager to have their baby speak that they may intimidate their child. Don't pressure your child, but provide verbal stimulation with books, singing, and repetitive rhymes.

## Language Milestones for the First 5 Years

By the end of the second year, your toddler should be able to speak in 2-word sentences and follow simple instructions and repeat words heard in conversation.

By the end of the third year, your child should be able to speak in 3-word sentences, follow an instruction with 2 or 3 steps, recognize and identify practically all common objects and pictures, and understand most of what is said to her. She should speak well enough to be understood by those outside the family.

By the end of the fourth year, your child should be using 4-word sentences. Your child will ask abstract (why?) questions and understand concepts of same versus different. She has also mastered the basic rules of grammar as she hears it around her. Although your child should be speaking clearly by age 4 years, she may mispronounce as many as half of her basic sounds; this isn't a cause for concern.

By the end of the fifth year, your child should be able to retell a story in her own words and use more than 5 words in a sentence.

| YOUR CONCERNS | POSSIBLE CAUSE | ACTION TO TAKE |
|---|---|---|
| Your child is making no effort to speak at 2 years. She is active and healthy. She understands you and communicates nonverbally. | Slower rate of speech development | Your child's speech may be slower than her motor skills. If she's surrounded by talkative siblings or others in child care, she may not feel the need to speak. Read and speak with her one-on-one, giving her plenty of opportunities to reply. |
| Your child responds to your voice only when he can see your face. | Hearing problem | Talk with your pediatrician, who will examine your child and test his hearing. Consultation with another specialist may be advised. |
| Your preschooler hesitates, stammers, repeats syllables, or confuses word order. | Normal period of dysfluency | Your child is learning to coordinate his thoughts with his motor skills. Speak clearly and read to your child. Don't overcorrect him or finish his sentences. This stage usually passes quickly. |
| Your preschooler still uses "baby" sounds, such as d- for th- or w- for l-. | Normal development | Many children don't master all consonants and blends until age 5 years. Speak clearly without drawing attention to the problem sounds; read to your child. |
| Your school-aged child speaks with a lisp or consistently mispronounces consonants. | Lisp or other speech impediment | If the impediment is very noticeable, ask your pediatrician to recommend a speech-language therapist for an evaluation. |
| Your school-aged child is stuttering or hesitating. He grimaces when trying to get words out. | Stammering or stuttering | Talk with your pediatrician, who may recommend an evaluation by a speech-language therapist. |
| Your school-aged child often repeats phrases or odd sounds. He sometimes repeats "bad words" aloud. He also makes unusual movements. | Tourette syndrome (a disorder marked by tics and involuntary utterances) Another neurologic condition | Talk with your pediatrician, who will examine your child and provide a referral to a neurologist, if necessary. |
| Your child avoids communicating with and without words. He is between 2 and 5 years old. He seems to be in a world of his own. He may have lost skills he used to have. | Communication disorder or autism (See page 68.) | Talk with your pediatrician, who will evaluate your child and recommend referral to appropriate specialists. |
| Your child's motor skills are also delayed. | Developmental motor problem with many possible causes | Talk with your pediatrician, who will evaluate your child's development and recommend referral to another specialist, if necessary. |

## IN GENERAL

The color, consistency, and frequency of stools can vary widely in the same child as well as among children of similar ages who are eating almost identical diets. Babies' and toddlers' stools may vary from several movements each day to only once every 2 or 3 days. Once children are eating the same food as the rest of the family, however, they generally settle into a routine of 1 or 2 daily bowel movements. As long as the stools are soft and well formed—not liquid diarrhea (see "Diarrhea in Infants and Children," page 70) or hard, dry pellets from constipation (see page 54)—your child's bowels are functioning normally, and he's simply following his own timetable.

The color of stools isn't usually important. But if they are blood streaked or black and tarry, your child may have gastrointestinal bleeding. If stools are excessively pale, your child may have a liver disorder.

. . . . . . . . . . . . . . . . . . . . . . . . . . . . . . . . . . .

### Call your pediatrician if your child is passing

- Tarry-looking stools
- Blood in the stool
- Very pale stools and has a yellow cast to the skin
- Bulky, greasy stools that float and are foul smelling

. . . . . . . . . . . . . . . . . . . . . . . . . . . . . . . . . . .

### WARNING!

The stools of toddlers and older children may contain fragments of undigested food. This is usually because of incomplete chewing and doesn't signal a serious problem like malabsorption. Stools that are bulky or greasy or float in the toilet, on the other hand, are signs of possible malabsorption.

## Stool Color and Consistency

Day-to-day changes in stool show what a child has been eating. A breastfed baby passes soft, almost runny stools that resemble light mustard. They may even contain seedlike particles. In formula-fed babies, normal stools are tan to yellow and somewhat firmer than in breastfed babies. But they should still be no firmer in consistency than peanut butter. If stools are hard or very dry, your baby may not be getting enough fluids or may be losing too much fluid through perspiration, fever, or illness. Hard stools in a baby eating solid foods can be a sign that the diet contains foods that he's not yet ready to handle, except in small quantities. When a baby has had a large serving of cereal or another food that takes an effort to digest, the process may slow down and the stools, when they pass, will be greenish. Iron supplements can turn stools black.

After a meal including beets, gummy candies, fruit chews, or food or drink containing red dye, a child's stools may be tinged an alarming red. Some children also pass pinkish urine. Stools of a brilliant blue, purple, or other rainbow hue probably show that your child taste-tested her crayons. Don't be alarmed; in all these cases, the color will disappear as soon as the food or crayon has left your child's digestive tract. It's reassuring to know that manufacturers of crayons as well as foods have to meet strict safety standards when using dyes in products meant for children.

| YOUR CONCERNS | POSSIBLE CAUSE | ACTION TO TAKE |
|---|---|---|
| *Your child has streaks of fresh blood on the toilet paper or around her anus. You see blood on the stool or in the toilet bowl. Your child has rectal pain. She is constipated but otherwise healthy.* | Anal fissure (See "Rectal Pain/ Itching," page 128.) | Talk with your pediatrician, who will examine your child and, if the diagnosis is confirmed, recommend measures to heal the fissure. |
| *Your child has been passing watery stools since starting a prescription medication, such as an antibiotic.* | Medication side effect | Call your pediatrician, who will review the medication and prescribe an alternative, if appropriate. |
| *Your child's stools are extremely dark in color. She has been taking iron supplements or eating large servings of blueberries or dark-green, leafy vegetables. She is otherwise healthy.* | Normal effects on the stool of diet or medication | No action is necessary; your child is healthy. |
| *Your child's stools are unusually pale. There is a yellow tinge to his skin and the whites of his eyes.* | Viral hepatitis (See "Jaundice," page 10.) Congenital malformation (atresia) | Call your pediatrician, who will examine your child and recommend appropriate treatment. |
| *Your child has been passing stools that are pale, bulky, and unusually foul smelling.* | Malabsorption disorder | Talk with your pediatrician, who will evaluate your child and recommend management. |
| *Your child has red or maroon blood in her stool. She says she feels unwell. She has a fever.* | Inflammatory disorder of the digestive tract causing bleeding (hematochezia) | Call your pediatrician right away; your child needs an examination and treatment. |
| *Your child's stools are black and tarry looking. They contain material resembling coffee grounds.* | Bleeding in the digestive tract causing blood in the stool (melena) | Call your pediatrician at once for an examination, diagnostic tests, and appropriate treatment. |
| *Your child has white or clay-colored stools and brownish urine.* | Liver problem | Contact your pediatrician immediately. Your child may have a liver problem. |

## IN GENERAL

Approximately 1.5% of young school-aged children have stool incontinence or fecal soiling. The problem affects boys 6 times more often than girls. Some children who have always soiled and have never been successfully toilet trained are said to have primary encopresis, which is more common. Children who have secondary encopresis, by contrast, start soiling again after they have been trained for months or years. When a child older than 4 years repeatedly passes stool in his underwear or other inappropriate places, he may be undergoing unusual emotional stress, which could be causing him to lose control. In many cases, the cause is a physical disorder. Whatever the reason for soiling may be, children rarely soil themselves on purpose, and they need help to achieve control. Unless he gets help, a child who has encopresis may become socially isolated and develop emotional difficulties.

Encopresis sometimes begins when a child repeatedly ignores the urge to defecate and holds the stool back. Gradually, the nerve sensations in the area grow weaker and the intestines become less able to contract. The stools become larger, harder, and more painful to pass, which makes the child afraid to have a bowel movement. Eventually, hardened feces block the passage, but liquid stool occasionally leaks around the solid mass and stains the underwear and bedsheets. The child may not be aware that he's passing liquid stools, but parents see the stains and wrongly believe their child has developed diarrhea (also see "Constipation," page 54). A child with encopresis needs help immediately. The longer the problem goes on, the harder it may be to deal with.

### Talk with your pediatrician if your child

- Is older than 4 years and hasn't yet learned to control his bowel movements
- Has started soiling his pants after a period of apparent control

### WARNING!

Enemas and medications such as stool softeners are sometimes needed to empty impacted stools and help a child retrain his bowels. Use only the medications your pediatrician prescribes; taken without a pediatrician's supervision, over-the-counter products may make the problem worse and even harm your child's health.

## Managing Stool Retention and Soiling

Stool holding is a fairly common phenomenon among young children. If this becomes a problem, your pediatrician can recommend a plan with the following goals: to help your child set regular bowel habits, to help your child recognize and respond to the urge to defecate and to hold stool only until the right time and place for a bowel movement, to lessen the family's concerns, and to provide a diet that will promote normal movements.

Pediatricians usually begin treatment with medication to help your child pass impacted feces. This lets the bowel shrink to a normal size. In the next phase, your child takes daily doses of medication to ease stool passage. Your pediatrician will review your child's diet to make sure it includes fiber in the form of vegetables, fruits, and whole-grain cereals and breads together with plenty of fluids. Air-cooked popcorn without butter is a high-fiber snack that promotes regular bowel function.

If soiling is the problem, a reward system can encourage your child, especially if he really wants to succeed. You could try gold-star stickers on a calendar for "accident-free" days or a toy or book to mark a week without an accident. Relapses are common, and treatment may take months or years. Reassure your child that you know he's trying and in time he'll reach his goal.

| YOUR CONCERNS | POSSIBLE CAUSE | ACTION TO TAKE |
|---|---|---|
| *Your child regularly soils his clothing or has bowel movements in inappropriate places. He is older than 4 years. He resists efforts to start toilet training.* | Primary encopresis | Talk with your pediatrician, who will examine your child and recommend a plan for management. |
| *Your school-aged child often a has diarrhea-like movement. He has stains on his clothing or sheets.* | Fecal retention, impaction, and leakage (See "Diarrhea in Infants and Children," page 70, and "Constipation," page 54.) | Talk with your pediatrician, who will examine your child and may prescribe treatment including medications and retraining. |
| *Your child has been soiling occasionally since having a bout of diarrhea or gastroenteritis.* | Upset of normal bowel habits | Remind your child to take regular breaks to go to the toilet. Her normal schedule should return within a week. If it doesn't or your child has other symptoms, talk with your pediatrician. |
| *Your formerly toilet-trained child started soiling since beginning or changing school. She is otherwise active and doing well.* | Behavioral response to difficult situation | Your child may dislike the school toilets, or the schedule may not mesh with her usual rhythms. Ask that school toilets be repaired or cleaned, if necessary. Encourage regular toileting at home to establish a routine and allow extra time to ensure complete movements. |
| *Your child began soiling after a period of control. He is under unusual stress. He is having learning or social difficulties at school.* | Stress | If your family is going through a trying time, explain the situation, but don't overburden your child. Talk with teachers to identify and deal with problems. Talk with your pediatrician about how to help your child retrain his bowels and manage stress. |
| *Your child is impatient or impulsive.* | Impulsiveness Lack of concentration | Encourage your child to spend enough time in the bathroom; use a reward system if it helps. Seek your pediatrician's advice if the problem doesn't improve. |

## IN GENERAL

When a child has an isolated bump or swelling confined to a small area, the most likely causes are infection, which can be tender to the touch, or a cyst, which is usually not tender. Trauma can also lead to swelling around an injured area, and bruising can be felt as a lump under the skin with overlying purple discoloration. From time to time, some children develop the acute, lumpy swellings of angioedema (a deep hive in the skin) because they are highly sensitive to a food, cold, or other stimulus. In this case, if the child has hives on the surface of her skin as well (see "Allergic Reactions," page 26), it's a further sign that the reaction is allergic in nature. This kind of reaction can also occur in response to a viral infection. (For swollen glands, see page 154.)

**Talk with your pediatrician if your child develops**

- A painful lump
- A red, warm, and tender lump
- A persistent and growing lump that can't be explained

> ### WARNING!
> If your child has a lump that can't be explained, bring it to your pediatrician's attention. Although tumors in children are rare, it's better to err on the side of caution than to ignore a possible warning sign.

## Lumps on the Wrist

Some children develop a fluid-filled cyst called a *ganglion* (Figure 2-17). A ganglion forms when synovial fluid—the lubricant that makes our joints work smoothly—leaks through a perforation in the capsule surrounding a joint and builds up in the tendon sheath. The joint most often involved is the wrist, and the ganglion is usually seen on the back of the hand or wrist.

Most ganglia are harmless and not painful; they gradually disappear without treatment. If, however, your child has a ganglion that is unusually large or painful or that keeps the child from fully using his wrist, your pediatrician may recommend treatment. A ganglion that interferes with proper hand function can be treated with surgery to cut out the cyst and seal off the fluid leakage. Don't attempt to treat a ganglion yourself.

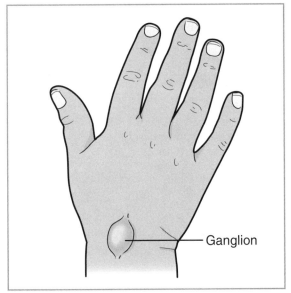

**Figure 2-17.** A ganglion (plural, ganlia) is a firm, smooth lump, usually about the size of a pea, just under the skin surface. A ganglion most often develops on the back of the wrist but may also occur on an ankle joint or a finger.

| YOUR CONCERNS | POSSIBLE CAUSE | ACTION TO TAKE |
|---|---|---|
| Your child has one or more painful, red, warm lumps under the skin anywhere on the body. A lighter area is visible at the top of each swelling. | Boils (infected hair follicles) | Apply warm compresses to relieve pain and swelling. Don't squeeze the boil to draw out the contents. Cover it with an adhesive bandage if it's open or exposed. If it fails to heal or more boils appear, your pediatrician will examine your child and may prescribe an antibiotic and additional treatment. |
| Your child has several painless, rough-surfaced lumps on her hands, feet, or elbows. | Warts | Warts, which are caused by human papillomavirus, eventually disappear without treatment. If the warts make it difficult for your child to use her hands, are disfiguring, or seem to be spreading, talk with your pediatrician, who may advise to treat by removal. |
| Your child has a soft, painless swelling in the groin. It disappears when lightly pressed. | Inguinal hernia | Talk with your pediatrician, who will examine your child and provide a referral to another specialist for further treatment, if necessary. (Also see "Abdominal Swelling," page 24.) |
| Your son has a soft, painless swelling on one side of his scrotum. One testicle appears a lot larger than the other. The swelling looks smaller when he lies down. | Hydrocele Hernia | Talk with your pediatrician, who will examine your child to determine whether he has a hydrocele, a minor inborn condition that allows fluid to accumulate in the scrotum. If your child has a hernia, your pediatrician will provide referral to another specialist for treatment. |
| Your child has a lump on the sole of his foot. There is a small opening in the swelling. It hurts a bit when he walks on it. | Plantar (sole of the foot) wart, also called *verruca* | Talk with your pediatrician, who will prescribe treatment. |
| Your child has swellings that look like bruises over the lower part of his legs, although he can't remember injuring himself. He recently had an upper respiratory infection. Your child has a weakened immune system. | Erythema nodosum, an inflammatory skin disorder caused by an immunologic reaction to a viral or bacterial infection | Call your pediatrician, who will examine the child and perform diagnostic tests. |
| Your child is complaining of a painful swelling over a bone. | Infection Tumor or other condition requiring diagnosis and treatment | Call your pediatrician for a consultation as soon as possible. |

## IN GENERAL

Children's lymph glands lie close to the surface of the neck, armpit, and groin. When they become swollen, it's usually because the child has developed an infection. In toddlers and older children, the swelling usually doesn't require treatment and disappears once the illness is over. If your child has swollen glands that are tender, persist for more than a few days or get larger, or aren't related to a recent infection, your pediatrician should examine them. Don't feel your child's glands more than once or twice a day. Excessive rubbing can make glands more tender and swollen.

### Call your pediatrician if your child has

- Swollen glands and is 12 months or younger
- Swollen glands for 7 days or longer
- Swollen glands together with a temperature above 101°F (38.3°C) for 5 days or longer
- Swelling of glands throughout the body
- Rapidly enlarging glands along with a color change in the overlying skin

> **WARNING!**
> Swollen glands in babies younger than 1 year aren't always easy to classify and should be brought to your pediatrician's attention.

## The Lymphatic System

The lymphatic system (Figure 2-18) is the body's major line of defense against invasion by infecting bacteria and viruses. The system consists of the spleen (the largest organ in the lymphatic system) and groups of smaller lymph glands or nodes linked by separate vessels called the *lymphatic system*. The lymph glands, found in the neck, armpits, groin, and many other parts of the body, act as barriers against the spread of germs. The lymphatic system carries lymph, the watery fluid that transports disease-fighting white blood cells known as *lymphocytes*. Produced in the spleen, lymph glands, and bone marrow, lymphocytes recognize foreign cells and germs and take part in the body's immune reaction to these and other unwelcome substances. Lymphocytes produce antibodies to disarm or destroy infecting germs; the antibodies stay in the bloodstream for long periods and help the body resist future invasion by the same agent. At times when the body is under attack by germs, the lymph glands swell noticeably as the lymphocytes increase and produce antibodies.

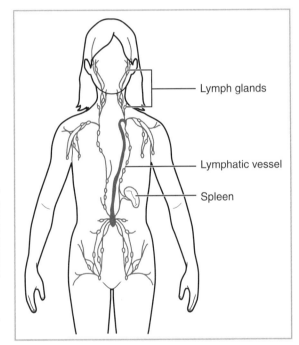

**Figure 2-18.** The main sites of the lymph nodes. Lymph circulates freely in the tissues of the body, and lymphatic vessels are present wherever there are blood vessels. Unlike the blood, lymph has no central pump, although valves in the large lymphatic vessels prevent backflow. The lymph nodes filter out germs and produce disease-fighting lymphocytes. The lymphatic system is also important in carrying fats, transporting nutrients and wastes, and preserving the fluid balance throughout the body.

| YOUR CONCERNS | POSSIBLE CAUSE | ACTION TO TAKE |
|---|---|---|
| Your child has painless swellings at the front and sides of the neck. She recently had a temperature of at least 100.4°F (38°C) as well as a runny nose, sore throat, or other symptoms of a respiratory infection. | Viral infection<br>Infectious mononucleosis<br>Tonsillitis | If your child is feeling better, check the size of the swellings in a day or two to make sure they're going down. If the swelling is unchanged after a week, talk with your pediatrician. |
| Your child has swelling just under her jawbone. She has pain in a tooth or elsewhere around the mouth. | Infection in the tooth, gum, or cheek | Talk with your pediatrician, who will examine your child and prescribe therapy, if needed. If the infection appears to be in the teeth or gums, your pediatrician will refer you to your child's dentist. |
| Your child has swollen glands only in the groin or armpit. He has a sore, a boil, or redness, pain, and warmth suggesting infection in the leg or arm on the same side of the body. | Infection (probably bacterial) | Call your pediatrician, who will examine your child and provide necessary treatment, including an antibiotic, if required. |
| Your child has developed swollen glands while on medication for a chronic condition such as epilepsy. | Side effect of medication | Talk with your physician, who may adjust the medication. |
| Your child has developed tender, swollen glands since being scratched or bitten by a cat. She also has a mild fever and headache. She is not her usual self. | Cat-scratch disease, an infection contracted through a scratch or bite from a (usually) healthy cat | Call your pediatrician, who will examine your child and prescribe any treatment required. Warm compresses and children's acetaminophen or ibuprofen can help alleviate discomfort. |
| Your child has swollen glands all over his body. He also has a temperature above 100.4°F (38°C) or other symptoms of illness. | General illness, most often a viral or another infection requiring diagnosis and treatment | Call your pediatrician, who will examine your child to determine whether diagnostic tests and treatment are required. |
| Your teen has swollen glands just above the collarbone. He has swollen glands elsewhere on his body. | Condition such as chest infection or tumor requiring prompt diagnosis and treatment | Call your pediatrician to arrange an examination as soon as possible. |

## IN GENERAL

At around age 2 years, a toddler's confusion about his growing independence often leads to crying and full-blown tantrums. During these outbursts, the child may fling himself on the floor, kick and fight, bang his head, and even hold his breath until he passes out (see "Dealing With Breath-holding," page 44). Parents may be confused because the triggers for outbursts are often trivial events. A toddler may throw a tantrum when he's asked to wear a hat outdoors or to try a different kind of cereal. When your toddler has a tantrum, remind yourself that this is part of normal development and doesn't reflect badly on your ability as a parent.

While tantrums are normal between about 18 months and 4 years, frequent emotional storms in a child of elementary school age may be a cause for concern. Children who are socially immature may express their negative or hostile feelings by being destructive (see "Behavioral Concerns," page 38). This kind of behavior is a red flag for adjustment problems later on. A child with such problems should be evaluated and treated by a specialist in behavioral and emotional disorders.

Yelling, losing your temper, or spanking your child won't help and may make the situation worse. When your child has a tantrum, it's best to ignore it if you can or lead your child to his room for a time-out. If a child still has tantrums after age 4 years, your pediatrician may recommend a consultation with a child psychiatrist or psychologist. A parent education group may be helpful for further support.

**Talk with your pediatrician if your child has tantrums involving any of the following:**

- Breath-holding and fainting
- Outbursts lasting and growing more intense after age 4 years
- Injury to himself or others or damage to property
- Frequent nightmares, severe problems with behavior and toilet-training, tearfulness, or overdependence

**WARNING!**
Try to keep toddler tantrums within manageable limits by seeing that your child doesn't get overtired, overstimulated, or needlessly frustrated. Set reasonable guidelines for behavior; children are more likely to have frequent tantrums if parents are too strict or fail to set any limits at all.

## Coping With Tantrums

When your toddler starts to get worked up, try a diversionary tactic: "Let's see what's in this storybook," or "Did you hear the doorbell?" If storm clouds continue to gather, it may help to leave the room or just ignore the behavior. It's best to let a tantrum run its course, then be ready to cuddle the child and resume interrupted activity as soon as she has cooled off. Don't put up with physical assaults; however, if your child lashes out, let her know that smacking and kicking are unacceptable. If a tantrum happens away from home, calmly carry your toddler to another room or outside so she can weather the storm away from onlookers.

While some tantrums are normal when children are younger than 4 years, there's no need to trigger extra outbursts by subjecting your toddler to unbearable indecision or making unrealistic demands. Give her reasonable freedom in making decisions, but keep choices simple. Let her choose between 2 items, not several—an apple or a banana, for example, but not the whole fruit bowl. Above all, choose your battles and make it clear that you can't negotiate issues relating to health and safety, such as going to bed or riding buckled up in the car seat. Once a choice has been made, stick to it and be consistent but not rigid. Soften your discipline with a joke or whimsy, and keep in mind that toddler tantrums are a phase that will pass.

After a show of temper in an older child, suggest alternative ways of behaving. Show that while you disapprove of the behavior, you still love your child.

Time-out in the child's room may help with cooling off. Be fair; watch your children to make sure that an apparently nonaggressive sibling isn't secretly teasing or physically hurting another.

If your child is past the preschool years and still having tantrums and you're afraid of losing your self-control when she does, talk with your pediatrician. Many community organizations, including churches, temples, and parent-teacher associations, sponsor parent-effectiveness training courses and support groups.

| YOUR CONCERNS | POSSIBLE CAUSE | ACTION TO TAKE |
|---|---|---|
| Your toddler or preschooler respond to almost every question with "No!" He is refusing foods he used to like. He sometimes does the opposite of what you tell him. He often cries for no apparent reason. | A normal phase of development lasting from about 18 months (and even younger) to 4 years | Help your child become increasingly independent by letting him choose between 2 acceptable options. Don't punish these outbursts; generally, if you ignore them, they'll grow less frequent over time. Provide playthings so he can work out his frustrations; be ready to comfort and joke with him when he's back to his normal, happy self. |
| Your child older than 4 years is having tantrums. She has day-time soiling. She finds it hard to get along with other children. | Behavioral disorder | Talk with your pediatrician, who will determine whether a consultation with a children's mental health specialist is advisable. Your pediatrician may suggest that you join a parent support group. |
| Your child is having tantrums at school. He is aggressive toward teachers or other children. | Behavioral disorder Learning difficulty | Talk with your child's teachers to identify problems that are causing frustration. Talk with your pediatrician, who should do vision and hearing tests to uncover hidden problems causing learning difficulties. Teach your child to resolve conflicts with words, and review the behavior he sees within the family. Your pediatrician may advise consultation with a behavioral specialist. |

## IN GENERAL

Tics are coordinated movements of the voluntary muscles. Transient tics are surprisingly common; it's estimated that 10% of the population has a tic that lasts a month or more but eventually disappears without treatment. Habit tics stem from a compulsion to repeat certain movements and are made consciously, at least initially. Common examples include sniffing, grimacing, blinking, neck stretching, and shoulder shrugging.

Rhythmic tremors, particularly of the chin or leg, that resemble spasms are normal in healthy newborns. This jitteriness, which is most noticeable when the baby is crying or being examined, disappears after the second week of life. Older children may have inherited tremors that can be severe enough to interfere with writing and other motor activities. Some medications may cause tremors. Spasms may involve jerking of the whole body, often during sleep. These benign movements often occur just as a child is falling asleep. Some spasms are caused by metabolic diseases that prevent the body from processing a substance such as copper or iron. Others are the result of rare inherited disorders. A child who develops rheumatic fever after having strep throat may have Sydenham chorea, a tic disorder formerly known as *St Vitus dance*. Prompt antibiotic treatment of a streptococcal sore throat is important to prevent these complications.

• • • • • • • • • • • • • • • • • • • • • • • • • • • • •

### Talk with your pediatrician if your child

• Is making sounds along with repetitive movements
• Becomes anxious when prevented from carrying out apparently meaningless rituals

• • • • • • • • • • • • • • • • • • • • • • • • • • • • •

### WARNING!

Certain medications may trigger or unmask tics in susceptible children, especially those with attention-deficit/hyperactivity disorder. If your child is being treated with a stimulant medication, bring any unusual movements or sounds to your pediatrician's attention.

## Tics as Signs of Obsessive-compulsive Disorder

In many cases, actions and habits thought to be tics are later recognized as signs of obsessive-compulsive disorder (OCD). While able to suppress the actions for a short time, a person with a compulsive disorder feels a buildup of emotional pressure that eventually erupts in a flurry of tics. A biochemical problem may be at the root of this disorder, and, in many cases, other family members have similar symptoms.

Children with OCD usually observe repetitive rituals as a protective mechanism. They may be obsessed with bodily wastes and contamination or a need to keep things the same. Eventually, the ritualistic behavior crowds out normal activities.

Although distressed by their compulsions, children may try to get their parents to join in the rituals. Features of an OCD are often present at the time tics first appear, and they become more pronounced in adolescence and early adulthood. In recent years, several medications have been developed to help control tics, attention difficulties, and OCD. Medication generally needs to be taken for a while before real improvement can be seen. Occasionally, the symptoms of a tic disorder may emerge after a child has begun treatment with a stimulant medication for attention-deficit/hyperactivity disorder (see page 30). At times, medication may need to be changed. In addition, there has been recently recognized association with OCD and strep infections. This condition, called PANDAS (pediatric autoimmune neuropsychiatric disorder associated with streptococcal infections), remains controversial, but experts recently concluded that this condition does exist. Speak to your pediatrician if you're concerned about this condition.

| YOUR CONCERNS | POSSIBLE CAUSE | ACTION TO TAKE |
|---|---|---|
| Your child's limbs jerk once or twice as she's falling asleep. | Nocturnal myoclonus | These normal muscle jerks require no treatment. They may persist into adulthood. |
| Your child has a recurrent twitch in the eyelid or another muscle. | Fatigue<br>Stress | The twitching is annoying but harmless; it disappears as your child gets over his fatigue or stress but may often recur. |
| Your child makes repetitive movements or sounds. He has a cough that disappears during sleep. He can't suppress the actions when asked. They are stronger or more frequent when he's under stress. | Transient tic of childhood or habit spasms | Transient tics of childhood usually disappear without treatment within several weeks but may last up to a year. If the movements become more marked or new ones develop, talk with your pediatrician to schedule an examination. |
| Your child makes repetitive movements for up to 30 seconds at a time. She is unable to suppress these actions. She is awake and aware. | Simple partial seizures (See "Convulsions," page 222.)<br>Tourette syndrome<br>Habit spasm. | Consult your pediatrician, who will examine your child and may recommend treatment or consultation with another specialist. |
| Your child repeats movements involving 3 or more muscle groups at once. Other family members have movement disorders. | Chronic motor tic disorder | Check with your pediatrician, who will examine your child to rule out any physical problems and may recommend treatment. |
| Your child developed movements since starting medication for hyperactivity. | Side effect of medication | Call your pediatrician to report the side effect and ask for a reevaluation of treatment. |
| Your child makes unusual movements and sounds that change from time to time. They are worse under stress. They have been present for a year or more. Other family members have movement disorders. | Tourette syndrome, a neurologic disorder | Talk with your pediatrician, who will examine your child and may recommend consultation with a pediatric neurologist. |
| Your child is making involuntary jerking movements. She is weak. She is having mood swings. She had a sore throat weeks or months ago. | Sydenham chorea, a complication of rheumatic fever | Call your pediatrician, who will examine your child and prescribe treatment, including an antibiotic |
| Your child has difficulty sleeping because of a "crawly" feeling in his legs. | Restless legs syndrome | Talk with with your pediatrician. Restless legs syndrome may be present in some children with iron deficiency anemia. |

## IN GENERAL

Many typically developing children have occasional wetting accidents for 6 months to a year after toilet training. By age 5 years, daytime accidents are rare, although some children still wet the bed periodically at night (see "Bedwetting," page 36). A few children older than 5 years have wetting problems during the daytime. Daytime incontinence is much less common than nighttime wetting and usually requires your pediatrician's attention. When it recurs after a long period of being dry, your child may be under emotional stress or have an acute infection or other medical problem. Your child should be seen by his pediatrician.

### Talk with your pediatrician if your child

- Complains of pain on urination
- Passes cloudy or pinkish urine
- Is passing an unusually large volume of urine and looks thin, pale, and tired
- Wets again after achieving a pattern of daytime and nighttime dryness

**WARNING!**
During the summertime, chlorine in swimming pool water may irritate the urethra, making a child feel like he has to urinate frequently.

### Developing Bladder Control

Before they can learn how to control passing urine or bowel movements, children have to be able to recognize what a full bladder or rectum feels like. They also have to be able to hold on to the contents and control their release (Figure 2-19). It's very unusual for a typical child to develop this complicated skill until well into the second year of life; many typically developing children and those with developmental delays achieve this skill later (see "Steps to Toilet Training," page 36). Between the ages of 3 and 4, most children learn to control their bladder and bowel functions while awake, but accidents—especially wetting—can still happen occasionally. Nighttime control of urinary function usually develops between 2½ and 3½ years. Bedwetting, however, is fairly common up to age 5 and isn't at all rare in typically developing, healthy children for several more years (see page 36).

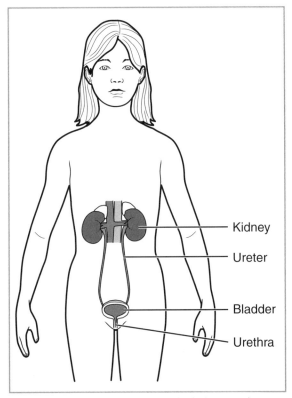

**Figure 2-19.** Urine is produced in the kidneys and passes through the ureters to collect in the bladder. From there, it's released at intervals through the urethra.

| YOUR CONCERNS | POSSIBLE CAUSE | ACTION TO TAKE |
|---|---|---|
| Your child often has a wetting accident when caught up in play or on outings. | Excitement Distraction Putting off going to the toilet | Train your child to take notice of his urge to urinate. Remind him to go to the bathroom at intervals and before outings. If he looks as if he needs to go, don't let him delay. If he's in an unfamiliar place, show him where the bathrooms are. |
| Your child is wetting herself frequently after a long period of dryness. She is having accidents or frequent dribbling of urine. She has pain or burning on urination. | Urinary tract infection Emotional stress | Call your pediatrician. A urinary tract infection must be treated promptly. If the family is under stress, discuss important changes with your child but don't overload her with details. Try to uncover sources of stress at school. Encourage regular bathroom breaks. |
| Your child is badly constipated in addition to having urinary troubles. | Pressure on bladder due to full rectum (See "Stool Incontinence," page 150.) | Talk with your pediatrician, who will examine your child and recommend a treatment plan. Dietary changes may include extra fiber and fluids. |
| Your child is urinating very often or having occasional accidents. He is on medication for asthma. | Side effect of medication | Call your pediatrician, who may wish to modify your child's prescription. |
| Your child is constantly dribbling urine. Your child has previously been diagnosed with a spinal disorder or other chronic illness. | Neurogenic bladder | Discuss the problem with your pediatrician, who will suggest ways to keep your child's bladder functioning as best as possible. |
| Your child is passing unusually large volumes of urine day and night. He is overly thirsty even though he is drinking plenty of fluids. He is looking tired and thin. | Diabetes mellitus | Call your pediatrician, who will examine your child and perform diagnostic tests. If diabetes is confirmed, your child will need lifelong treatment. |
| Your child with epilepsy and developmental disabilities cries with wetting and has a lot of debris in the diaper after urinating. | Bladder stones, related to medication and metabolic effects | Talk with your child's pediatrician, who will likely test the blood and urine for stones; neurology consultation on seizures may be needed. |

## IN GENERAL

Children usually need to pass urine more often than adults because their bladders are smaller and they tend to drink more fluids relative to their size. In addition, young children may feel the need to pass urine more urgently because it takes a long time—several years—to develop mature control of the muscles that open and close the bladder. If a child has pain on urination, a urinary tract infection is the most likely reason, but several other conditions can also cause pain.

### Call your pediatrician right away if your child

- Cannot pass urine
- Is passing bloody urine
- Has a swelling in the abdomen and difficulty urinating
- Has pain on urination
- Is urinating with unusual frequency
- Is having daytime or nighttime wetting after achieving a pattern of dryness

### WARNING!

Some children who have pain from recurrent urinary tract infections are in the habit of passing urine infrequently. They may also be severely constipated. Train your child to respond promptly when she feels the urge to use the bathroom.

## Preventing Urinary Tract Infections

Pain on urination is most often caused by infection. Girls are particularly susceptible to urinary tract infections because their urethras are very short and germs from the bowel can easily pass along this route to the bladder. To reduce the risk of infection, girls should always wipe from front to back after bowel movements. A popular home remedy for infections is drinking cranberry or blueberry juice. Studies show that these fruits contain substances that make the urine more acidic and stop bacteria from growing. However, drinking plenty of plain water to flush out the bladder may be just as effective. Other helpful measures include the following:

- Wear cotton underpants and avoid very tight-fitting jeans and other pants.

- Avoid bubble baths, perfumed soaps, and other substances that can irritate the genitals and urethra.

- After swimming, change into dry clothes instead of sitting around in a wet suit.

- Avoid foods and beverages that can cause bladder irritation. Common offenders include colas and other caffeinated drinks, chocolate, and some spices.

| YOUR CONCERNS | POSSIBLE CAUSE | ACTION TO TAKE |
|---|---|---|
| *Your toilet-trained child is urinating often or with greater urgency. She has started wetting her bed or underclothes after a long dry period. She is having abdominal pain. Her urine smells bad. She has blood in her urine. She has pain or burning on urination.* | Urinary tract infection | Call your pediatrician. If a bacterial infection is present, it must be treated promptly to prevent complications. If the infection is caused by a virus, antibiotics won't help, but the infection should clear up by itself in about 4 days. In the meantime, your pediatrician will recommend ways to keep your child comfortable. |
| *Your baby's urine has an unpleasant smell. She is feverish and fretful.* | Urinary tract infection | Call your pediatrician, who will examine your baby, perform diagnostic tests including a urine culture, and prescribe appropriate treatment. |

| YOUR CONCERNS | POSSIBLE CAUSE | ACTION TO TAKE |
|---|---|---|
| *Your daughter is complaining of pain in the genital area. There is a discharge or redness around the vaginal opening.* | Foreign object in the vagina (Also see "Vaginal Itching/Discharge," page 164.) | Children sometime push foreign objects into their vaginas, causing pain and irritation. Call your pediatrician, who will examine your daughter, remove the object, and prescribe treatment if needed to prevent infection. |
| *Your son has signs of swelling or irritation at the tip of his penis. He is having difficulty passing urine and emptying his bladder.* | Inflammation of the glans penis (balanitis) Narrowing of the urethral opening (meatal stenosis) | Irritation can be caused by infection or, in circumcised boys, the growth of scar tissue at the opening (meatus) of the urethra. Talk with your pediatrician, who will examine your child and provide appropriate treatment. |
| *Your daughter is having difficulty passing urine. She feels irritation in her vaginal area.* | Labial adhesions | Occasionally, a girl's genital folds (labia) grow together and close off the vaginal and urethral openings. Talk with your pediatrician, who will examine your child and provide any necessary treatment. |
| *After a bath, your child complains of a burning sensation when he urinates.* | Soap in the urethra | Show him how to rub soap into a lather on his hands instead of rubbing it directly on his skin. Have him use a washcloth and rinse thoroughly with clear water. |
| *Your child is having difficulty passing urine. You can feel a lump on one side of his abdomen. He has blood in the urine. He has vomiting or pain.* | Wilms tumor (a type of kidney tumor) or another condition requiring immediate diagnosis and treatment | Call your pediatrician at once for an examination and diagnostic tests. Your child may have to be hospitalized for more extensive tests and treatment. |
| *Your child has redness, bruises, or other marks around the anus or vagina. There are unexplained marks elsewhere on the body. He is unwilling or too young to tell you where they came from. There are signs of urinary infection.* | Sexual abuse | Call your pediatrician, who will examine your child, determine the likely cause of the condition, and advise a plan for management. |

## IN GENERAL

Normal vaginal discharge is made up mostly of cells and secretions shed from the vaginal walls. It is white or colorless, has no unpleasant odor, and varies in consistency from water to a thick mucus. This discharge increases in quantity as your daughter nears her first period, and it changes after that according to each stage of her menstrual cycle. In a girl of any age, vaginal itching or pain, along with a discharge of unusual odor or color, may signal that she has inflammation of the vagina, called *vaginitis*. You should call your pediatrician if you suspect your child has vaginitis and get treatment.

School-aged and adolescent girls sometimes have vulvovaginitis—inflammation of the vagina *and* external genitalia—because the vagina and the bladder opening can easily be contaminated with fecal bacteria from the anus. Young girls are especially susceptible to infections of the genital area because the mucous membranes of their vulva and vagina are immature and lack the protection that comes with higher levels of estrogen that starts to rise in puberty. During puberty labial fat pads and pubic hair will develop over the external genitalia and provide yet another layer of protection.

Common causes of vulvovaginitis include irritating chemicals or allergens in soaps and lotions, along with germs carried by pinworms (see "Rectal Pain/Itching," page 128). Irritation may be caused by foreign objects inserted into the vagina, including tampons that adolescent girls may forget to remove. The overgrowth of yeasts may occur in girls with a chronic illness such as diabetes. Antibiotics and other medications can also upset the normal vaginal environment and allow bacteria or yeasts to spread (also see "Preventing Vulvovaginitis").

**Talk with your pediatrician if your daughter has**

- Recurrent vaginal itching, pain, and irritation
- An unusual vaginal discharge

### WARNING!

Don't buy over-the-counter antifungal or anti-yeast medications to treat your daughter's vaginitis. These products won't help if her condition is either noninfectious or caused by a different type of germ. Your pediatrician will prescribe appropriate treatment.

## Preventing Vulvovaginitis

To prevent vulvovaginitis, girls should practice healthy hygiene habits. Girls who often get irritations should use hypoallergenic soaps and avoid bubble baths and scented or deodorant soaps. It's important to change underwear daily and perhaps more often during menstrual periods. Tight clothing—such as pantyhose, tights, or form-fitting jeans—and underwear made of synthetic fabrics can form a warm, damp environment in which germs readily grow. Tight-fitting garments, such as swimsuits, should be washed after each wearing, and girls should wear loose-fitting cotton underwear and pantyhose with a cotton crotch. Adolescents should understand that shaving the area increases the chance of irritation.

| YOUR CONCERNS | POSSIBLE CAUSE | ACTION TO TAKE |
|---|---|---|
| *Your newborn daughter has a clear, white, or blood-tinged discharge from her vagina.* | Effects of withdrawal of the mother's hormones | This is normal and will stop after a few days. |
| *Your daughter has redness around her vulva and vagina. She also has a thick, white, curd-like discharge.* | Yeast infection | Talk with your pediatrician, who will examine your child and prescribe treatment. Use only the treatment your pediatrician prescribes. |
| *Your infant daughter has a diaper rash. She has a white discharge too.* | Monilial (yeast) diaper rash | Call your pediatrician, who will examine your baby and prescribe treatment. |
| *Your daughter has a foul-smelling discharge from her vagina.* | Foreign object in the vagina Infection | Call your pediatrician; your daughter may need treatment for an infection or removal of a foreign object. |
| *Your daughter is passing urine more often than usual. She also has redness and irritation around her vulva and vagina.* | Vulvovaginitis | Talk with your pediatrician, who will prescribe any necessary treatments. |
| *Your daughter aged 9 to 10 years complains of an increase in secretions from her vagina.* | Effects of hormones with approaching puberty | This effect is normal if the discharge is white or colorless and free of unpleasant odor. Talk with your daughter about the changes in her body that she's about to experience. |
| *Your preadolescent daughter has a blood-tinged discharge.* | Foreign object in the vagina Infection | Talk with your pediatrician, who will examine your child and determine whether treatment is required. |
| *Your daughter has bruises or other marks in addition to redness and discharge around her vulva, vagina, or anus.* | Sexual abuse | Consult your pediatrician, who will treat the symptoms and determine the cause, and may be able to find out what's happening with your daughter. |

## IN GENERAL

Your pediatrician checks your child's eyes routinely at regular well-child visits. Provided his eyes are developing normally and you have no family medical history of serious eye disorders, formal vision testing isn't usually done until 3 years of age, when a child is capable of following directions and describing what he sees. Your pediatrician may also use a specially designed camera to look for potential eye problems that can affect vision even before 3 years of age. If screening tests show defects in vision or signs of eye disease, your pediatrician will recommend further evaluation by a pediatric ophthalmologist.

Despite what many people believe, the common vision problems—nearsightedness, farsightedness, and astigmatism—aren't made worse by reading too much or sitting too close to the television (Figure 2-20). Nor does wearing glasses weaken the eyes. A tendency to these vision problems usually runs in the family. (For problems with the alignment of the eyes or diseases that affect the eyes, see "Cross-eye, Wandering Eye," page 60, and "Eye Problems," page 80).

### Talk with your pediatrician if your child

- Squints a lot in an apparent effort to see more clearly
- Bends her head unusually close to her work
- Complains of headaches, eyestrain, or blurry vision after reading or doing close work
- Cannot see close-up objects clearly
- Regularly twists her head to view objects
- Sees distant objects in a blur

> **WARNING!**
> Nearsightedness often emerges when the eye structures change in size and shape during the growth spurt at puberty.

### Dealing With Color Blindness

Color blindness is a common visual defect that's rarely a significant handicap, although people who are color blind can't pilot aircrafts or hold other jobs where the inability to perceive colors could be hazardous. Those who are color blind see colors but not of the same hue or intensity as others.

| YOUR CONCERNS | POSSIBLE CAUSE | ACTION TO TAKE |
|---|---|---|
| *Your child is having trouble seeing distant objects. He squints a lot. He holds a book very close to his face. He bends very close to the surface he's writing on.* | Myopia (nearsightedness) | Talk with your pediatrician, who will examine your child and determine whether referral to an ophthalmologist is warranted. |
| *Your child complains of sore eyes or headaches after reading. Objects that are close look blurry to him.* | Hyperopia (farsightedness) | Most children are born with some degree of farsightedness that gradually resolves itself, but ask your pediatrician to examine your child and determine whether he should be seen by an ophthalmologist. |
| *Your child is complaining of blurry vision at any distance.* | Astigmatism (a condition in which the eye's refractive surfaces are curved in such a way that light isn't sharply focused inside the eye) | Your pediatrician will examine your child and may provide a referral to an ophthalmologist for further examination. |
| *Your child is seeing double. She covers one eye or tilts her head to focus on objects.* | Disorder that requires diagnosis and treatment | Talk with your pediatrician promptly to arrange an examination and possible referral to another health specialist. |

Most color-blind people can't tell red from green; some with a mild form of the condition have difficulty only in dim light. A more unusual defect is the inability to distinguish yellow and blue.

Color blindness is inherited, usually passed from mother to son; few females are affected. Parents may suspect color blindness when their child doesn't learn to name certain colors; other cases are diagnosed at about the time the child starts preschool or kindergarten. While the condition can't be cured, wearing color-filter glasses or contact lenses can improve some your child's perception of contrasts, although they don't help your child see colors normally.

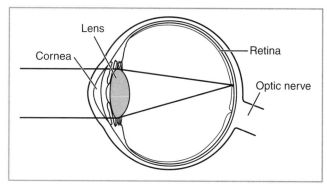

**Figure 2-20.** How the eye sees. Rays of light pass through the cornea and lens to the retina. From there, the light impulses are sent to the optic nerve and then to the visual cortex; the area of the brain that interprets what we see.

When our eye focuses on an object, the image is projected through the pupil (the black spot at the center of the eye) to the retina, which is a multilayered structure on the inside of the eyeball. The image is received upside down, but the brain's visual cortex interprets the message and lets us perceive the image correctly.

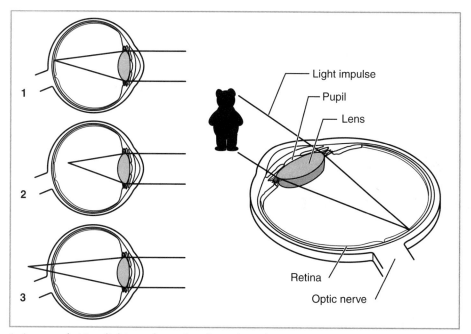

1. In normal vision, light rays focus sharply on the retina.

2. In nearsightedness (myopia), light rays from a distance come to a sharp focus in front of the retina. Blurry vision caused by this condition can be corrected by wearing glasses with concave lenses.

3. In farsightedness (hyperopia), light rays from close objects come to a sharp focus behind the retina. People with this condition can see clearly if they wear glasses with convex lenses.

## IN GENERAL

In children, vomiting is a common response to various events or stimuli, including illness, ingestion of toxic substances, or emotional stress brought about by pressure at school or tension at home. An isolated vomiting episode is not a cause for concern. Vomiting that happens again and again, however, may be a sign that your child needs medical attention, especially if she also has abdominal pain, fever, or headache.

Forceful vomiting in babies is quite different from the normal developmental phase of spitting up (see page 16). To learn more about the special problem of induced vomiting in teens, see "Eating Disorders," page 184).

### Call your pediatrician right away if your child is vomiting and has

- Swelling and sharp pain in his abdomen
- Blood or bile (green material) in his vomit
- Confusion, lethargy (a lack of energy), or irritability
- Diarrhea for more than 12 hours
- Signs of dehydration such as dry lips and a very small amount of urine

### WARNING!

Occasional vomiting isn't a cause for worry, but if your baby vomits after every feeding in a 12-hour period, call your pediatrician.

## Feeding a Vomiting Child

Vomiting is common and uncomfortable. Fortunately, it's usually not serious and quickly passes. While a child is vomiting, care should be taken to prevent dehydration due to fluid loss, especially if she also has a fever or diarrhea. She will probably be able to drink fluids before she feels well enough to eat again. Encourage her to drink frequently, even if she can manage only a few sips at a time.

Let your child choose the drinks he enjoys. For a toddler or preschooler, a commercial rehydrating solution is suitable. A school-aged child may prefer popsicles that contain electrolytes. When giving your child fluids, encourage him to start slowly by taking a couple of small sips and waiting 20 minutes before taking another drink. Avoid beverages high in sugar of caffeine, which may make the fluid loss worse.

If your child vomits after drinking, the best course is 1 or 2 hours with no food or fluids—not even water. Your child may be able to take just spoonfuls of a liquid or prefer to suck on ice chips for a while. Call your pediatrician if the vomiting continues for more than 6 hours or your child has a stomachache and fever. Don't give your child any medications to stop vomiting except as prescribed by your pediatrician.

When your child hasn't vomited for several hours and can keep fluids down, let her try a small helping of any food she chooses from her usual diet. Good choices to begin with might be toast, oatmeal, a soft-boiled egg, bananas, applesauce, or other cooked fruits. Don't give your child milk, dairy products, and foods containing large amounts of insoluble fiber—such as raw fruits and vegetables and bran cereals—until your child's stomach feels settled. Get her back on a normal diet as soon as possible.

| YOUR CONCERNS | POSSIBLE CAUSE | ACTION TO TAKE |
|---|---|---|
| Your toddler or older child who is vomiting also has diarrhea and mild fever. | Gastroenteritis (inflammation of the stomach and intestinal lining) Food poisoning | Withhold solid foods, but give your child an electrolyte replacement fluid as soon as she can keep it down. Give her small amounts, no more than 1 ounce, every 15 minutes or so. As the symptoms improve, have her resume a normal diet. If the symptoms last longer than 12 hours, call your pediatrician for advice. |
| Your child has symptoms of an infection such as a sore throat, earache, or burning on urination. | Infection | Seek your pediatrician's help for treatment of the underlying infection. Vomiting will stop as the symptoms improve. |
| Your child seems tense or upset. He has no other symptoms of illness. | Stress, anxiety | Let your child talk about what's bothering him. If no cause is obvious and vomiting continues or becomes more frequent, talk with your pediatrician. |
| Your child feels nauseated and vomits when riding in cars, boats, or elevators. | Motion sickness | Ask your pediatrician how to prevent motion sickness (also see "Dizziness," page 72). |
| Your baby younger than 2 months vomits forcefully after every feeding. | Pyloric stenosis (a narrowing of the passage between the stomach and small intestine) or another condition that requires treatment | Call your pediatrician, who will examine your baby and advise on treatment. |
| There is blood or greenish bile in your baby's vomit. She is crying, pulling her legs up, distressed, and in pain. | Gastrointestinal blockage that requires diagnosis and treatment (eg, folding of the intestine called *intussusception*) | Call your pediatrician right away. Your baby needs urgent medical attention. |
| Your child's vomiting comes after a fall or head injury. Your child becomes more and more sleepy or less responsive. | Head injury | Call your pediatrician without delay. |
| Your child is irritable or drowsy. He has complained of a headache. He has a fever. | Meningitis or another serious disease of the nervous system | Call your pediatrician without delay. |

## IN GENERAL

Most children take their first steps around their first birthday, although some perfectly healthy children don't walk independently until about 18 months of age. The developmental stages leading up to the first steps follow a recognized sequence, starting with rolling over and progressing through sitting up, crawling, and cruising to walking unaided (see "Developmental Milestones for the First 3 Years," page 66). A few independent children, however, skip over the crawling stage; they go directly from scooting about on their bottoms to walking. No matter what style of locomotion your baby prefers, what's important is that he uses each arm and leg equally and coordinates the two sides of his body.

In the first stages of walking, a toddler will plant her legs wide apart, point her toes outward, hold her arms bent at her elbows, and rock from side to side as she moves along (Figure 2-21). Although she trips and falls a good deal at the beginning, once she's been walking for a few months she'll be confident enough to carry out complicated maneuvers, such as stepping sideways and backward, stooping to pick up and carry a toy, or throwing a ball while on the move. As your child continues to gain experience, she will experiment with running, which will again lead to falling. This is normal, to fall safely, and it will be important to your future athlete, to fall safely with sports.

· · · · · · · · · · · · · · · · · · · · · · · · · · · · · · · · · · · · ·

### Talk with your pediatrician if your child is

- Not walking by 17 months of age
- Still walking on the balls of his feet by 3 years of age
- Not using both arms and legs symmetrically

· · · · · · · · · · · · · · · · · · · · · · · · · · · · · · · · · · · · ·

### WARNING!

Baby walkers are a serious safety hazard. They often put young children in danger of falling down open stairways and get them into dangerous places that would otherwise be out of their reach. The American Academy of Pediatrics strongly urges parents not to use baby walkers.

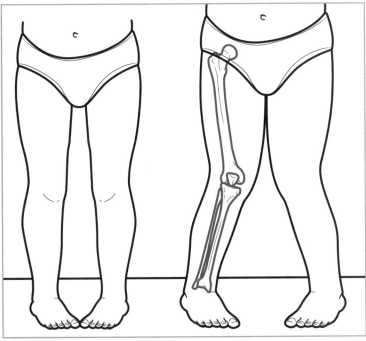

**Figure 2-21.** The typical bowleg and intoeing of the early months gradually straighten out over the first 3 years. As the child begins to walk, however, the inward curve of the lower leg (left) may turn to mild knock knee between ages 2 and 3 (right). The legs generally straighten out by about 10 years without treatment. Braces and corrective shoes are rarely helpful. Most youngsters have straight legs by adolescence, although a tendency to intoeing or out-toeing may run in some families.

## Shoes for Active Toddlers

In the early months, babies' feet develop best if they're not confined in shoes; socks are all that's needed to keep their feet warm; however, once children start walking outdoors, they need shoes for protection. Look for comfortable shoes with nonskid soles, such as sneakers, that will help keep your toddler steady on slippery floors. Buy well-made shoes, but don't spend a lot of money. At this stage, your child's feet grow so rapidly that the first pair of shoes won't last more than 2 or 3 months. You should check the fit about once a month; the top of your child's big toe should be about finger-width distance from the inside edge of the shoe. It's better to have no shoes at all than shoes that are too tight.

| YOUR CONCERNS | POSSIBLE CAUSE | ACTION TO TAKE |
|---|---|---|
| Your toddler aged 15 months is showing no signs of getting ready to walk. He shows little interest in moving about. | Developmental delay (See page 64.) | Talk with your pediatrician to arrange an evaluation of your toddler's development. |
| Your child turns her toes noticeably inward when she walks. | Normal developmental stage | This tendency usually disappears as your child matures. It rarely interferes with mobility (see "Bowleg, Knock Knee, Intoeing," page 46). |
| Your child is limping. She is complaining of pain. | Injury Infection Arthritis Another condition that requires treatment | If you can't see and remove an obvious source of pain, such as a splinter, ask your pediatrician to determine the cause of the limp. |
| Your child limps but isn't complaining of pain. He walks with a waddling gait. | Neuromuscular weakness Hip joint disorder | Talk with your pediatrician, who will examine your child and determine whether he should be seen by another health specialist. |
| Your child often walks on the balls of her feet after many months of walking. | Habit Neuromuscular problem | Although normal during early walking, walking on the toes or the balls of the feet after 2 years of age should be evaluated. Ask your pediatrician to determine whether your child has a problem that requires treatment. |
| Your toddler has difficulty walking. He falls a lot and has trouble getting on his feet again. He uses his hands to climb up his legs when trying to stand. He tends to waddle when he walks. | Muscular dystrophy or another neuromuscular condition that requires diagnosis and treatment | Call your pediatrician, who will examine your child and may refer you to another health specialist. If the diagnosis is confirmed, your child will need long-term treatment. Your pediatrician will also help you find support groups for children and parents. |

## IN GENERAL

Many short-term illnesses can leave a child feeling weak and shaky, especially if she has a fever and stays in bed for a few days. Most of the time she will quickly get her strength back once she's on her feet again, eating and exercising normally; however, weakness that doesn't go away or gets worse requires medical attention.

The term *congenital* refers to symptoms that are present at birth or appear soon after birth. Some children are born with congenital weakness, whereas others develop weakness later in childhood or adolescence. Certain forms of muscle weakness are progressive; a child loses strength and mobility slowly over time and may eventually lose the ability to walk. Others come on suddenly and severely—sometimes due to infection or another illness—and the subsequent course of the weakness depends on the cause and whether treatment is available.

The outward appearance of a child's muscle isn't always a good sign of strength. Children with certain forms of muscular dystrophy—a progressive muscle disease—have calf muscles that look large and overdeveloped, although they are actually weak. On the other hand, many young children with scrawny-looking limbs have normal strength.

Your pediatrician will determine whether your child has weakness based on a thorough evaluation. The physical examination typically includes an evaluation of muscle strength and motor function. Your pediatrician will also check your child's muscle bulk and tone (the resistance of the resting muscle), as well as posture (see "Posture Defects," page 126), movement, reflexes, and range of motion. Signs of problems include weakness, low muscle tone, postural problems, abnormal reflexes, and contractures (shortening of muscles). Your pediatrician may also examine your child for subtle signs in her eye muscles, face, and other areas depending on the circumstances.

### Talk with your pediatrician if

- Your baby uses his arm and leg on only one side to crawl.
- Your child is more and more clumsy and fatigued.
- Your child lacks energy, despite plenty of food and rest.

### WARNING!

Don't use honey when preparing food for your baby younger than 1 year. Honey may harbor *Clostridium botulinum* spores, which can cause life-threatening food poisoning known as botulism, with severe muscle weakness and difficulties in breathing and feeding.

## Diagnosing Muscular Dystrophy

One example is Duchenne muscular dystrophy, an inherited muscle disorder that begins in early childhood. Without treatment, Duchenne muscular dystrophy in a person is usually fatal by the second or third decade of life, but currently available therapies can extend the life expectancy into the fourth or even fifth decade. At the moment there is no definitive cure, but doctors are continually researching possible treatments.

Like hemophilia (see "Bleeding and Bruising," page 42) and color blindness (see page 166), Duchenne muscular dystrophy is linked to the X chromosome and is thus passed from mothers to sons. Only boys are usually affected; some girls develop muscle weakness and cardiac problems. Thanks to our expanding knowledge of genetics, a woman with a family medical history of Duchenne muscular dystrophy can often find out whether she's a carrier and her risk for passing it on to her children. Genetic counselors can inform prospective parents of their risks of having an affected child and families of technologies such as preimplantation genetic diagnosis that involves genetic screening of embryos prior to implantation in an in vitro fertilization procedure.

| YOUR CONCERNS | POSSIBLE CAUSE | ACTION TO TAKE |
|---|---|---|
| Your baby is slower than others her age in reaching her motor (movement) milestones (see "Developmental Delay," page 64). Her limbs and muscles feel oddly soft and mushy. | Hypotonia (which can be caused by problems with the central or peripheral nervous systems) Benign congenital hypotonia (a neuromuscular disorder that does not get worse but often results with delays in achieving developmental milestones) | Talk with your pediatrician, who will evaluate your child's development and may advise you to see another specialist, if necessary. |
| Your baby feels weak and listless. He is falling behind in developmental milestones (see "Developmental Delay," page 64). He gets tired quickly. His face looks swollen. | Thyroid disorder | Babies are generally checked at birth to make sure their thyroid glands are working properly. Talk with your pediatrician, who will examine your child and order laboratory tests if a thyroid problem is suspected. |
| Your son is having difficulty walking or standing again after he falls. He uses his hands to climb up his legs when trying to stand. He falls unusually often or has a waddling walk. Other family members have had muscular dystrophy. | Muscular dystrophy (a genetic disorder) or another neuromuscular condition that requires diagnosis and treatment | Call your pediatrician, who will examine your child and may refer you to another specialist. If the diagnosis is confirmed, your child will need long-term treatment. Your pediatrician will also help you find support groups for parents and children. |
| Your older child or teen has been unusually tired since recently having a sore throat. | Infectious mononucleosis ("mono," a viral infection) Rheumatic fever or heart muscle disease (rare) | Talk with your pediatrician. There is no specific treatment for mononucleosis, and most children are back to normal in 4 to 6 weeks. Your pediatrician will evaluate your child's general health and advise you about rest and recovery. |
| Your school-aged child or teen is lacking energy as the day wears on. Her eyelids droop in the morning. She reports double vision sometimes and has a nasal voice. | Myasthenia gravis (an illness that affects the nervous system, which causes weakness in certain muscles) | Call your pediatrician, who will examine your child and provide a referral, if needed, to a pediatric neurologist. |
| Your child has weakness that started in his legs and now affects his arms as well. He had a viral (respiratory or gastrointestinal) infection in the last 10 days or so. He is irritable. | Guillain-Barré syndrome (a nerve condition that may follow a viral illness) | Call your pediatrician, who will examine your child and may recommend hospitalization. Most children get better in 2 to 3 weeks, but a few may have long-term effects. |

## IN GENERAL

Your child's exact weight is less important than the rate at which she's growing and gaining weight. Still, a child's loss of or inability to gain weight is worrisome at any stage, except in the first week of life, when most healthy babies lose up to 10% of their birth weight. Babies generally start to gain weight on the fifth day of life and are back to their birth weight by about 10 to 14 days of age. From then on weight gain should continue until growth is completed. Good nutrition is essential in a child's first year because that's when the rate of growth is greatest. An unusual slowing down in a baby's or toddler's growth rate may signal failure to thrive (see "Growth Problems," page 92), which may have both physical and emotional roots. This condition requires a pediatrician's attention to determine the cause and treatment.

The rate of weight gain isn't steady; children typically grow in spurts, with a noticeable gain in height/length often followed by a coming-together phase when their weight catches up to their height.

After a period of rapid growth in the first 12 months of life, your child will undergo a relative slowdown in his growth rate, which is offset by a decrease in his appetite. This cycle recurs to some degree throughout childhood, culminating in a noticeable growth spurt during adolescence. At that time your child will have a huge appetite as he starts to fill out. Although obesity is one of the leading health problems in the United States, unhealthy weight loss due to eating disorders is also a major problem, especially in teenaged girls (see page 184).

**Talk with your pediatrician if your child is**

- Losing or unable to gain weight
- Gaining weight out of proportion to her height

### WARNING!

Overweight children often are troubled by their weight problem but find it impossible to slim down without professional help. It's hard for your child to change his diet if you're overeating, and crash diets can be physically and emotionally harmful and unsustainable. Sensible family eating habits and exercise are the keys to successful weight control and are healthy for the whole family.

## Helping Your Child Lose Weight

Childhood obesity has become a more and more common problem. In fact, over the past 2 decades it has doubled in children and tripled in teens in the United States. Throughout a child's lifetime, chronic obesity can lead to serious health problems, including diabetes, cirrhosis of the liver, and high blood pressure. It also can cause psychological stresses associated with feeling different from peers and being bulled and teased, which can lead to depression and low self-esteem.

The American Academy of Pediatrics believes that both parents and pediatricians need to take steps to prevent the development of overweight problems in children. Your pediatrician can monitor your child's weight gain from birth at each visit and help make sure that it remains within normal guidelines as he grows. Your doctor can calculate your child's body mass index (BMI). To calculate BMI, take your child's weight in pounds, divide by the height in inches squared, and then multiply by 703. You can also find an online calculator on the Centers

Disease Control and Prevention Web site. A child with a BMI at or above 85th percentile for age and sex is considered overweight; when the BMI is at or above the 95th percentile, he's considered obese.

You can help your child lose excess weight by watching his portion sizes and limiting foods that contain excess calories with little nutritional value. Among those are cakes, cookies, candy, ice cream, and sweetened drinks (including juice). Cut down on the amount of saturated fat in your child's diet, and increase your child's intake of fresh fruits, vegetables, and whole grains. Offer your children water instead of sodas or juices, and encourage exercise, such as family walks or bike rides, as well as healthy eating for the whole family.

| YOUR CONCERNS | POSSIBLE CAUSE | ACTION TO TAKE |
|---|---|---|
| *Your baby is lethargic (lacking energy) or fretful. She is feeding unusually slowly. She seems to be ill.* | Underlying illness | Call your pediatrician, who will evaluate your baby's health. |
| *Your breastfed baby is losing or unable to gain weight, despite feeding eagerly.* | Insufficient calories | Talk with your pediatrician promptly. If your baby is 6 months of age, he may be ready for solid foods. Your pediatrician may recommend seeing a breastfeeding consultant. |
| *Your formula-fed baby is losing or unable to gain weight. She drains every bottle.* | Insufficient calories | Talk with your pediatrician. Be careful to mix formula according to the directions. Increase the amount you offer in the bottle, and let your baby stop when she's ready. If your baby is 5 months or older, ask whether it's time to try solids. Don't give her juice. |
| *Your bottle-fed baby is gaining weight too fast.* | Overfeeding | Discuss your concerns with your pediatrician. Don't offer food every time your baby cries; he may simply want attention, changing, or distraction. The crying may also signal a change in sleep pattern or that your baby is ready for solid foods. |
| *Your school-aged child is overweight and has almost always been chubby.* | Excess weight in this age group is frequently due to physical inactivity and overeating. The whole family should work together to encourage more healthful habits. | Cut down on fats, and don't serve a lot of sweets and other high-calorie, low-nutrient foods. Encourage more physical activity. Serve meals at the dining table, not in front of the television. Stop juice completely or at least dilute it (half juice, half water). If your child is grossly overweight, ask your pediatrician for diet and exercise guidelines. Lead by example. Healthy food is good for the whole family regardless of weight. |
| *Your toddler or school-aged child has lost weight. She is pale or unusually tired.* | Illness that requires diagnosis and treatment | Call your pediatrician without delay to schedule an examination. |

## IN GENERAL

Children breathe quietly and with little to no effort when their airways are working normally. But if the tubes that carry air into your child's lungs are blocked, you'll hear a high-pitched sound as air forces itself through them. *Wheezing* is the whistling sound you hear when your child breathes in and out through narrowed airways. Common causes of air-flow blockage include airway swelling due to infection, blockage by a foreign object, or inflammation and bronchial muscle spasms due to asthma. Some airway problems cause noisy breathing or wheezing only as a child breathes in; this sound, called *stridor,* is a symptom of croup (see "Dealing With Croup," page 58).

............................................

### Call 911 or your local emergency number right away if your child is wheezing and

- Has severe difficulty in breathing
- Has bluish color around the lips
- Abnormal drowsiness
- Inability to speak or make normal sounds

............................................

**WARNING!**
A child may suddenly start wheezing when a harmful object gets lodged in his airway. Isolated bouts of mild wheezing may be caused by a minor respiratory infection. But if your child is wheezing all the time, bring it to your pediatrician's attention.

## Why Small Children Wheeze More

Wheezing is particularly noticeable in children younger than 3 years. This is because their airways are small and more prone to blockage caused by muscle spasms, inflammation that leads to swelling of the mucous membranes, and buildup of secretions.

Environmental pollution, including cigarette smoke caused by members of the household, is one of the factors known to cause airway disease and wheezing in young children. If any of your family members smokes, strongly encourage him or her to quit.

| YOUR CONCERNS | POSSIBLE CAUSE | ACTION TO TAKE |
|---|---|---|
| *Your infant makes loud wheezing sounds as she breathes in. She is eating and growing normally.* | Laryngomalacia or tracheomalacia (a short-lived, floppiness of the larynx [voice box] that is common in infants) | As long as your infant is feeding, growing, and playing well, action is unnecessary. The sounds will lessen and taper off by about 18 months of age. But bring the wheezing to your pediatrician's attention. |
| *Your child also has a runny nose or cough.* | Common cold | Give your child liquids to thin his secretions, and keep your child comfortable. If his symptoms get worse or don't clear up within a week, ask your pediatrician for advice. |
| *Your infant is also coughing. Her wheezing came on 3 to 4 days after a cold. She is breathing fast and having difficulty feeding.* | Bronchiolitis (viral infection) | Viral infections can occur at any time but are very common in winter and spring. Keep your infant comfortable. If her symptoms get worse or don't improve in 3 days, call your pediatrician. |

| YOUR CONCERNS | POSSIBLE CAUSE | ACTION TO TAKE |
|---|---|---|
| Your child coughs repeatedly or has difficulty breathing, especially at night. Your family has a history of allergies or asthma. | Asthma | Call your pediatrician, who will examine your child. If your pediatrician confirms this diagnosis, he or she will prescribe treatment. |
| Your child is having trouble catching his breath. He has a barking cough and hoarseness. His symptoms are worse at night. He recently had a respiratory infection. | Laryngotracheobronchitis (croup) | Give your child acetaminophen or ibuprofen to relieve his discomfort, and use a cold mist vaporizer at night. If symptoms persist, call your pediatrician (also see "Dealing With Croup," page 58). |
| Your child is having severe difficulty breathing. Her wheezing came on suddenly. She may have choked on a bit of food or a small object. | Foreign object in airway (most common in children between 6 months and 2 years of age) | This may be an emergency. If your child is younger than 1 year, follow the first aid guide for choking (see page 215). For an older child, try the Heimlich maneuver (see page 216) to dislodge the object. If your child is turning blue or having trouble breathing, have somebody call 911 or your local emergency number while you keep trying to clear her airway. |
| Your child has a deep, chesty cough and a fever. He is breathing rapidly. The space between his ribs appears to suck in every time he takes a breath. | Pneumonia | Call your pediatrician (see "Breathing Difficulty/Breathlessness," page 50). Acetaminophen or ibuprofen may soothe your child's discomfort. |
| Your child snores and breathes through her mouth. She has a runny nose. Sometimes she gets an earache. Her voice sounds blocked when she speaks. | Adenoidal hypertrophy (enlarged adenoids [tonsils in the pharynx]) (The enlargement may be due to allergies or colds, or your child may be born with large adenoids.) | Consult your pediatrician, who will examine your child and determine whether treatment is needed (also see "Runny/Stuffy Nose," page 132). |

**CHAPTER 3**

# Common Physical and Mental Health Symptoms in Teenagers

## THE CHALLENGES OF ADOLESCENCE

While teenagers are brimming with health, energy, and strength, several concerns, problems, and disorders can make their first appearance in the teen years or reach a peak during these years. The physical developmental, psychosocial, and mental health changes and growth that occur during adolescence have a bearing on the development and progression of various physical and mental health concerns and conditions, as well as typical pubertal development.

As your teenager grows up, he may be less open to sharing concerns with you about his physical and mental health. However, during the school-age and teenage years, it is important for you to try to keep the lines of communication open. It is also important to continue to bring your child in for annual well-child visits with his pediatrician. Your teen can benefit from the open, trusting relationship he establishes with his pediatrician over the years. In addition, ongoing and regular screening for physical, psychosocial, and mental health concerns using evidence-based tools and strategies in your pediatrician's office as part of the well-child visit is effective and important to try to address early or prevent physical, mental, emotional, and behavioral health disorders.

Pressure and stress to perform more independently at school, among peers, and within the family can present symptoms of anxiety, depression, performance anxiety, mood swing, fatigue, substance abuse, and eating disorders in some teens. Red-flag symptoms for possible mental health concerns may or may not become apparent in some cases, and they may only emerge as physical ailments or as worsening symptoms of chronic conditions that are already present.

It is a good idea for teenagers to take an increasingly more active role in caring for and understanding their body and physical and mental health well-being over time as is developmentally appropriate. This also helps teens to prepare and plan for their transition to the adult health care system. Several of the symptoms in this chapter may appear in younger children but more often appear in teenagers. However, at any age, significant concerns always need to be addressed early in partnership with your child's pediatrician.

Your teen is at a good age to start figuring out his interests (eg, art, drama, mentoring, volunteering, sports). As his parent, help him find activities that most appeal to him. Teenagers who participate in activities of interest are more confident, manage their time better, and do better in school than those who do not. Such activities can nurture your teen's strengths and assets, which will help him successfully navigate this developmental stage.

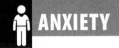 

## IN GENERAL

Every child has occasional short-lived and situational anxiety symptoms when apprehension may be intensified by fight-or-flight primitive symptoms such as dry mouth, racing pulse, sweating, tremors, and "butterflies in the stomach." As toddlers and preschoolers grow, a period of separation anxiety is a normal developmental stage (see "Fears," page 84). In later years, anxiety symptoms often occur in anticipation of or during known, short-lived stressful situations, such as a test or speech, to help deal with the tension. Fortunately, the anxious feeling evaporates and may turn into relief as soon as a taxing event is over.

However, some teenagers have anxiety symptoms when there is a significant event that they are unable to effectively cope with. After the event, the teen returns to his baseline low level of stress. In some teens, anxiety may also occur when there is no one precipitating event. In these teens, anxiety may be the result of a chronically stressful situation, such as family tension, financial strains, a relative with alcoholism, or illness. Viewed in this light, anxiety is a response to events beyond a teen's control or ability to effectively cope with one or more stressors. For many of these teens, anxiety becomes a chronic condition that interferes with school, friendships, and work. Some teens experience anxiety symptoms when faced with the typical challenges of adolescence because of their temperament, skills, and limited social supports. According to recent national studies, about 5% to 8% of teenagers have an anxiety disorder.

An anxiety disorder can take on various forms in response to varying perceived stressors, and it will cause serious difficulties in daily living if not recognized and treated. Examples of anxiety disorders include obsessive-compulsive disorder, post-traumatic stress disorder, panic disorder, social and specific phobias, and generalized anxiety disorder. Some teens have panic attacks, a manifestation of several anxiety disorders that may occur several times a day without warning. During an attack, fearfulness is worsened by symptoms such as a pounding heart,

clammy skin, trembling, diarrhea, and nausea. Many teens hyperventilate (fast and shallow breathing), leading to light-headedness or fainting; some teens actually fear that they are about to die. The pediatrician will ask you or your child screening questions and may recommend counseling or referral to a psychiatrist or psychologist. A course of medication may be helpful in addition to counseling if your teen is found to have an anxiety disorder. Additional strategies to help a teen reduce her anxiety symptoms include regular aerobic exercise, meditation, and biofeedback.

### Talk With Your Teen's Pediatrician If Your Teen

- Refuses to go to school
- Routinely avoids family and social activities and spends his time alone
- Becomes upset if kept from a set routine or doing things his way
- Has noticeable weight loss or gain along with a change in behavior
- Appears more anxious or fearful than his siblings or peers

> **WARNING!**
> Certain medications used to relieve anxiety may produce additional symptoms, especially if not used exactly as prescribed. Follow the pediatrician's instructions and call right away if new symptoms appear during therapy.

## Procrastination and Performance Anxiety

"Stubborn," "lazy," "inattentive," "puts everything off until tomorrow": a child who hears himself described in these harsh terms often enough will eventually incorporate them into his own self-image. He fails to try because that's what he thinks others expect. The effects can be disastrous.

The procrastinating teenager may fail to hand in his homework because he was afraid to ask how to go about it. Chores don't get done because he'd rather be called lazy than fail to reach the standards he thinks his parents expect. Because he has a poor sense of organization, he can't break down a task into manageable components. When he fails to begin, he is accused of not trying or caring.

A teen can benefit from help with organization—an orderly space where he can keep necessary items used for school, sports, and free time; a desk or table that is kept clear for homework; a daily checklist of essential tasks; and a calendar marked with future assignments. Steady encouragement and positive reinforcement are essential; parents should show they're pleased if a job is done—not perfectly, but well enough and on time. What's important is that parents help their teen see that completing large tasks begins by simply putting one foot in front of the other. There are some teens who have performance anxiety and who fail to complete certain tasks that require them to get up in front of a group for a speech or complete an examination. These concerns need to be addressed and may require counseling with a mental health professional recommended by your pediatrician.

| YOUR CONCERNS | POSSIBLE CAUSE | ACTION TO TAKE |
|---|---|---|
| Your teenager is complaining of palpitations or chest pain. She has vague symptoms such as a headache or stomachache. She uses these symptoms as an excuse to avoid difficult tasks or going to school. | Anxiety Hyperventilation syndrome Physical illness Manipulative behavior | Question your teen about situations that may be bothering her. Make an appointment with her pediatrician, who will rule out physical illness and suggest ways to help her learn how to develop coping strategies, or refer her to a mental health provider for counseling. |
| Your teenager is refusing to go to school or is playing hooky. | Anxiety (school phobia) Boredom Negativism Bullying Abuse | Talk with your teen's teachers and include your teen to identify school-related problems. Work with your pediatrician and teen to develop coping strategies. Make an appointment or ask your teen's pediatrician to recommend a mental health professional. Find ways to involve your teen in making and implementing decisions that affect him. |
| Your teen has abruptly developed signs of anxiety. She is having problems at school. Her behavior has changed for the worse. You suspect she may be using drugs. | Effects of illegal drugs | Talk with your teen about legal and health implications of drug use. Let her know where you stand on this issue. Talk with your teen's teachers to identify problems at school. Talk with your teen's pediatrician or schedule a visit for your teen. Ask your pediatrician's advice for dealing with the situation. |
| Your teenager is having attacks of rapid breathing with other symptoms. He is intensely fearful during these episodes. | Panic attacks | Ask your teenager whether specific situations or people are the source of his worry. Schedule an appointment with your pediatrician. Your pediatrician may do screening and may recommend counseling, mental health referral, and, in some cases, medication to treat your teen's anxiety. |
| Your teenager is having problems with schoolwork. He is disruptive in class. He fails to hand in assignments and acts like the class clown. | Learning difficulty Behavioral problem Performance anxiety/ procrastination Attention-deficit/ hyperactivity disorder (ADHD) | Talk with your teen's teachers, including your teen, to identify specific problems. Help him to organize his study space and work habits at home. Your pediatrician should perform an evaluation including a thorough history and physical examination. Behavioral rating scales, examining issues at home and school, may be needed. |
| Your teen is having symptoms such as frequent urination, fatigue, weight loss, or eye problems. | Physical illness mimicking anxiety, such as diabetes mellitus or thyroid disorder | Talk with or schedule an appointment with your child's pediatrician, who will examine your child to determine whether a medical problem exists and prescribe appropriate treatment. These symptoms could also be manifestations of anxiety. |

## IN GENERAL

Teenagers, like adults, have short-lived mood changes; they can be elated today but down in the dumps tomorrow. However, there is an important difference between feeling sadness (reactive depression) and having the emotional illness called clinical depression. If occasional periods of sadness (especially after a temporary setback) lift after a few days, there is no cause for concern. But teens who persist for weeks in feelings of hopelessness, worthlessness, futility, and anger need help to improve their mental health and well-being.

Although clinical depression can affect children in all age groups, teens are particularly vulnerable. A teenager who suffers from depression is at greater risk for suicide, the most serious consequence of depression.

### Call Your Teen's Pediatrician Right Away If Your Teen

- Is preoccupied with death or expresses a wish to end his life
- Seems to improve from depression by giving away treasured possessions
- Attempts to set his affairs in order
- Hints he has the means to end his life, should he decide to do so

### WARNING!

Depression tends to run in families. The causes may be rooted in brain chemistry and behavior. If you recognize symptoms of depression in any family members, try to persuade them to seek medical help. Although depression tends to happen again in the future, people with depression usually respond well to treatment.

| YOUR CONCERNS | POSSIBLE CAUSE | ACTION TO TAKE |
|---|---|---|
| Your teenager is extremely solitary and withdrawn almost all the time. She is overly concerned about aspects of her appearance. | Teenage behavior<br>Shyness<br>Self-consciousness about a perceived physical or social problem (ie, bullying)<br>Abuse<br>Depression<br>Also see "Eating Disorders," page 184. | Provide opportunities for socialization to extend but not overwhelm her capabilities. Talk with your pediatrician to determine what can be done to cope with a problem such as acne, obesity, abuse, or bullying. Ask your teen's pediatrician to do a formal screening for depression or refer to a mental health professional if needed. Reassure but don't patronize. |
| Your teen's behavior has undergone a marked change since a major family upheaval, such as a death or divorce. | Reactive depression<br>Anxiety<br>Significant clinical depression | Talk about the situation with your teen. Be patient while your teen adjusts to conditions. Keep teachers informed to help them understand unusual behavior. |
| Your teen has a chronic illness. | Adjustment to managing illness | If your teen is ill, let him take part in decisions affecting his treatment. If there's no improvement in a month, talk with your pediatrician about doing a formal screening. |
| Your teenager complains of vague symptoms such as headaches or stomachaches. She sometimes misses school. She drives or handles dangerous items carelessly. You suspect she is using drugs or alcohol. She is sullen or exhibiting regressive behaviors. | Depression<br>Acting out<br>Anxiety over school or social problems<br>Family tension<br>Substance abuse disorder<br>Bipolar disorder | Talk with your teen's pediatrician, who will determine whether your teen should be referred for a mental health evaluation. The pediatrician might screen for substance use or depression. |

| YOUR CONCERNS | POSSIBLE CAUSE | ACTION TO TAKE |
|---|---|---|
| Your teen is disinterested in activities such as sports or hobbies. He has low energy and trouble sleeping. He is often irritable. | Depression<br>Depressive reaction to unsatisfactory family dynamics or other overpowering situation | Ask your teen's pediatrician to evaluate his overall health, including screening for depression. His pediatrician may recommend therapy for him and possibly the entire family. |
| Your teenager has lost interest in schoolwork. His concentration is poor. He often expresses feelings of worthlessness and incompetence. | Learning disability<br>Attention-deficit/ hyperactivity disorder (ADHD)<br>Depression and substance abuse | Talk with your teen's teachers to identify specific difficulties. Schedule an appointment with his pediatrician to discuss possible medical conditions. Your teen may require an evaluation by the educational system or mental health specialist. |
| You notice cuts on your teen's arms, tomach, and thighs. She seems stressed and upset. | Self-injury by cutting | Schedule an appointment with your teen's pediatrician to find out why she is cutting and for a referral to a mental health specialist. |
| Your teen shows interest in things and wears clothes typical of the opposite gender. Your teen recently expressed sexual interest in someone of the same gender. | Depression caused by conflicts around gender identity and sexual orientation<br>Gender dysphoria | Start with talking to your teen about these feelings. Bring him in for a private discussion with his pediatrician about sexual orientation, including sexual behavior and safe-sex practices. Families can find support with http://pflag.org or other parent and youth organization Web sites. |
| Your teen has a marked change in appetite, with weight loss or gain. She is sleeping much more or less than usual. She lacks faith in her ability to succeed and has lost interest in pleasurable activities. | Major clinical depression | Call your teen's pediatrician for advice and urgent referral to a mental health specialist. It is important to make sure your teen is not thinking about suicide. |
| Your teenager is acting erratically. He is unusually talkative or having trouble sleeping. His activities include unrealistic ideas and plans and are a source of concern. If he had a similar episode, it was followed by a slump. | Bipolar disorder/manic depression or other severe mental illness<br>Substance abuse | Talk with your teen's pediatrician, who will do an evaluation and may refer your teen to a mental health consultant. |

## Living With a Diagnosis of Depression

Depression is often triggered by an event such as academic failure, death in the family, or romantic disappointment. Certain medications may cause depression as a side effect. However, in many cases, there is no identifiable cause. Depression often results from a chemical imbalance in the brain, which can run in families.

Ask your teen's pediatrician to evaluate your teen if you spot a sign of depression, such as

- Reduced interest in normal activities; lack of pleasure in daily life

- Fatigue, restlessness, trouble concentrating
- Withdrawal, lack of sociability
- Change in appetite; marked weight loss or gain
- Sleeping much more or less than usual
- Acting out, reckless behavior
- Vague but troubling physical symptoms

Physicians may choose to use medications or counseling to relieve clinical depression. Regular, moderate exercise can also be beneficial because it stimulates the production of endorphins—natural mood enhancers that can help reduce depression symptoms.

## IN GENERAL

Eating disorders continue to be a problem among teenagers in the United States and other affluent countries. Although teenaged girls are by far the most often afflicted, boys and girls in all age groups may develop an unhealthy preoccupation with food, dieting, and body image. Disordered eating ranges from picky eating to self-starvation (anorexia nervosa) and from occasional overeating and weight problems to the binge eating of bulimia. There are 3 major groups of disorders that demand medical attention: anorexia nervosa, bulimia nervosa, and eating disorders not otherwise specified (EDNOS). Patients with EDNOS may not meet all criteria for anorexia or bulimia but may still need medical attention.

Anorexia nervosa is characterized by a markedly distorted body image in which a teen perceives herself as fat when she is not. Although young women are often preoccupied with food, teens with anorexia nervosa refuse to eat, or they eat very little. Some girls with anorexia nervosa exercise for hours on end to burn up the few calories they consume. By contrast, a teenager with bulimia gorges on abnormally large quantities of food and then ends the binge with laxatives, self-induced vomiting, intense exercise, or a period of starvation to avoid gaining weight. Those with bulimia are usually a normal weight or overweight. Some teens exhibit a combination of behaviors, including eating less than they need to maintain their weight and periods of bingeing and purging, but they may not yet meet criteria for anorexia or bulimia.

An eating disorder has many serious effects on a teen's health. Girls with anorexia nervosa often fail to menstruate and risk long-term problems such as premature bone loss (low bone density).

Those with bulimia nervosa who force themselves to vomit have a high rate of dental caries because regurgitated stomach acids erode their tooth enamel. They also often have severe reflux esophagitis and are at risk for abnormal blood chemistries. Both conditions can be life-threatening. Without professional help, it is almost impossible to get teenagers with eating disorders back to healthy habits and a healthy weight. Some require nasogastric feeding, and all require treatment with a team approach involving a physician, mental health professional, and nutritionist.

For feeding problems involving babies and young children, see pages 6 and 28.

**Call your pediatrician at once if your teen has previously been diagnosed with an eating disorder and has any of the following:**

- Unusually slow or irregular heartbeat
- Chest pain
- Frequent dizziness; fainting
- Continuing weight loss or failure to maintain previous weight goals, despite treatment
- Cessation of menstrual periods

### WARNING!

Ask your teen's pediatrician's for advice if your preteen or teenager insists on an extreme diet that may be deficient in important nutrients. Many teens today eat alternative diets such as vegan or vegetarian, but no matter what the diet, it is important that it is nutritionally complete.

## Identifying Those at Risk for Eating Disorders

Experts have not yet found a way to predict which teens are likely to develop an eating disorder. However, in many cases, the eating problem develops after a girl embarks on a rigid weight-loss diet.

There may be a demanding, perfectionist home environment in which achievement or external appearances are overemphasized. Eating disorders do run in families; there may be a genetic predisposition. Teens involved in highly competitive athletic activities, where attention is focused on weight and form, are especially prone to eating disorders (eg, ballet, gymnastics). Boys who wrestle competitively sometimes try to meet their weight groups by fasting, dehydration (for losing weight), and bingeing (to gain weight).

## Feeding Teenagers

Teenagers, already highly susceptible to peer pressure, face daily pressure to conform to artificial standards of appearance and behavior that are dreamed up as marketing ploys. Waif-thin models in fashion magazines make poor role models for teens who need a balanced diet to support the many changes of puberty along with exercise for healthy bones and strong muscles.

Many teenagers diet to lose weight. Idealistic teens also often renounce meat and poultry for humanitarian reasons. Omitting meat or another specific food will not take away essential nutrients as long as the overall diet is well balanced and the teen is getting enough daily calories—about 3,000 for a boy and 2,200 for a girl at the peak of the growth spurt (which usually peaks around 13.5 years for boys, and 11.5 years for girls).

Nutritionists recommend that complex carbohydrates—whole-grain cereals and breads, pasta, beans and other legumes—make up 50% to 60% of a teenager's daily calories. Not only

are these foods good sources of energy, but they also provide protein and important vitamins and minerals. Vitamin supplements are rarely needed. With plenty of fresh fruits and vegetables and low-fat dairy products, the diet should provide adequate nutrients for growth metabolism. If a teenager dislikes milk or has trouble digesting it, yogurt, cheese, lactose-free milk, and soy milk can supply essential calcium and vitamins. For further information on appropriate portion sizes and food groups at mealtime, please refer to Figure 3-1 on page 187.

If a teenager's busy schedule means that many meals include hamburgers or pizzas eaten on the run, he should learn to make healthier choices. Choose low-fat foods and beverages when dining at a fast-food restaurant. Get in the habit of splitting high-fat options like french fries with a friend. Balance high-fat options with low-fat foods such as fruit slices or a salad. A diet that includes lots of fast foods can still be based on the right proportions of carbohydrates, protein, and fats and include dairy products, fruits, and vegetables for calcium, folic acid, and other vitamins and essential nutrients.

Foods rich in fat, sugar, and salt—french fries, chips, candies, and sugary drinks, among others—contribute little that's useful other than calories and may actually interfere with the absorption of essential nutrients. Soda is one example. Too much phosphorous in a diet means that less calcium can be absorbed. A teenager who drinks a lot of soda during her peak bone-building years risks decreasing the amount of calcium her body absorbs.

| YOUR CONCERNS | POSSIBLE CAUSE | ACTION TO TAKE |
|---|---|---|
| *Your teen refuses to eat with the rest of the family. She seems overly concerned with losing or gaining weight. You are worried that she's not eating enough.* | Anorexia nervosa<br>Other eating disorder<br>Teenage preoccupation with diet and appearance | If your teen's weight, appearance, or diet is causing worry, discuss your concerns with her pediatrician and have your teen seen (and weighed). |
| *Your son refuses family meals because he's following his own diet for sports or another reason. He is trying to gain or lose weight for a sports competition. You are concerned about his nutrition.* | Normal behavior<br>Personal preferences<br>Food fads | Review training with your son's coach to make sure his advice is sound; discuss any concerns with your teen's pediatrician. As long as your teenager's diet is healthy, respect his preferences. |
| *Your teen spends long periods in the bathroom after eating. She tends to skip family meals and instead eats large amounts of snack foods, cereal, or other foods. She complains that her weight goes up and down.* | Eating disorder (bulimia nervosa; eating disorder not otherwise specified) | Talk with your pediatrician, who may want to examine your teen. With sensitive questioning, your pediatrician may be able to obtain information that your teen is uncomfortable discussing with those close to her. |
| *Your daughter lost a lot of weight in a short time. She looks gaunt and her hair is thin. She developed downy hair on her face and arms. She tries to cover her thinness with bulky clothing.* | Anorexia nervosa<br>Metabolic disorder<br>Depression | Talk with your teen's pediatrician without delay; your daughter's condition should be diagnosed and treated promptly. |
| *Your daughter started exercising for hours and gets upset if anything interferes with it. She follows dieting fads or a strict diet.* | Anorexia nervosa<br>Compulsive exercise | Evaluate your teenager's diet over several days to assess her calorie and nutrient intake. Discuss your concerns with her pediatrician. |

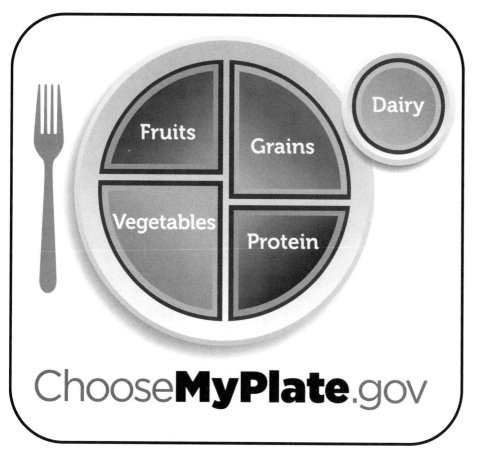

**Figure 3-1.** This illustration from ChooseMyPlate.gov demonstrates the 5 food groups that are the building blocks for a healthy diet, using a familiar image—a place setting for a meal. Fruits and vegetables should compose half of the plate, and the meal should be rounded out with grains (using whole grains whenever possible), a small amount of protein, and dairy. Monitor portion sizes, avoid oversized portions, and use fat-free or low-fat (1%) milk.

## IN GENERAL

Fainting is brought on by a sudden decrease in the flow of blood to the brain. This may occur for a number of reasons, but the result is that blood pressure rapidly drops and the brain is temporarily deprived of blood and oxygen. Your teen will feel light-headed and perhaps nauseated, her skin will feel cold and clammy, and she will lose consciousness. Fainting is in some ways the body's protective mechanism: When the fainting person lies flat, blood can flow more easily to the brain, so she quickly recovers consciousness. In almost all cases, she's awake again and aware of her surroundings within a minute or less, although she may continue to feel weak and wobbly for a while longer.

Fainting is unusual in a child younger than 10 years. The breath-holding spells that cause children to pass out during the terrible 2s (see "Dealing With Breath-holding" page 44) are different from fainting, although the underlying reflex mechanism is similar. However, it's fairly common for teens to faint. Girls tend to faint more often than boys.

An occasional fainting spell is not usually a sign that something is seriously wrong. Fainting is often triggered by stress, excitement, overexertion, fear, hunger, or being confined in a hot, stuffy atmosphere. Certain odors may cause faintness.

A surprising number of people faint at the sight of blood. Most people recover quickly. Even so, if a fainting spell occurs in a teen who has not had one, you should talk with your pediatrician. Your pediatrician will examine your teenager to make sure that the loss of consciousness was caused by fainting and not a more serious, treatable condition such as a seizure (see page 134) or an irregular heartbeat (see page 100).

**Call 911 or your local emergency number right away if your teen faints and**

- She isn't breathing.
- Her limbs, face, and body are jerking.
- Her skin is turning bluish.
- Her breathing is shallow and her pulse is weak.
- She is still unconscious after more than 2 minutes.

## WARNING!

If a teen feels faint, don't splash cold water on her face. If possible, have her lie on her back with her legs and feet slightly raised. In this position, the blood can flow more easily to her heart and brain. If she cannot lie down, have her sit with her head lowered. Loosen any tight clothing and make sure she can breathe freely. She should rest for at least 5 minutes or until she feels well enough to get back to normal activities.

| YOUR CONCERNS | POSSIBLE CAUSE | ACTION TO TAKE |
|---|---|---|
| Your teenager complains of feeling faint when she stands up suddenly. She is tired and pale at times. | Orthostatic hypotension (a momentary drop in blood pressure when abruptly changing position) Iron deficiency anemia | The faint feeling is not unusual or serious; it just means that the reflexes controlling your teen's blood pressure are acting slowly. This can often be prevented by having your teen drink plenty of fluids throughout the day. If your teen is unusually tired and pale, her pediatrician will examine her to determine whether treatment is needed. |
| Your teen was breathing rapidly before becoming faint. It occurred during an emotional upset. She has had other episodes of anxiety with rapid, shallow breathing, | Hyperventilation (rapid, shallow breathing) Panic attack Anxiety (See page 180.) | Talk with your teen's pediatrician, who can suggest ways to deal with anxiety and may recommend counseling. |

| YOUR CONCERNS | POSSIBLE CAUSE | ACTION TO TAKE |
|---|---|---|
| Your teenager fainted after standing a long time in strong sunshine. Or, he was confined to a warm, stuffy environment such as a crowded school assembly or church. He is usually active and healthy. | Heat exhaustion<br>Dehydration<br>Lack of fresh air | Let your teen rest until he feels well enough to resume his activities. Offer water or a drink containing sugar as soon as he's well enough to take it. The pediatrician may want to examine your teen if this was his first fainting episode. |
| Your teen faints when he gets his blood drawn. He sometimes faints when he gets upset. | Vasovagal syncope | Call your pediatrician if it's the first time your teen fainted. |
| Your teen fainted during a coughing bout. He often coughs and wheezes, especially at night. He was diagnosed with asthma. | Asthma | Call your pediatrician who will examine your teen and make a diagnosis. If your child has asthma, your pediatrician can adjust his medication, prescribe different treatment, or refer him to a pulmonologist. |
| Your teenager is feeling weak, faint, clammy, or shaky. He has not eaten in several hours. Your teen may be generally healthy or has a diagnosis of type 1 diabetes. | Low blood sugar or hypo-glycemia | Give your teen a drink that contains sugar for immediate energy. Encourage your teen to eat regularly to maintain a steady supply of energy; provide a balance of starches, protein, and a small amount of fat at each meal. If your teen fainted and has type 1 diabetes, call 911. Call your pediatrician and schedule an examination. You will need to talk about adjusting your child's medication. |
| Your teen suddenly became ill and fainted. He has swelling around his mouth. He is having trouble breathing. He might have been stung by a bee or other insect. He is allergic to a food. Or, he is taking a medication such as an antibiotic. | Severe allergic reaction (anaphylaxis) | Call 911 or your local emergency number at once; this is an emergency. Give CPR (see Chapter 4, pages 215–216) if necessary while you're waiting for help. |
| Your teenager had one or more fainting spells after exertion or emotional upsets. She complains that her heart is racing or skipping beats. | Long QT syndrome (type of irregular heart-beat; see page 100)<br>Other abnormal heart rhythm<br>Other dysrhythmia, including Wolff-Parkinson-White syndrome | Talk with your pediatrician, who will perform a physical examination and further evaluation to determine whether treatment is warranted. |
| Your teenaged daughter has been faint and nauseated for several days in a row. She seems worried or withdrawn. You believe she may be sexually active. | Pregnancy | Talk with your daughter. If you have reason to think she could be pregnant, talk with your pediatrician without delay. |

## IN GENERAL

Fatigue includes feeling tired and sleepy, but it is also a temporary loss of energy and heaviness in the muscles. Fatigue can be a warning to slow down and let the body repair itself. It's normal to feel fatigued after physical activity or a period of intense pressure at school. Fatigue is also a common symptom of illness. Even a mild cold may temporarily rob a teenager of energy and make him want to sleep longer than usual. Healthy teenagers rapidly return to normal once an illness is over. However, when fatigue is unusually severe or prolonged, it may be because of a chronic disorder such as iron deficiency anemia. It may also reflect an emotional problem such as depression (see page 182). In rare cases, it may be related to a viral infection of the heart, resulting in reduced heart function.

The tendency to sleep more is normal during adolescence. Also, teenagers tend to be most sleepy in the morning, making it difficult for them to concentrate during early morning classes. This sleepiness is partially due to the rapid growth rate and hormonal changes that come with adolescence, and partially due to the fact that teenagers lose sleep at both ends. They get up progressively earlier as they advance from elementary to middle school and then to high school. Meanwhile, they stay awake longer and often self-medicate with caffeine and stimulants to compensate for the daytime sleepiness, making it worse.

A sudden attack of extreme drowsiness may signal a need for medical attention, especially if there are other symptoms such as fever, vomiting, and confusion. In very rare cases, irresistible daytime drowsiness that occurs with certain other symptoms is caused by narcolepsy, a rare condition that can be managed with medication. You should talk with your child's pediatrician if your teen has fatigue that isn't relieved by rest, complains of muscle weakness, or hasn't recovered his energy weeks after the end of an illness.

**Talk with your pediatrician if your teen's fatigue lasts more than a week or two or is accompanied by**

- Fever, a persistent sore throat, muscle and joint aches, and swollen glands
- Constant thirst and nagging hunger, frequent urination, weight loss, numbness or tingling in the hands or feet, blurred vision, and anxiety
- Unusual pallor, bruising in places not following injury, loss of appetite and weight, bone pain, night sweats, swollen glands, and fever

> **WARNING!**
> Unusual fatigue may be a signal that your child is abusing substances, particularly if she is not participating in family activities, her grades have slipped, and she doesn't answer your questions about the time she spends with friends. It may also be a symptom of pregnancy.

## Chronic Fatigue Syndrome

If your teenager suffers severe fatigue that lasts for weeks and occurs for no apparent reason, he may be diagnosed with chronic fatigue syndrome (CFS). Unlike healthy people who can often beat fatigue with regular, moderate exercise or a good night's rest, people with CFS remain exhausted. The cause of CFS is unknown.

Chronic fatigue syndrome is not infectious, although it may follow a viral illness. Those affected often report having felt nonspecific symptoms such as sore throat, fever, swollen lymph glands, muscle pain, and diarrhea for weeks or months before. Their energy level gradually declines, they have trouble concentrating, and they lose interest in activities they used to enjoy. However, there is no sign of physical illness, and laboratory tests are normal.

To confirm a diagnosis of CFS, symptoms must be present for 6 months or more. Although not common in children, CFS can occasionally affect older teenagers and young adults.

Time seems to be the only proven treatment. A regular schedule for sleep, rest, exercise, and meals is usually beneficial. Recovery may be helped along by medications to relieve specific symptoms such as depression and muscle aches.

| YOUR CONCERNS | POSSIBLE CAUSE | ACTION TO TAKE |
|---|---|---|
| Your teenager has been tired since having a sore throat, swollen glands, or an upper respiratory infection. | Infectious mononucleosis Other viral infection Reduced heart function | Talk with your pediatrician, who will examine your teenager and advise on treatment. |
| Your teen feels tired all the time, is irritable, and has trouble falling or staying asleep. | Teen insomnia Depression Anxiety Excess caffeine intake Substance abuse | Try to eliminate sources of stress. Encourage your teenager to eat right and exercise regularly. If insomnia persists, talk to your teen's pediatrician. |
| Your teen has been feeling unusually tired since starting medication for allergies or another condition. | Medication side effects | If your teen takes an antihistamine, have him take it at night so he sleeps well and is less tired during the day. If he is taking another medication, tell his pediatrician about the side effects and ask whether the prescription should be changed. |
| Your teenager feels nervous or anxious for no reason. She is pale and her weight has changed noticeably. | Iron deficiency anemia Thyroid disorder Unhealthy dieting Pregnancy Other conditions requiring diagnosis and treatment | Talk with your teen's pediatrician, who will examine your teen and perform diagnostic tests as necessary. If your teen wants to lose weight, ask her pediatrician to recommend a plan for steady weight loss. |
| Your teen is often fatigued only 3 or 4 hours after waking. He snores and awakens often during the night. He is having difficulties at school. | Sleep apnea Oversleeping (hypersomnia) | Talk with your teen's pediatrician, who will examine him and determine if diagnostic tests and treatment are needed. |
| Your teen often falls asleep during the day and is having problems with that during school. She has a short attention span, reports seeing vivid images while falling asleep, and feels weak when upset. | Narcolepsy | Talk with your teen's pediatrician, who will examine her and may recommend a special kind of sleep study (ie, multiple sleep latency test). |
| Your child's eyelids look droopy. He has fatigue that gets worse as the day goes on and is having vision problems. | Myasthenia gravis (a disorder of the nervous system) or another condition requiring diagnosis and treatment | Talk with your teen's pediatrician, who will examine him and order diagnostic tests. |

## IN GENERAL

The long-term effects of high blood pressure (hypertension) are serious and include heart attacks, strokes, and kidney failure. Fortunately, treatment to lower even mildly elevated blood pressure can reduce the risk of long-term effects. The sooner treatment is started, the better. That's why your teen's pediatrician regularly checks your teen's blood pressure. The top number measures systolic pressure, which is the pressure exerted on the arteries as the heart pumps blood out to the body. The bottom number measures diastolic pressure, which is pressure in the arteries when the heart relaxes in between the beats. In adults, optimal blood pressure is 120 (systolic) over 80 (diastolic), measured in millimeters on a mercury gauge. In children, blood pressure is lower and evaluated according to age and height. If blood pressure is high, treatment is required, including dietary changes, regular exercise, and medication, if necessary.

Hypertension is unusual among young children but sometimes develops during adolescence. Children with blood pressure in the high-normal range are more likely to develop hypertension during adulthood. Children of parents with hypertension are also more likely to develop high blood pressure. High blood pressure is more common in African Americans than other ethnic groups. It becomes more severe with age and gets worse with a diet high in sodium.

Other factors such as genetics, obesity, and stress also play a part in the development of hypertension. High blood pressure caused by an underlying illness is called secondary hypertension. Severe hypertension in children is usually caused by an illness such as kidney disease, a tumor, and narrowing of the aorta or abdominal levels of certain hormones in the body.

Children with hypertension rarely have symptoms unless their blood pressure is extremely high because of an underlying condition. High blood pressure is often discovered during routine examinations.

The only way to identify the condition is by using a blood pressure gauge.

**Call your teen's pediatrician right away if your teen has high blood pressure and develops any of the following:**

- A persistent or severe headache
- Dizziness
- Shortness of breath
- Visual disturbances
- Unusual fatigue

### WARNING!

Help your teen avoid unnecessary sodium by seasoning dishes with herbs and spices instead of salt. Keep salt off the table. Don't buy heavily salted snacks; if you're buying commercially prepared foods, look for unsalted and low-salt versions. Learn to recognize sodium in all its forms on ingredient lists. Any ingredient with "sodium" or "Na," the chemical name for sodium, in its name contains the substance. Sodium might also be labeled as baking soda, baking powder, monosodium glutamate (MSG), disodium phosphate, or salt.

## How Salt Affects Blood Pressure

Table salt is a compound of sodium and chloride, 2 chemicals that are essential for health but in small amounts. In fact, sodium and chloride occur naturally in so many foods that we don't need to add them. Salt is hardly needed to preserve foods any more since refrigeration and newer technologies now do this job better. The real reason we add salt to foods is habit; we've developed a taste for it. In reality, health experts recommend that adults consume no more than about 1,500 to 2,300 milligrams of sodium a day; children need even less. Eating too much salt is an important factor in raising blood pressure in people who are extra sensitive to sodium.

Salt concentrations help regulate the amount of water in the body. In a healthy person, the kidneys retrieve sodium from blood, conserving and recycling sodium as a valuable resource. In people who are sodium sensitive, the kidneys retain more sodium than the body needs, which throws their sodium-water concentration off balance. The body tries to dilute the sodium by increasing the amount of fluid circulating in the bloodstream; the excess fluid eventually shows up as puffiness, especially in our hands, feet, and legs. The increased fluid volume makes blood vessels oversensitive to nerve stimulation and they constrict, causing blood pressure to rise. (Imagine how water pressure changes when you bend and choke off a garden hose.) As a result, the heart has to work harder to keep the blood

moving through tight vessels. The constant high pressure stiffens blood vessel walls. This effect is often first noticed in eye and kidney vessels. Reducing salt consumption helps to lower the sodium concentration and eases pressure on the heart, kidneys, and blood vessels.

If you have hypertension or know you are salt sensitive, cut down on salt in your family's diet now to help your children avoid high blood pressure later.

| YOUR CONCERNS | POSSIBLE CAUSE | ACTION TO TAKE |
|---|---|---|
| Your teenager's blood pressure is in the high-normal or mildly elevated range. There is a family history of high blood pressure. | Essential hypertension (high blood pressure without an obvious physical cause) | Monitor your teen's weight and food intake. Encourage regular exercise. Ask your pediatrician to check your teen's blood pressure at regular visits. Keep tabs with a home monitor. Find out whether any further action is advisable. |
| Your teen was diagnosed with hypertension. There is blood in his urine. His blood pressure is higher in his arms than in his legs. He has trouble sleeping and is anxious and irritable. | Kidney disease (causing renal hypertension) Coarctation of the aorta (an inborn condition affecting the artery that arises from the heart) Tumor Hyperthyroidism | Your pediatrician will perform tests to determine the cause and recommend treatment accordingly. |
| Your teen is overweight or obese. | Obesity-related hypertension | Ask your teen's pediatrician for advice about helping her to lose weight while providing the calories and nutrients necessary for growth. Discourage eating salty foods. |
| Your teenager is unusually irritable but has no other apparent symptoms. Or he suddenly develops headaches, dizziness, or a change in vision. | Severe hypertension | Call your pediatrician at once. Your teen must be evaluated and diagnosed. |

## IN GENERAL

Most knee pain in teenagers is caused by minor accidents, sports injuries, or overuse. However, occasionally childhood knee pain can be caused by serious conditions such as arthritis, auto-immune diseases, infections, tumors, and blood disorders.

The kneecap (patella) is linked to the thighbone (femur) at the patellofemoral joint by the strong patellar ligament (above the kneecap) and the patellar tendon (below the kneecap). This joint is stabilized by the combined force of ligaments and muscles, as well as the fit of the bony structures. The base of the kneecap is V-shaped and slides through a matching groove (trochlea) in the thigh-bone. The kneecap does not slide straight but slight-ly shifts sideways as it moves, as force is exerted by the muscles and tendons. A slight irregularity in the bone or unevenness in the strengths of the muscles, tendons, and ligaments can make the kneecap move abnormally; this causes knee pain that gets worse with strenuous activity.

Injuries to the knee ligaments are common in adults but less so in children because a child's immature ligaments are stronger than the bone to which they are attached. On forceful impact, the bone will often break before the ligament can tear, especially from near where the bone grows. However, as the bones harden during adolescence, injuries to the knees and ligaments become more like those in adults. Skiers and in-line skaters and tennis, basketball, soccer, and football players are particularly vul-nerable. Young athletes should always wear appropriate protective gear for games and practice.

### Talk with your teen's pediatrician if

- Knee pain or swelling lasts more than 3 days or gets worse
- Pain or rapid swelling follows a knee injury
- The knee joint is tender, red, and warm to the touch, whether or not an injury occurred
- Your teen complains of knee weakness or instability

### WARNING!

Although conditions directly affecting the knee are the usual cause of pain, knee pain may also be a symptom of a hip disorder.

## Preventing Knee Injuries

The most common cause of knee pain is overuse, in which repeated, low-grade injury causes a progres-sive loss of strength in the entire limb. Conditioning exercises are essential for preventing joint and muscle injuries in children. Coaches and school athletic directors should stress the importance of warm-ups and stretching exercises before sports.

Most acute, minor muscle injuries can be managed by applying cold compresses right away after the injury, taking acetaminophen or ibuprofen for pain, and resting for 1 to 2 days. If your teenager has severe or persistent pain related to exercise, or pain over a specific location in the bone or knee joint, call your teen's pediatrician for an evaluation or referral to a sports medicine specialist or an orthopedic specialist. After assessing the injury, your teen's physician may suggest exercises to improve strength and function. Your teenager should not play sports again until his doctor gives the go-ahead.

| YOUR CONCERNS | POSSIBLE CAUSE | ACTION TO TAKE |
|---|---|---|
| *Your teen has tenderness, redness, warmth, or swelling over the knee.* | Infection<br>Trauma<br>Arthritis | Call your teen's pediatrician, who will examine her and refer her to a specialist if necessary. |
| *Your teen has pain and tender swelling at the top of his shin. The symptoms came on when he started participating in a sport.* | Bruising<br>Muscle strain<br>Osgood-Schlatter disease (a common, painful, but benign condition in teens) | Ask your teen's pediatrician to examine him. If Osgood-Schlatter disease is confirmed, treatment usually involves rest, decreased participation in sports, and pain medication as required. |
| *Your teen complains that her knee feels "out of joint." The feeling occurred following an injury.* | Dislocation of the kneecap<br>Ligament tear<br>Chondromalacia patellae (softening of the kneecap cartilage) | Call your pediatrician, who will determine whether your teen's knee is injured. Treatment may involve rest followed by isometric exercise. Teens rarely need surgery. |
| *Your son limps from pain after strenuous activity. He complains of stiffness, buckling, or locking in the knee joint. The knee makes an audible click and is swollen.* | Osteochondritis dissecans (possibly due to trauma; much more common in boys)<br>Discoid meniscus (a malformation of the knee cartilage) | Your teen's pediatrician will examine your son and advise on management of this common condition, which results from separation of a small bone section and causes cartilage inflammation and splitting. Your teen's pediatrician may refer him for evaluation by an orthopedic specialist. |
| *Your teen is complaining of vague knee pain, especially after vigorous activity. The knee looks normal and seems to function without locking or giving way.* | Patellar maltracking<br>Knee pain of unknown cause<br>Slipped capital femoral epiphysis (dislocation of the thighbone head) | Talk with your teen's pediatrician, who will examine your daughter to rule out serious causes of knee pain and may recommend isometric exercises to improve strength and flexibility. Ice packs can be used to relieve discomfort. The pain usually disappears with time. Slipped capital femoral epiphysis is a true emergency and may require surgical pinning. Slipped capital femoral epiphysis may lead to early arthritis and the need for joint replacement at an early age. |
| *Your teen has swelling at the back of her knee.* | Baker cyst (popliteal cyst), a benign condition in school-aged children | Ask your pediatrician to examine your teen. Most Baker cysts are best left alone because these benign swellings normally disappear without treatment. Surgery is necessary only if there is severe discomfort or the swelling increases. |
| *Your teen's knee pain awakens him from sleep.* | Overuse<br>Tumor<br>Blood disorder (ie, leukemia)<br>Arthritis or another systemic condition | Call your pediatrician if your teen has pain in the daytime or is limping, or if the pain lasts more than a few days. |
| *Your teen's knee is painful and slightly swollen. There is a loud click or "clunk" as the knee is bent.* | Discoid lateral meniscus, a rare condition in which the meniscus, a pad of cartilage at the top of the shinbone, is round instead of half-moon shaped | Talk with your teen's pediatrician, who may recommend a consultation with an orthopedic specialist. |

## IN GENERAL

Most teenagers are growing up immersed in all things media. As young children, they played computer games, watched DVDs of their favorite shows and movies, and made phone calls to Grandma on Mom's cell phone. Now, as teenagers, their media use has grown exponentially. They post pictures on Instagram, engage with peers on Facebook, and compose short snippets of their lives on Twitter. They send text messages all day long, watch YouTube videos on the Internet, and play all sorts of electronic games.

No doubt, the explosion in media has benefits. For starters, it provides teens and tweens with an easy mode for communicating. Many students also use social media to connect with each other for homework assignments and group projects. In addition, media provides teens and adults alike with seemingly endless amounts of entertainment and news.

But, like most things, it is possible to get too much of a good thing, and media use is no exception. Children who spend too much time in front of the screen often do not get enough exercise. Those who watch too much violence are at risk for becoming aggressors themselves and desensitized to the effects of violence as a whole. In addition, too much media time exposes your child to images featuring sexual activity and drug and alcohol use. Girls, in particular, may develop body image issues from seeing celebrities who are excessively thin.

Excessive media can also cause sleep problems. Children who watch more TV at night tend to fall asleep later. Research links unlimited cell phone use, in particular, to sleep problems. Studies also show that teens are often awakened by text messages and calls on cell phones, causing fatigue and trouble concentrating the next day.

Although we can no longer escape media, it's important to teach teens how to use it appropriately and safely.

**WARNING!**

Research has found that 1 in 5 children have sent a third party nude or seminude photos of themselves or someone else in a text message. This practice, known as sexting, is a form of pornography and is illegal. Sexting is a crime in all 50 states, and your child can be charged as a sex offender. It is also a form of harassment and cyber-bullying that can humiliate the person in the photo. If and when you give your child a cell phone that allows him to text, make sure he knows the ramifications of sexting.

## Know Your Digital Footprint

Every time you do a Google search, post a comment, or create a profile online, you are adding to your digital footprint. Your digital footprint is the trail of data you leave behind in the digital world (ie, the Internet). Setting up an online account adds to your digital footprint, as does writing a blog or posting a photo or video—images that can create lasting and powerful impressions. And a Web site that copies and stores your information is also contributing to your digital footprint.

A digital footprint doesn't just make you findable; it also makes you knowable. But surveys show that most adults aren't that concerned, so they aren't diligent about teaching their children what it means to have a digital footprint. In fact, one study found that teens are actually more private than their parents about what they post on their social media profiles and more selective about who views them.

Still, it's important that teens understand that what they post online can create a lasting impression. Lengthy political tirades, personal attacks, and tasteless jokes are probably best left off-line.

To help your teen gauge what he should or shouldn't post, ask him to consider whether he'd want another parent to see it or whether his posts would make a good impression on a college admissions officer or future employer. You can also ask him to remember RITE, which stands for

- **R**eread the message you wrote to make sure it sounds OK.
- **I**magine how you'd feel if you got the message. Would you be hurt or angry?
- **T**hink about whether it needs to be sent now or if it should wait.

- **H**it the Enter button if the message is OK, is harmless, and can be sent now.

A good thing to remember: what happens in cyberspace stays in cyberspace.

| YOUR CONCERNS | POSSIBLE CAUSE | ACTION TO TAKE |
|---|---|---|
| *You suspect your tween or teen is engaging in sexual activity. She often dresses in provocative clothing and seems preoccupied with boys.* | Excessive exposure to sexual imagery in media | Talk with your teen about the movies and TV shows she is watching. Encourage her to pursue other interests. Talk with her pediatrician for advice if you suspect she is sexually active. |
| *Your teen is withdrawn and often sad. She seems consumed with texting. She is having trouble getting along with classmates.* | Cyberbullying | Talk with your teen about the messages, texts, and postings she receives. Follow and "friend" her on social media sites. Contact her school for guidance. If your teen's safety is at risk, call the police. Talk with your daughter's pediatrician if she starts experiencing other symptoms such as insomnia (see "Sleep Problems," page 142), loss of appetite (see page 28), or depression (see page 182). |
| *Your teen no longer enjoys doing things with friends and family. He is skipping other activities to sit with his texting device or play games. He is frequently moody. He gets defensive when you ask him about his social media activities. You've caught him engaging in risky behaviors like drug use.* | Excessive use of social media or gaming | Ask your teen's pediatrician for a referral to a licensed psychiatrist. Talk with your teen about your concerns. Search his computer, cell phone, and other devices to check text messages, Web search and browsing histories, friend lists, and e-mail messages. Find ways to reduce his use of social media. |
| *Your teenager is engaging in frequent fights, some of them physical. He is irritable and aggressive when confronted.* | Overexposure to violent media | Set limits on your teen's media use. Talk with him about what concerns you in violent movies and games. Ask his pediatrician for a referral to a psychiatrist, if necessary. |
| *Your teen is gaining weight. He is prone to injury whenever he exercises.* | Lack of activity from too much media time | Find ways to restrict your teen's media use. Encourage him to exercise by finding a sport or engaging in fitness activities such as walking or biking. |
| *Your teenager is preoccupied with her body and frequently says she is fat when she is not. She often binges and then disappears for a while in the bathroom.* | Anorexia or bulimia resulting from too much exposure to media (See "Eating Disorders," page 184.) | Talk with your teen's pediatrician for advice and guidance on treatment. Limit your teen's exposure to celebrity magazines, movies, and television. |

## IN GENERAL

Children at either end of the age spectrum may have mood swings. During the terrible 2s, children experience complex feelings toward their parents: love, jealousy, frustration, fear of a parent's displeasure, or abandonment. A preschooler's moods may switch from sunny to thunderous and back again in the space of a few minutes until she is better able to express herself and outgrows tantrums as a way to cope with angry or frustrated feelings (see "Temper Tantrums," page 156). Adolescence unleashes a new set of mood swings due partly to hormonal changes and partly to the challenges, growing responsibilities, and uncertainties of the teen years (see "Anxiety," page 180).

Mood swings are especially common in children with chronic illnesses. Teens who have endocrine or hormonal disorders, such as diabetes mellitus or thyroid problems, are especially vulnerable to mood swings. Teens with motor disabilities may have feelings of frustration and helplessness. Counseling and participation in a peer support group may help a teenager see that others share her difficulties and help her learn ways to cope with similar problems.

Extreme emotional volatility may signal a serious psychiatric disorder, poor impulse control, abuse, an underlying personality disorder, or drug or alcohol use. In some teenagers it may signal the onset of mental illness. At the very least, a teen who has extreme, unpredictable mood swings is hard to get along with at home and is likely to run into difficulties with schoolmates, teachers, and other authority figures. A teen with extreme mood swings usually needs professional help.

Emotional problems sometimes become apparent with weight gain or loss (see "Depression," page 182, and "Eating Disorders," page 184). Be alert to signs of trouble. If your teen gets careless about his appearance and hygiene, stops seeing friends, or his grades drop, you should talk to his pediatrician. You should also talk to his pediatrician if mood swings interfere with family life, social relationships, and

school performance. Your teen's pediatrician can refer him to a mental health professional for an evaluation.

In addition to professional help, it is important to encourage your teen to exercise regularly. People who exercise regularly maintain a steady output of endorphins—the brain's natural mood-enhancers—which may help promote a more balanced emotional state.

### Talk with your teen's pediatrician if your teen

- Has a noticeable weight change due to a lack or increase of appetite
- Loses interest in activities she formerly enjoyed
- Sleeps much more or much less than usual
- Expresses feelings of worthlessness or guilt
- Has a marked change in energy level, becoming listless or overactive

### WARNING!

Don't ignore severe mood swings, especially if they involve cycles of deep depression and extreme elation. Simply hoping your teenager will "snap out of it" is not enough. Your teen may need medical help and needs to be evaluated by her pediatrician, who can decide if a referral for mental health counseling is needed.

## Temperament and Moodiness

Teenagers are often characterized as having an easy, a withdrawn, or a difficult temperament. An *easy* teen has a positive outlook, takes changes and new situations in stride, and meets challenges with good humor and minimal anxiety. A *withdrawn* teen adapts more slowly, is less outgoing, and tends to be more anxious when confronted with new people and situations. A *difficult* teen may have tantrums and adjustment difficulties. Within these categories, teens are adaptable according to activity level, regularity of habits, sensory threshold, setting, situation, and mood (the degree of pleasantness in communications and actions). Parents shouldn't hurry to label a teen as difficult or moody if the teen has had stresses that can temporarily affect behavior. What's more, a teenager may seem difficult only when his personality and behavior differ from those of his parents and teachers. Be sensitive to your teen's temperament and emotional makeup in dealing with conflicts.

Help your teen to make the best of his basic characteristics. Your pediatrician can offer advice and referral.

| YOUR CONCERNS | POSSIBLE CAUSE | ACTION TO TAKE |
|---|---|---|
| *Your teenager is sometimes moody, feeling up one minute and down the next. But she is generally well and happy.* | Normal teenage behavior | Try to keep your sense of humor in dealing with teenage moods. This behavior is a normal phase. |
| *Your teenage daughter becomes tearful, oversensitive, and moody for several days each month.* | Premenstrual syndrome (PMS or premenstrual dysphoric disorder) | Explain to your daughter that her difficult feelings are part of the natural hormonal cycle. Premenstrual syndrome isn't disabling, and she can learn to anticipate it and plan her activities accordingly. Talk with her pediatrician if her moodiness is adversely affecting her life. |
| *Your child has been irritable and moody since a recent viral illness.* | Gradual recovery from a viral illness | Irritability is not unusual following a viral illness. If your teen isn't back to normal in a week or two, talk with his pediatrician. |
| *Over a period of days or weeks, your teenager has become sad, tearful, irritable, and withdrawn. The mood change was set off by an identifiable event.* | Reactive depression, a normal response characterized by feelings of sadness (See "Depression," page 182.) | Discuss the events with your teen, as well as practical solutions to problems. If the mood lasts longer than 3 weeks or is getting worse, talk with your teen's pediatrician, who may recommend counseling or medical therapy. |
| *Your teen has low moods lasting weeks at a time, alternating with normal moods. There is a family history of depression.* | Mild chronic depression (dysthymic disorder) | If low moods are interfering with family life, schoolwork, or your teen's happiness, talk with his pediatrician. Your teen may need further evaluation and treatment. |
| *Your teen has a chronic illness. You are concerned that he may neglect to take medication or perform monitoring tests.* | Anxiety, depression, resentment, and denial related to chronic illness Effects of the medication or illness | Talk with your teen's pediatrician, who may refer him to a counselor as well as a peer support group. |
| *Your teen's low moods alternate with periods when she is erratic, hyperactive, argumentative, and sleeping little.* | Bipolar disorder (manic depression) | Talk with your pediatrician; your teenager may need medication to settle her moods and psychotherapy to deal with her feelings. |

## IN GENERAL

Adolescence is a time to plan for transition from childhood to adult independence. Although parents often find this a trying time, most teenagers with appropriate and early support and guidance will move to adult mastery in relationships, health care responsibilities, education, work, and recreation with only minor problems or none at all. But for some, the transition is hampered by mental or physical health problems.

Teens having a difficult adolescence who are unable to effectively cope with the different stressors present in their lives (which may include typical and unusual stressors as well as significant ongoing adverse experiences) may become clinically depressed. Others seek escape in self-destructive behavior or physical symptoms that cover up clinical depression (see "Mood Swings," page 198). For many parents, the first clue that their teenager needs help from a mental health professional is a significant change in his personality. Different from the normal ups and downs of a teenage personality, the change is a deep-rooted, often negative shift in attitude and behavior. A change in personality shouldn't be written off as teenage moodiness. Occasionally, a personality change follows serious accidental head injury or results from a rare physical condition such as a metabolic disorder or brain tumor. In many teens, a marked personality change is a signal that they are taking part in risky behavior such as substance abuse and other self-destructive acts. Early risky and unprotected sexual experiences can lead to or manifest as a form of a personality change too; these risky behavioral changes can result in pregnancy; sexually transmitted infections, including AIDS; and long-term mental health problems.

Because the results of risky behavior are potentially tragic, parents should be alert to warning signs of personality change indicating that a teenager needs help from a mental health professional. Whether the personality change is a symptom of depression, conduct disorder (see Chapter 2, "Behavioral Concerns," page 38), physical condition, or emerging mental illness, the teen needs to be evaluated. Your teen's pediatrician will guide you in choosing suitable treatment and may also recommend a family support group.

**Talk with your teen's pediatrician and your teen if his personality has changed and**

- He misses school repeatedly or his grades drop.
- You believe he may be using alcohol or illegal substances.
- He is withdrawn, reclusive, and uncommunicative.
- He is often hostile and aggressive.
- He is acting in a way that may endanger his health or even life or risk confrontation with the law.
- He also has symptoms suggesting a physical illness.

> **WARNING!**
> If your teenager makes offhand remarks about suicide, don't ignore them. Direct questioning may show you that he wants to talk about his problems. He should be evaluated by his pediatrician without delay.

## Teenage Suicide

Suicide ranks third—after accidents and homicide—among causes of death in American teenagers. Although girls attempt suicide more often, boys outnumber girls in suicide deaths because they are more likely to choose a lethal method.

Teens try to kill themselves primarily because of undiagnosed or untreated depression, serious conflicts with family and friends, physical and sexual abuse, victimization or conflicts around sexual orientation or gender identity, or problems with school and the law. Many teens attempt suicide while under the influence of alcohol or drugs. It's impossible to draw a clear line between some accidents and suicide attempts because many fatal accidents occur when teenagers use alcohol or drugs. The substance loosens teens' inhibitions and makes them more likely to be impulsive and not think through self-destructive behavior, such as driving while intoxicated or performing dangerous stunts on a dare. Experts calculate that only about one-third of those who attempt suicide really intend to kill themselves; the others are looking for attention, love, acceptance, or escape from situations and feelings with which they are unable to effectively cope. A recent report from the Centers for Disease Control and Prevention, "Mental Health Surveillance Among Children–United States, 2005–2011," found that nearly 30% of teens made their intent known before they died and 21% had made a previous suicide attempt.

A teen who is unable to cope well with ongoing stressors and who has ongoing depressed or angry feelings as a result of problems in the family, at school, or with the community may be harboring ideas of suicide. At the very least, he may be risking injury to himself or others because of impulsive behavior. His pediatrician should evaluate him as soon as possible to rule out physical problems and determine whether he should be referred to a psychiatrist or another mental health professional.

| YOUR CONCERNS | POSSIBLE CAUSE | ACTION TO TAKE |
|---|---|---|
| *Your teen is hostile and aggressive. He is having problems at school.* | Learning problem<br>Behavioral problem | Talk with your teen's pediatrician, who will evaluate your teen and may recommend treatment or referral. If the level of hostility is frightening to family members, your teen may need a quicker referral. |
| *Your teen is secretive about how he spends his time. He has money or possessions for which he can't account.* | Substance use, including dealing in illicit drugs | Discuss your concerns with your teen's pediatrician, who may suggest how to approach and talk with your teen. |
| *Your teen is missing school. Her grades have plummeted.* | Truancy<br>School difficulties<br>Substance use<br>Acting out<br>Pregnancy | Talk with your teen's teachers to identify specific problems and get recommendations. Talk with your teen's pediatrician for an evaluation and to discuss counseling as soon as possible. |
| *Your teenager's erratic behavior is interfering with family life. He has mood swings with prolonged ups and downs. He is also having difficulties at school.* | Emotional disorder<br>Mental illness | Talk with your teen's pediatrician right away for an evaluation. |
| *Your teen has bouts of trembling. She is panicky and short of breath during attacks. Her heart races and she has trouble concentrating.* | Anxiety attacks<br>Early sign of diabetes | Talk with your pediatrician, who will perform an examination to rule out physical conditions and may prescribe treatment, including counseling or referral to a mental health specialist. |
| *Your teenager has become aggressive or forgetful. He gets headaches that are worse when he lies down. He has double vision, muscle weakness, or nausea and vomiting.* | Tumor or another condition requiring diagnosis and treatment | Talk with your teen's pediatrician as soon as possible. |

## IN GENERAL

Secondary sexual characteristics emerge under hormonal control at puberty. In girls, the first sign of sexual maturation is breast development, which begins somewhere between 8 and 13 years of age. Boys generally commence puberty a year or so later than girls, as the testes and penis begin to grow between ages 10 and 14 years. Even before the earliest physical signs appear, parents usually notice that their child needs more food to keep up with his rapidly accelerating growth rate. With the teenage growth spurt that follows about 2 years after the early signs, your child's height increases by about 25%, while his weight may almost double.

On average, girls begin to menstruate at about 12 to 13 years of age. Studies in ballet dancers, athletes, and girls with eating disorders (see page 184) show that those who are at a very low weight or have an abnormally low percentage of body fat tend to have their first menstrual period (menarche) later than average. Irregular periods are common during the first 2 to 3 years after menstruation starts. More regular, ovulatory cycles then occur in most teens.

In boys, ejaculation first occurs somewhere between 11 and 15 years, although the range of 8 to 17 years is considered normal. Growth of the larynx (Adam's apple) and deepening of the voice coincide with the first appearance of facial hair, and the increase in height is matched by a corresponding increase in muscle mass.

In girls, growth gradually stops within a year or so after menarche. In boys, full height is usually reached by age 17 or 18 years, although young men may continue to grow until 21 years of age and many keep on filling out their lanky frames with muscle bulk into their early 20s.

**Talk with your teen's pediatrician if you notice**

- Signs of sexual development in your daughter if she is younger than 8 years or your son if he is younger than 9 years

> **WARNING!**
> The timing of sexual maturation varies widely and is influenced by a host of factors, including genetic background, nutrition, and body mass. But talk with your teen's pediatrician if there is no sign of sexual development in your 13-year-old daughter or 14-year-old son.

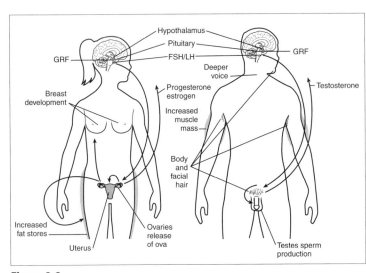

**Figure 3-2.**

## Hormonal Control of Puberty

In boys and girls, puberty begins when a part of the brain called the hypothalamus (Figure 3-2) secretes a gonadotropin-releasing hormone (GnRH). This hormone prompts the nearby pituitary gland to release a follicle-stimulating hormone (FSH) and luteinizing hormone (LH).

In girls, FSH and LH act on the ovaries, stimulating them to produce progesterone and estrogen, which are female hormones that are instrumental in regulating the menstrual cycle and monthly release of egg cells (ova). Also under hormonal control are the secondary sexual characteristics, including breast development, pubic and armpit hair, and the increased fat stores that give a girl a womanly figure. The increase in estrogen can cause vaginal discharge in prepubescent girls (see page 164).

In boys, the pituitary hormones act on the testes to produce testosterone, which stimulates growth of the genitals and production of sperm. Secondary sex characteristics under testosterone control include growth of facial and body hair, enlargement of the larynx with deepening of the voice, and increase in muscle mass.

| YOUR CONCERNS | POSSIBLE CAUSE | ACTION TO TAKE |
|---|---|---|
| *Your preteen daughter has painful swelling underneath each nipple.* | Normal development | Your daughter is experiencing a normal phase of breast development; the tenderness will decrease in time. |
| *Your 13-year-old daughter is showing no signs of physical maturation, such as breast development, pubic hair, or increased growth.* | Delayed puberty | Discuss your concerns with your teen's pediatrician. Your daughter may be following a family pattern, but the pediatrician will evaluate her status and determine whether further evaluation is required. |
| *Your son shows no signs of development by his 14th birthday.* | Delayed puberty | Your pediatrician should examine your teen to determine whether a problem exists and treatment is necessary. |
| *Your school-aged child (younger than 8 years) is starting to show enlargement of one or both breasts or growth of pubic hair.* | Precocious puberty Premature adrenarche or thelarche (See Chapter 2, "Breast Swelling," page 48.) | Talk with your pediatrician, who will determine whether your child should be tested and seen by a specialist. |
| *Your teenaged son is developing at a normal rate but worried that his breasts are growing.* | Breast enlargement (gynecomastia) Fatty tissue | Breast swelling is normal and temporary and usually disappears without treatment. If breast enlargement persists or if your son is embarrassed by his appearance, he should be seen by his pediatrician, who will examine him and, if indicated, reassure him that he's normal. Very rarely, your pediatrician may refer your son for a surgical consultation. |
| *One of your daughter's breasts is larger than the other, but her development is otherwise normal.* | Normal asymmetric breast development | Reassure your daughter that many women have somewhat asymmetric breasts. The difference may become less obvious, but if it remains very marked after she attains her full growth, surgical treatment is possible when she gets older. |

## IN GENERAL

Throughout childhood and adolescence, children need straightforward information about the changes occurring in their bodies and related behavioral and emotional aspects of sexual development. They need to know about erections, nocturnal emissions ("wet dreams"), masturbation, the menstrual cycle, sexual feelings and behavior, and pregnancy, as well as abstinence, contraception, and sexually transmitted infections (STIs), including HIV/AIDS. Some schools teach the biology of sex, but parents should make sure their children understand that sexuality is also tied to emotions, responsible behavior, and moral choices based on their own values as well as those of others. Teenage sexuality and sexual behavior is influenced by a teen's cultural and religious beliefs, as well as by peers and the media.

Early sexual experience in teenagers tends to be associated with other high-risk behaviors, including multiple sexual partners, unsafe sexual behaviors, alcohol and drug use, school problems, and delinquency. Teens need guidance in developing self-control, commitment, and responsible sexual attitudes. Many parents are uncomfortable discussing sexual issues. Your teen's pediatrician can provide impartial advice, suggest reading material, and refer your teen for further counseling, if needed.

If you have strong views about teen sexual activity, be sure to let your teenager know what you consider acceptable behavior and why. While you can educate, you cannot always enforce your rules. If your teenager chooses differently, let him know you're available to listen when he needs to talk and that you are concerned about anything that can affect his health.

• • • • • • • • • • • • • • • • • • • • • • • • • • • • • • • •

### Talk with your teen's pediatrician if you find it difficult to communicate with your teen and you are concerned that he is

- Having unprotected intercourse (sex)
- Taking part in high-risk behavior, including unsafe sexual activity, drug and alcohol use, or truancy
- Confusing public and private sexual behaviors (ie, masturbation) in the context of developmental disabilities

• • • • • • • • • • • • • • • • • • • • • • • • • • • • • • • •

> **WARNING!**
> If your teen is involved with an adult partner in a position of relative authority, you should question if the relationship is abusive. Direct action may only drive a wedge between you and your teen. Your pediatrician may recommend consultation with a family counselor.

## Gender Identity and Sexual Orientation

The teen years are tough enough, but they can be excruciating for teenagers who are sexual minorities (lesbian, gay, bisexual, transgender, questioning [LGBTQ]) or who have questions about their sexual orientation. Gender identity confusion isn't just about boys who don't like sports or girls who prefer football to dolls. Children with gender identity confusion actually identify with members of the opposite sex and may cross-dress and prefer to adopt roles of the opposite gender. They often do not accept their biological sex and prefer playing with children of the opposite gender. Unfortunately, LGBTQ youth are often bullied or isolated from peers at school, which may lead to mental health problems, substance use, and high-risk sexual behaviors.

Children and teens who display or express an interest in members of their own sex may be homosexual, bisexual, or even heterosexual. Although you may wonder if you can influence your child's orientation, an individual's physical and emotional attraction to a member of the same sex, opposite sex, or both is a biological and environmental phenomenon that cannot be changed. But the pressure to behave heterosexually, and the discrimination and victimization LGBTQ youth often experience, can be isolating and lead to serious mental health problems. It can also affect self-esteem and self-confidence.

As a parent, your most important role is to offer understanding, respect, and support to your teen. A nonjudgmental approach will gain your teen's trust and put you in a better position to help him through these difficult times. If your teen is lesbian, gay, bisexual, or transgender, or has questions about his sexual orientation, talk with his pediatrician, who may refer your teen to a mental health specialist to help him during these difficult years. There are organizations that provide information and support to parents as they face the fact that their child is different from them (eg, Parents, Families and Friends of Lesbians and Gays [PFLAG]).

| YOUR CONCERNS | POSSIBLE CAUSE | ACTION TO TAKE |
|---|---|---|
| *You have found items in your teenager's bedroom or backpack or within his social media use that suggest he is sexually active.* | Normal teenage sexual activity<br>Exploration and curiosity<br>High-risk sexual activity | Let your teenager know your views on commitment and respect. Make sure he understands the importance of contraception, as well as the prevention of sexually transmitted infections (STIs). If you find it hard to talk with your teenager, arrange an appointment with your pediatrician. |
| *Your teenaged daughter has pain when she urinates. She urinates frequently or has blood in her urine. She is sexually active.* | Inflammation of the bladder (cystitis)<br>STI | Talk with your teen's pediatrician. Your daughter may need antibiotics. She may also need advice about contraception and disease prevention. |
| *Your daughter complains of heavy bleeding during her periods. She is frequently exhausted and has severe cramps and headaches. Occasionally, she has bleeding between periods.* | Heavy menstrual flow<br>Dysfunctional uterine bleeding<br>Cervicitis<br>Pregnancy | Talk with your teen's pediatrician, who will perform blood tests. Your daughter may need medications to treat her symptoms or hormone treatments to control the bleeding. If she has anemia, she may require iron supplements. |
| *Your teenager asked you for contraceptives.* | Sexual activity | If you do not approve, say so. But if you believe she'll continue without your approval, arrange a talk with her pediatrician, who can give impartial advice and discuss effective contraception. |
| *Your teenager suggested that he is physically attracted to members of the same sex.* | Normal same-sex attraction<br>Homosexuality<br>Lesbian, gay, bisexual, transgender, or questioning youth | It's not unusual to question your sexual orientation during adolescence. Your local library will have age-appropriate books on this issue. If your teenager wants to discuss these concerns in depth, his pediatrician can talk to him and recommend resources such as http://pflag.org. |
| *Your sexually active daughter missed a period. She is having nausea or faintness.* | Pregnancy | Discuss your concerns with your daughter. If you have reason to think she may be pregnant, talk with your pediatrician right away. |
| *Your daughter, who is developmentally disabled, recently started crying with diaper changes, which were usually not stressful before.* | Sexual abuse | Children with disabilities are twice as likely to be sexually abused as typically developing children. Talk with your teen's pediatrician for further evaluation. |
| *Your daughter is unusually upset or withdrawn. She got upset after she accepted a date or a ride with someone. Or she just abruptly broke up with a boyfriend.* | Forced sexual activity<br>Date rape<br>Rape | Try to get the facts without making your daughter overanxious. Give her tips about resisting pressure; tell her you support her and that she can always call you for a ride. If she was forced into having sex, call her pediatrician right away for an examination, treatment for potential STI/HIV or pregnancy prevention, and advice about taking legal action, if necessary. |

| YOUR CONCERNS | POSSIBLE CAUSE | ACTION TO TAKE |
|---|---|---|
| *Your teenager has an unusual discharge from her vagina or his penis and is complaining of low abdominal pain, difficulties urinating, or itching and discomfort in the genital area. Your teen may also have a fever and fatigue.* | STI, including complications, such as pelvic inflammatory disease | Call your teen's pediatrician as soon as possible if you suspect an STI. The pediatrician will do an evaluation and diagnostic (STI) tests and prescribe medications, if needed. |
| *Your teenager has a persistent fever, frequent diarrhea, swollen glands, and fatigue. He recently lost weight and has little appetite. He may have had a series of infections and might have white spots in his mouth. You suspect your teen is engaging in risky sexual behaviors.* | HIV infection or AIDS | Call your teen's pediatrician, who will do a blood test to confirm diagnosis and refer if needed. Discuss safe-sex practices and other ways to prevent the spread of HIV. Early treatment is essential to staying healthy. |
| *Your teen insists he is of the other gender. He expressed a desire for treatment to change his body. These ideas have been present since early childhood.* | Transgender Gender dysphoria | Talk with your teen's pediatrician. People with this condition believe that their anatomic sex does not match how they really feel. Some choose to take hormones or undergo sex reassignment surgery. |

## IN GENERAL

Skin problems are common in teens, and the most common is acne. About 85% of teenagers have acne to some degree. The lucky ones—about three-quarters of those with acne—have nothing more troubling than a few whiteheads, known medically as closed comedones, caused when sebaceous glands become blocked. These glands are attached to hair follicles, through which they secrete a greasy substance, called sebum, to lubricate and protect the hair and skin. Mild acne blemishes generally clear up with little or no scarring, provided they are left alone, not picked, and don't become infected. In severe cases, inflamed pustules and cysts may cause scarring on the face, back, and chest. This severe form, known as *nodulocystic acne,* is more common in boys and is generally managed by dermatologists. Most other acne care in the United States is provided by pediatricians.

The tendency to develop acne runs in families, but skin eruptions are triggered by increases in the levels of male hormones—androgens—that occur in both sexes at puberty. Under the influence of these hormones, the sebaceous glands enlarge and increase sebum output. Girls who have acne may break out because of a surge in hormone levels in the week or so before each menstrual period.

Acne can be very upsetting to teenagers, who are often self-conscious and concerned about their appearance. However, in many cases, parents are more concerned than their children. Safe, effective treatment is now available. Your teen's pediatrician may recommend an over-the-counter lotion or cream to deal with mild or moderate acne. Many teenagers find they have fewer blemishes if they avoid soaps (which are harsh and alkaline) and use a water-rinsable cleansing lotion or soap substitute (which is mildly acidic and less irritating) to wash their faces once or twice every day. But it's important to avoid over-washing and vigorous scrubbing, which can irritate the skin and worsen acne. For more severe outbreaks, treatment may include a prescription medication as well. Teenagers with acne should avoid oil-based skin creams and cosmetics.

### Talk with your teen's pediatrician if

- Your teen has several painful, warm, reddened swellings with pus visible at the peak (these may be boils).
- Your teen compulsively picks at skin blemishes (your teen may benefit from counseling for an underlying emotional problem).
- You are concerned about acne.

### WARNING!

Picking at blemishes can make the skin vulnerable to infection, which may result in permanent scarring. Left alone, most acne lesions heal and don't leave a permanent mark.

## Effects of Diet on Acne

Despite old wives' tales, there is no proven link between acne outbreaks and a diet that includes liberal amounts of chocolate, candy, or fried foods. Acne is not caused by dirty skin, sexual activity, or constipation. Nevertheless, some acne sufferers find that pimples regularly appear after they eat certain foods. Researchers theorize that in such cases, it's not the foods themselves that trigger the outbreak. Instead, they suspect that the real culprit may be stress. It's well known that stress can trigger or worsen acne, perhaps by altering hormone levels. In some people, hormonal changes seem to stimulate food cravings, especially for chocolate and other sweets. So the person may wrongly blame sweets for the acne when the real cause is stress. Exercise, coupled with a diet that balances carbohydrates, protein, and a small amount of fat with plenty of fresh vegetables and fruits, benefits the entire body, including the skin.

The only known cause and effect between diet and acne is an acne-like flare-up that some people get after eating foods high in iodine. A number of medications, especially steroids and other hormone preparations, anticonvulsants, and lithium, can cause acne. Kelp supplements sold in health food stores have been linked to acne. But remember that the levels of iodine in fish and shellfish are unlikely to cause acne in teenagers.

| YOUR CONCERNS | POSSIBLE CAUSE | ACTION TO TAKE |
|---|---|---|
| *Your teen is getting occasional whiteheads or small pustules.* | Teenage acne | To reduce skin oiliness, encourage your teen to clean her face with a mild soap-free cleanser. If pimples are troubling, your teen's pediatrician may recommend an over-the-counter wash or lotion with benzoyl peroxide. Most acne can be managed by your teen's pediatrician. |
| *Your teenager has acne in large bumps or cysts spreading over his face, shoulders, chest, or back.* | Severe acne<br>Cystic acne | Talk with your pediatrician, who will examine your teen and may refer him to a dermatologist for treatment. Left untreated, this condition can lead to painful cysts, unsightly scarring, and severe distress. |
| *Your teenager has a burning or itching feeling in his feet. The skin between his toes is whitish and moist. His toenails may even look yellow.* | Athlete's foot<br>Fungal infection (tinea pedis) | Talk with your teen's pediatrician, who will recommend an antifungal treatment. Encourage your teen to thoroughly dry after baths and showers, use cotton socks, and wash his sneakers. |
| *Your teenager has itching in his crotch area.* | Jock itch (tinea cruris)<br>Intertrigo (inflammation in skin creases and folds)<br>Crabs (sexually transmitted pubic lice) | Talk with your teen's pediatrician, who will evaluate the problem and recommend appropriate treatment. Encourage your child to wear loose-fitting cotton underwear, avoid tight pants, and thoroughly dry himself after baths and showers. When in the pubic hair area, lice are usually spread by close, sexual contact. They can be eradicated with special shampoos, creams, or lotions that contain chemicals to kill the parasites. Talk with your pediatrician for advice on which one to use. |
| *Your teen develops a rash with pale reddish, scaly spots over her trunk and upper arms.* | Pityriasis rosea | Pityriasis rosea is common in teenagers and generally clears up in 6 to 12 weeks. Its cause is unknown. The rash is itchy but harmless and leaves no scars. Talk with your pediatrician, however, to make sure that the rash is not caused by a fungal infection. |

## IN GENERAL

Many people overlook the importance of a good night's sleep. Teenagers are no exception and may in fact have more difficulties when it comes to practicing good sleep habits. In reality, sleep needs do not drop significantly as children mature into teens. But the amount of sleep that teens actually get tends to decrease.

Numerous factors conspire to make sleep a challenge for teenagers. Delays in circadian rhythms (the body's "clock") associated with puberty (rather than actual age) and a decline in sleep drive cause most teens to fall asleep later and later. On top of that, teens face a barrage of competing priorities for sleep that help to further delay bedtime, including homework demands, sports, after-school jobs, dating, socializing with friends, electronics (eg, television, the Internet, texting, video games), and just hanging out. There aren't enough hours in the day for all of this and sleeping too.

At the same time, many schools have earlier start times, which require that teens wake up and function at significantly earlier hours than they did in elementary school. Squeezed between late bedtimes and early wake times, average teens get far less than the 9+ hours of sleep they need. Most teens actually sleep only about 7 hours a night, a number that often dwindles as they get older. Because the teen's normal circadian rhythm changes, weekend "catch-up" sleeping may do more harm than good in maintaining adequate sleep (the teenager may experience something similar to jet lag if he sleeps in too late). Many beverages, supplements, and even lip balm contain caffeine that may temporarily assist the sleepy teenager but worsen sleep issues.

Lack of adequate sleep can affect your teenager's ability to concentrate. It can impair performance academically and in sports (increased injuries). It can also reduce her alertness during waking hours and affect her mood. When your teen starts driving, the lack of sleep can become a safety issue. Recent studies link length of sleep to depressive disorders and even suicide in teens.

### Call your teen's pediatrician right away if she

- Has a dramatic change in sleep patterns
- Snores loudly when sleeping
- Has mood swings as well as sleep problems

**WARNING!**
If your teen sleeps a full night and snores loudly but wakes up exhausted, he may have sleep apnea, a condition in which he is not having proper exchange of gases during sleep. Snoring pauses may lead to frequent arousals from sleep. Sleep apnea can lead to difficulties with school performance. Talk with your pediatrician if you suspect your teen has sleep apnea.

## The Teen Sleep Quandary

Teenagers still need a solid 9 hours of sleep every night, but the ability to sleep is severely challenged at this age. Changes in the circadian rhythm—your body's natural clock—busy schedules, and early school start times can make it difficult for your teen to get the rest she needs.

As a result, many teens wind up sleeping until the late morning, even the early afternoon on weekends. While the goal is to make up for lost sleep during the week, sleeping in only makes things worse. If your teen wakes up more than 2 to 3 hours later than she does on weekdays, she may feel like she is jet-lagged. This makes it even harder for your teen to get up on weekdays.

To reset your teen's schedule, make it a rule that she cannot sleep later than 10:00 am on weekends. Make her responsible for getting up in the morning and not relying on others to wake her. Put a clock radio in her room, with a backup alarm away from her bed so she has to get up to turn it off. Discuss the plan with your teen and even have her sign a contract if it helps. Try to get your teen out into sunlight within 2 hours after she wakes up, which may also help reset her internal clock. If these measures don't help, talk with your teen's pediatrician about seeing a sleep specialist.

| YOUR CONCERNS | POSSIBLE CAUSE | ACTION TO TAKE |
|---|---|---|
| *Your teen is grumpy and has trouble focusing in school. She is tired almost all the time.* | Chronic insufficient sleep | Help your teen get on a consistent sleep schedule. Aim for her to get at least 9 hours of sleep. Practice good sleep hygiene by limiting caffeine, avoiding bright lights in the evening, turning off computers/TV/cell phones at night, and relaxing before bed. |
| *Your teen can't fall asleep at night. He has a hard time getting up for school and then sleeps in late on weekends.* | Insomnia<br>Anxiety | Practice the same suggestions for chronic insufficient sleep. Do not let your teen sleep more than 2 hours later than normal on the weekends. |
| *Your teen can't fall asleep until 2:00 am or later.* | Delayed sleep phase disorder<br>Anxiety | Have your teen go to bed and get up at the same time every day, even on weekends. In the evenings, your teen should try to avoid lights (including computers and tablets), which suppress melatonin, a hormone needed for sleep. Ask your teen's pediatrician for a referral to a sleep specialist. |
| *During sleep, your teen gets up and walks around. When you talk to her about it the next day she has no memory of it.* | Sleepwalking | Sleep-deprived teens are more likely to sleepwalk. Do not awaken your teen when she is sleepwalking; gently guide her back to bed. |
| *Your teen is sleeping much more or less than before. She is increasingly isolated and withdrawn. She often wakes up too early.* | Depression | Call your teen's pediatrician for an examination and possible referral to a mental health specialist. |
| *Your teen complains of sleeping poorly and is often tired during the day, even after a good night's sleep. He snores loudly. He is overweight or has allergies or asthma.* | Obstructive sleep apnea | Talk with your teen's pediatrician, who may recommend your teen receive an overnight sleep study for a diagnosis. If severe, your teen may require surgery to remove enlarged tonsils or adenoid or nasal continuous positive airway pressure. |
| *Your teen is sleeping in much longer than he did in the past. He often wakes in the middle of the night and can't get back to sleep. He is sometimes moody and over-sleeps, while other times he is hyperactive and argumentative and sleeps little.* | An emotional or mental health problem<br>Substance abuse | Talk with your teen's pediatrician, who may refer your teen to a mental health specialist. |
| *Your teen falls asleep in the middle of meals or during conversations. The muscles in her legs sometimes get weak. She says she has strange dreams just before she falls asleep or wakes up.* | Narcolepsy | Talk with your teen's pediatrician, who will refer your teen for an overnight sleep study. Narcolepsy often emerges in adolescence and requires lifelong management. |

## IN GENERAL

Teenage substance use is a major public health problem. Teens who use alcohol or drugs are more likely to do poorly in school, develop a sexually transmitted infection, and become pregnant. They are also at greater risk for suicide and homicide. All teens should be screened for substance use. About 10% of them will have substance abuse issues, and half of this 10% are likely to require treatment.

Some teens are at greater risk for substance abuse than others, including those who are impulsive, aggressive, and disruptive. Teens who have attention-deficit/hyperactivity disorder (ADHD) (see page 30) are also at greater risk; teens treated properly for ADHD may have a lower rate   of substance use later in life. In addition, the risk is higher in teens who lack parental monitoring or have a family history of drug or alcohol abuse. A preteen or teenager who begins experimenting with cigarettes between the ages of 12 and 14 years is at greater risk for a lifetime of substance use and abuse. Teens who report that their parents monitor them closely, praise them frequently, and strongly disapprove of drugs report lower rates of substance use.

If you suspect your teen is using drugs, trust your instincts and monitor your teen closely. During a calm moment, have a discussion with him about your concerns. Avoid direct accusations, but be specific. Remember to say, "We love you and are concerned. We hope you will be honest with us." Make it clear that you are strongly opposed to any form of drug use. Discuss your specific concerns with your pediatrician. Remember that concerns such as recent changes in academic performance, friends, appearance, and irritability can all be nonspecific signs of a substance use or other mental health disorder. The earlier a substance abuse problem is identified and treated, the less likely it is that your teen will suffer adverse consequences.

### Call your teen's pediatrician right away if

- You need to schedule an appointment with your teen's pediatrician because your teen is using drugs or alcohol regularly or getting into trouble because of his substance use.
- Your teen is using drugs or alcohol and displaying dangerous behaviors such as self-mutilation, threats of suicide or homicide, or driving under the influence.

### WARNING!

Do not dismiss your teenager's use of drugs or alcohol as a passing phase. Among US teenagers, substance use is associated with the leading causes of death, including unintentional injuries (eg, motor vehicle crashes), homicides, and suicides. More than 30% of all deaths from injuries can be directly linked to alcohol. Substance use also is associated with a wide range of nonlethal but serious health problems, including memory problems, vitamin deficiencies, balance difficulties, and high-risk sexual behaviors.

### Teens, Drugs, and the Media

As a society, we tell our children and teens to just say no to drugs. And yet we allow $20 billion of advertising for cigarettes, alcohol, and prescription drugs in movies, television, and other media. The average American teen sees 2,000 beer and wine commercials in a year, most of it during sports programming. On prime-time television, 71% of shows feature alcohol use.

It isn't easy to limit a teen's exposure to unhealthy advertisements. It starts with limiting how much media your teen gets in a day. The American Academy of Pediatrics recommends no more than 2 hours of media a day. It's also best to keep electronics like television, computers, cell phone, or any other device that provides access to the Internet out of the bedroom.

| YOUR CONCERNS | POSSIBLE CAUSE | ACTION TO TAKE |
|---|---|---|
| *Your teen smells like cigarettes. His teeth are stained and his breath is bad.* | Cigarette smoking | Discourage tobacco and other drug use by making your values clear to your teen. Ask his pediatrician to discuss the effect of tobacco on health. Provide your teen with ways to cope with peer pressure. Offer to enroll your teen in a smoking cessation program. Discuss the problem with his pediatrician. |
| *Your teen is nauseous and vomiting on arrival home after a party. You think you smell alcohol on her breath.* | Alcohol use | Make it clear that you do not tolerate alcohol use. Discuss the dangers of drug and alcohol use. Find teachable moments to discuss tragedies that result from alcohol use. Give your teen strategies for coping with peer pressure. Talk with her pediatrician for additional advice. |
| *Your teen often comes home smelling of alcohol and has slurred speech and poor coordination. He is often combative and was recently in a car accident.* | Alcohol and other drug use<br>More significant alcohol problem | Contact your teen's pediatrician for further evaluation and recommendations. Suspend driving privileges until your teen engages in treatment. |
| *Your teenager is often moody and grumpy. She doesn't care about school the way she used to, and she has been dropping out of activities. She comes home talkative and giggly and has red eyes.* | Marijuana use | Discuss the hazards of marijuana use with your teen. Help her deal with peer pressure and find positive interests. Be a positive role model in how you handle stress and pressure. Talk with your pediatrician for additional advice. |
| *Your teen often has a dazed look. His breath smells like chemicals. He has little appetite and appears anxious. He complains of nausea. You have found spray cans or rags soaked with solvents in his room. He has rings around his nose or mouth.* | Inhalants, such as solvents, nitrous oxide, and volatile nitrites found in air fresheners | Tell your teen that you do not tolerate drug use. Discuss the importance of a healthy lifestyle. Help your teen develop other interests and hobbies. Call his pediatrician for help. |
| *Your teen is often restless, hyperactive, and talkative. She is excitable and says her heart is racing.* | Use or abuse of stimulants such as ADHD medications, methamphetamines, ecstasy, and cocaine | Make clear that you do not tolerate drug use. Discuss the importance of a healthy lifestyle, which includes good nutrition. Help your teen develop other interests and hobbies. Call your teen's pediatrician for help. |
| *Your teen has strange symptoms such as paranoia, drowsiness, or slurred speech that you can't explain. You find pills in his bedroom that don't belong to him. Or one of your prescription medications is missing pills.* | Prescription pain medication | Talk with your teen's pediatrician for advice and potential referral to substance abuse professionals. Your teen may be abusing prescription drugs that he is obtaining from friends or the family medicine cabinet. Discuss the dangers of using medications that are not prescribed to him. |

**CHAPTER 4**

# Basics of First Aid

## ADMINISTERING FIRST AID

First aid involves giving immediate, often lifesaving care to a child who is injured or has a sudden illness. It demands fast thinking and action to provide needed care until you can obtain medical assistance. Train yourself to stay calm in emergencies: count slowly or breathe deeply if it helps keep you steady. You will be able to think more clearly, and your child will be less likely to get upset. Read this chapter several times so you'll know what to do in an emergency. Keep this book where it's easy to find.

Make sure to store 911 or your local emergency number in your cell phone as well as numbers for your pediatrician, dentist, nearest poison center, nearest emergency department, and next-door neighbor. Keep an up-to-date list of those emergency numbers in your home. Include any medical information your babysitter might need (eg, the names of all medications your child takes, any allergies your child has). Top the list with 911 or your local emergency number, and keep your own address and telephone number handy; stress can affect your memory in a crisis.

## LIFESAVING TECHNIQUES

Every parent and caregiver should know how to perform 2 very important lifesaving techniques: first aid for choking and first aid for cardiopulmonary resuscitation (CPR). The instructions written in this chapter should not take the place of an approved class in basic first aid, CPR, or emergency prevention. Contact your local American Red Cross office or the American Heart Association to find out about classes offered in your area. Most of the classes teach basic first aid, CPR, and emergency prevention along with what to do for a choking infant or child.

## THE IMPORTANCE OF PREVENTION

Each year millions of American children need medical care because of injuries. According to the Centers for Disease Control and Prevention, approximately 9 million children are taken to the emergency department each year for an unintentional injury, and more than 12,000 of them lose their life. In fact, unintentional injuries are the leading cause of death in children and teenagers younger than 19 years. While cars are involved in a large number of injuries and deaths, many injuries occur around our homes and may involve furniture or playground equipment designed for children. Being ready to manage injuries as they occur isn't enough to keep your child safe; instead, you must be alert to hazards related to the use of everyday objects, your environment, and your child himself. Chapter 5 ("Guide to Safety and Prevention"), which begins on page 229, can help you recognize potentially dangerous situations in your home. Refer to it frequently; you'll need to revise your safety procedures over time as your child grows older and faces new risks.

## First Aid Kit

You will find it easier to cope with an emergency if you have a few essential supplies on hand. The following items should be in every first aid kit:

- Acetaminophen or a nonsteroidal anti-inflammatory medication (such as ibuprofen)
- Sterile adhesive bandages (in various sizes)
- Adhesive tape (hypoallergenic)
- Scissors
- Gauze pads
- Petroleum jelly or another lubricant
- Tweezers
- Antibiotic cream or ointment
- Soap or another cleaning agent
- Moistened towelettes
- Thermometer

Keep one kit in your home and one in each family member's car. Store the items in a marked container, and place the container out of the reach of young children. Pharmacies also stock pre-packaged first aid kits. Check the supplies of your first aid kid from time to time so you can replace outdated items; replace other items as you use them.

## Choking

Many children die from choking each year. Most children who choke to death are younger than 5 years of age. It is a serious emergency that occurs when food or small objects get caught in the throat and block the airway. This can prevent oxygen from getting to the lungs and the brain. A child who is choking can't speak, cry out, or cough. Her face rapidly becomes flushed and turns blue.

### Prevention

Parents and other caregivers must be especially watchful of young children who are sampling new foods; food is the most frequent cause of choking.

- Cut food for infants and young children into pieces no larger than one-quarter inch for infants and one-half inch for toddlers, and teach them to chew their food well.
- Supervise mealtime for infants and young children.
- Small toys are also a common source of danger.

- Follow the age recommendations on toy packages. Age guidelines reflect the safety of a toy based on any possible choking hazard as well as the child's physical and mental abilities at various ages.
- Be aware that balloons pose a choking risk to children up to 8 years of age.

For further guidelines on safety and prevention, see Chapter 5, page 229.

### What You Can Do

Please take time to look over the "Choking/CPR" chart specific to your child's age on pages 215 and 216. If your infant or child is choking and unable to breathe, cannot cough or talk, or looks blue, you must act immediately. Shout for help and begin first aid for choking appropriate for your child's age. If possible, have someone nearby call for emergency assistance. If at any time an object is coughed up or the infant/child starts to breathe, stop rescue breaths and call 911 or your local emergency number. If your child is unconscious or unresponsive, you need to perform CPR appropriate for your child's age. The following instructions are choking and CPR procedures for infants younger than 1 year and choking and CPR procedures for children 1 to 8 years of age. Ask your pediatrician for information on choking/CPR instructions for children older than 8 years and for information on an approved first aid or CPR course in your community.

### Treatment

Once a blockage is cleared, most children are soon back to normal. A child who breathes on his own within 2 or 3 minutes is unlikely to have long-term damage. If your child isn't breathing by the time help arrives, the emergency medical team will attempt to dislodge the blockage. At the same time, they will prepare your child for transport to a hospital for further treatment, such as insertion of a breathing tube.

- If your child keeps on coughing, gagging, or drooling, or has trouble swallowing or breathing after a choking incident, it may mean that some of the foreign material is still partly blocking his airway. He should be transported to the emergency department for further treatment.

# CHOKING/CPR

## LEARN AND PRACTICE CPR (CARDIOPULMONARY RESUSCITATION).

### IF ALONE WITH A CHILD WHO IS CHOKING...

### 1. SHOUT FOR HELP.  2. START RESCUE EFFORTS.  3. CALL 911 OR YOUR LOCAL EMERGENCY NUMBER.

| START FIRST AID FOR CHOKING IF | DO *NOT* START FIRST AID FOR CHOKING IF |
|---|---|
| • The child cannot breathe at all (the chest is not moving up and down).<br>• The child cannot cough or talk, or looks blue.<br>• The child is found unconscious/unresponsive. (Go to CPR.) | • The child can breathe, cry, or talk.<br>• The child can cough, sputter, or move air at all. The child's normal reflexes are working to clear the airway. |

## FOR INFANTS YOUNGER THAN 1 YEAR

### INFANT CHOKING

If the infant is choking and is unable to breathe, cough, cry, or speak, follow these steps. Have someone call 911.

### INFANT CPR

To be used when the infant is **UNCONSCIOUS/UNRESPONSIVE** or when breathing stops. Place infant on flat, hard surface.

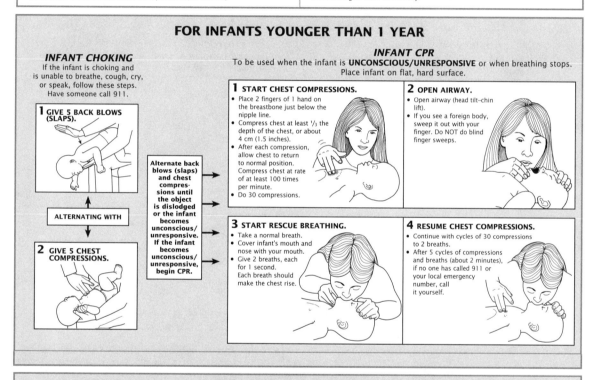

**1 GIVE 5 BACK BLOWS (SLAPS).**

**ALTERNATING WITH**

**2 GIVE 5 CHEST COMPRESSIONS.**

Alternate back blows (slaps) and chest compressions until the object is dislodged or the infant becomes unconscious/unresponsive. If the infant becomes unconscious/unresponsive, begin CPR.

**1 START CHEST COMPRESSIONS.**
- Place 2 fingers of 1 hand on the breastbone just below the nipple line.
- Compress chest at least $1/3$ the depth of the chest, or about 4 cm (1.5 inches).
- After each compression, allow chest to return to normal position. Compress chest at rate of at least 100 times per minute.
- Do 30 compressions.

**2 OPEN AIRWAY.**
- Open airway (head tilt–chin lift).
- If you see a foreign body, sweep it out with your finger. Do NOT do blind finger sweeps.

**3 START RESCUE BREATHING.**
- Take a normal breath.
- Cover infant's mouth and nose with your mouth.
- Give 2 breaths, each for 1 second. Each breath should make the chest rise.

**4 RESUME CHEST COMPRESSIONS.**
- Continue with cycles of 30 compressions to 2 breaths.
- After 5 cycles of compressions and breaths (about 2 minutes), if no one has called 911 or your local emergency number, call it yourself.

**If at any time an object is coughed up or the infant/child starts to breathe, stop rescue breaths and call 911 or your local emergency number.**

**Ask your pediatrician for information on choking/CPR instructions for children older than 8 years and for information on an approved first aid or CPR course in your community.**

# CHOKING/CPR

## LEARN AND PRACTICE CPR (CARDIOPULMONARY RESUSCITATION).

### IF ALONE WITH A CHILD WHO IS CHOKING...

### 1. SHOUT FOR HELP.  2. START RESCUE EFFORTS.  3. CALL 911 OR YOUR LOCAL EMERGENCY NUMBER.

| START FIRST AID FOR CHOKING IF | DO *NOT* START FIRST AID FOR CHOKING IF |
|---|---|
| • The child cannot breathe at all (the chest is not moving up and down).<br>• The child cannot cough or talk, or looks blue.<br>• The child is found unconscious/unresponsive. (Go to CPR.) | • The child can breathe, cry, or talk.<br>• The child can cough, sputter, or move air at all. The child's normal reflexes are working to clear the airway. |

## FOR CHILDREN 1 TO 8 YEARS OF AGE

### CHILD CHOKING (HEIMLICH MANEUVER)

Have someone call 911. If the child is choking and is unable to breathe, cough, cry, or speak, follow these steps.

1. Perform Heimlich maneuver.
   • Place hand, made into a fist, and cover with other hand just above the navel. Place well below the bottom tip of the breastbone and rib cage.
   • Give each thrust with enough force to produce an artificial cough designed to relieve airway obstruction.
   • Perform Heimlich maneuver until the object is expelled or the child becomes unconscious/unresponsive.

2. If the child becomes UNCONSCIOUS/UNRESPONSIVE, begin CPR.

### CHILD CPR

To be used when the child is **UNCONSCIOUS/UNRESPONSIVE** or when breathing stops.
Place child on flat, hard surface.

**1 START CHEST COMPRESSIONS.**
• Place the heel of 1 or 2 hands over the lower half of the sternum.
• Compress chest at least $^1/_3$ the depth of the chest, or about 5 cm (2 inches).
• After each compression, allow chest to return to normal position. Compress chest at rate of at least 100 times per minute.
• Do 30 compressions.

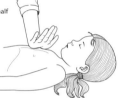
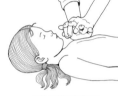

**1-hand technique**          **2-hand technique**

**2 OPEN AIRWAY.**
• Open airway (head tilt–chin lift).
• If you see a foreign body, sweep it out with your finger. Do NOT do blind finger sweeps.

**3 START RESCUE BREATHING.**
• Take a normal breath.
• Pinch the child's nose closed, and cover child's mouth with your mouth.
• Give 2 breaths, each for 1 second. Each breath should make the chest rise.

**4 RESUME CHEST COMPRESSIONS.**
• Continue with cycles of 30 compressions to 2 breaths until the object is expelled.
• After 5 cycles of compressions and breaths (about 2 minutes), if no one has called 911 or your local emergency number, call it yourself.

**If at any time an object is coughed up or the infant/child starts to breathe, stop rescue breaths and call 911 or your local emergency number.**

**Ask your pediatrician for information on choking/CPR instructions for children older than 8 years and for information on an approved first aid or CPR course in your community.**

# Drowning

Drowning is a leading cause of death in children, including infants and toddlers. A child can drown in only a few inches of water, whether on a lake-shore or in a bathtub, toilet, or bucket of water. A child drowns either because she ventures into water that's too deep, such as a pond, a river, or a lake, or because she's trapped in a position where her face is in water. Drowning occurs when a child inhales water and suffocates.

If a child is rescued before death occurs, the event is referred to as a *nonfatal drowning*. Recovery from a nonfatal drowning depends on how long the child is deprived of oxygen. A child who is submerged only momentarily is likely to recover completely. Every child who has a nonfatal drowning must be examined by a pediatrician, even if the child seems to have experienced no ill effects. A child who stops breathing, inhales water, or loses consciousness should remain under medical observation for 24 hours to make sure his respiratory and nervous systems are undamaged.

## What to Do in the Event of Drowning

If you see your child drowning, get him out of the water immediately and check to see if he is breathing on his own. If not, begin CPR immediately that is appropriate for your child's age (see page 215 or 216). If someone else is with you, ask that person to call 911 or your local emergency medical number immediately. Don't waste time looking for someone; instead, concentrate on giving him CPR until he's breathing on his own again. Your child may vomit swallowed water during CPR. Only when he's breathing again should you stop and get help. Once the paramedics arrive, they will give your child oxygen and continue CPR, if necessary.

A child's recovery from a nonfatal drowning depends on how long she's deprived of oxygen. If she's under water only briefly, she will most likely recover completely. If a child is without oxygen for longer periods, she may experience damage to her lungs, heart, or brain. A child who doesn't respond

quickly to CPR may have more serious injuries. It's important to continue CPR as sustained CPR has revived children who have appeared lifeless or who have been immersed in very cold water for lengthy periods.

## Prevention

Never leave an infant, toddler, or young child for even a moment when he's in a bathtub, pool, wading pool, spa, or another body of water. Practice "touch supervision," which means that a supervising adult should be within an arm's length of the child at all times. This adult's attention should be focused entirely on the child, not diverted by other distractions such as cell phones, conversations, or household chores.

Home swimming pools should be surrounded on all 4 sides by a fence that completely separates the house from the pool so your child can't leave the house and get inside of the pool. The fence should be at least 4 feet high, non-climbable, and 4-sided with a self-closing, self-latching gate. Every parent, caregiver, and pool owner should learn CPR and keep at the poolside a telephone and equipment approved by the US Coast Guard (ig, life preservers, life jackets, shepherd's crook).

Toddlers, children with developmental delays, and children with seizure disorders are particularly vulnerable to drowning, but *all* children are in danger if unsupervised in or near water. Even a child who knows how to swim may drown a few feet from safety. Remember, children should be supervised at all times. Swimming lessons should not be considered as a surefire way to prevent your child from drowning, but it's still essential for water safety.

Children need to learn to swim. The AAP supports swimming lessons for most children 4 years and older, and for children 1 to 4 years of age who are ready to learn how to swim. Keep in mind that because children develop at different rates, each child will be ready to swim at her own time. Some factors you may consider before starting swimming lessons for younger children include frequency of exposure to water, emotional maturity, physical limitations, and health concerns related to swimming pools (eg, swallowing water, infections, pool chemicals). Swim lessons don't provide "drown-proofing" for children of any age, so supervision and other layers of protection are necessary even for children who have learned swimming skills.

## Poisoning

Every year more than 2 million people swallow or come into contact with a poisonous substance. More than half of these exposures to poison occur in children younger than 6 years. Most children who swallow poison aren't permanently harmed, especially if they receive immediate treatment. If you think your child has been poisoned, stay calm and act quickly. You should suspect poisoning if you ever find your child with an open or empty container of a toxic substance, especially if he's acting strangely. Be alert for these other signs of possible poisoning.

- Unexplained stains on his clothing
- Burns on his lips or mouth
- Unusual drooling, or odd odors on his breath
- Unexplained nausea or vomiting
- Abdominal cramps without fever
- Trouble breathing
- Sudden behavior changes, such as unusual sleepiness, irritability, or jumpiness
- Convulsions or unconsciousness (only in very serious cases)

### Prevention

Store all medications and hazardous materials in locked cabinets out of the reach of children. Keep all medications in containers with child-resistant caps. Remember, these caps are child-resistant but not childproof, so keep them in locked cabinets. Safely dispose of leftover prescription medicines when the illness for which they were prescribed has passed. You can take them back to your pharmacy, where they can be safely discarded. Read the label, and follow dosing instructions every time you give a child medicine. For more detailed guidelines, see Chapter 5 page 229.

### What You Can Do

Anytime your child has ingested a poison of any kind, you should notify your pediatrician; however, your regional Poison Center will provide the immediate information and guidance you need when you first discover that your child has been poisoned. These centers are staffed 24 hours a day with experts who can tell you what to do without delay. Call the national toll-free number for Poison Help at 800/222-1222, which will provide you with immediate and free access around the clock to your regional Poison Center. *If there's an emergency and you can't find the number, dial 911 or your local emergency number, or dial Directory Assistance and ask for the Poison Help number.*

The immediate action you need to take will vary with the type of poisoning. The Poison Help number can give you specific instructions if you know the specific substance your child has swallowed. Don't try to make your child vomit unless the Poison Center staff advise you to do so, as this can be more harmful than helpful.

### Treatment

- Depending on the toxic substance and your child's condition, she may be placed in a hospital for treatment and observation. Most children don't need to be hospitalized.

*Everyday items that are hazardous to young children include*

- Detergents
- Drain cleaner
- Furniture and metal polishes
- Gasoline, kerosene, lamp oil
- Poisonous house plants (eg, jade plant, African violet)
- Insect sprays and pest repellents
- Mouthwash
- Nail polish remover
- Paints, thinners
- Rubbing alcohol
- Spot removers
- Tobacco products
- Vitamins, including prenatal vitamin pills

## FREQUENTLY USED FIRST AID MEASURES

There are dozens of situations that may require first aid; those covered in the following section are among the more common ones. Because there is no time to consult a book when an emergency arises, it's a good idea to frequently review the steps described here, so you'll know what to do if the need arises.

### Animal Bites

As many as 1% of all visits to pediatric emergency centers during the summer months are for human or animal bite wounds. Most are dog bites, but children are also bitten by cats, snakes, and other people.

It's important to keep your child safe around animals, including family pets. Most bites are inflicted by animals familiar to the child. Although the injury is often minor, biting does at times cause serious wounds, facial damage, and emotional problems. The risk of rabies is much higher in bites from wild animals (eg, skunks, bats, raccoons, foxes) than from pets, where it can be eliminated by having the animal properly immunized.

### Prevention

- Avoid rough play with animals to prevent scratches or bites.
- Do not allow your children to kiss pets on the mouth. Also, be sure children learn not to put their hands into their mouths after touching their pets.
- Keep your pet healthy with regular visits to the veterinarian. Keep your pet free of fleas and ticks.
- Follow leash laws and keep your pet under control at all times.

For more information, see "Preventing Injury From Animals," page 241.

### What You Can Do

- If the wound is bleeding, apply firm, continuous pressure to it for 5 minutes or until the bleeding stops.

- Wash the wound with soap, and rinse it with plenty of water. Call your pediatrician.
- Always call your pediatrician if a bite breaks your child's skin; your pediatrician will determine whether your child is adequately protected against tetanus, should you be concerned about rabies exposure or if your child needs to be seen.
- Capture or confine the animal only if you can do so without danger to yourself or others. Don't destroy the animal; call the police to handle it. If the animal has been killed, call your local animal control officer or veterinarian to find out how to preserve a specimen for rabies examination.
- In the days following the bite, call your pediatrician if you see any of the following signs of bacterial infection:
  - Pus or drainage from the wound
  - Increasing swelling or tenderness around the wound after the first 8 to 12 hours
  - Red streaks or an increasing red zone spreading out from the bite
  - Swollen glands above the bite
- If your child has suffered a snake bite, take her immediately to a emergency department right away if you're unsure of the type of snake or whether it's poisonous. Keep your child at rest. Don't apply ice. Loosely splint her injured area, and keep it at rest, positioned at or slightly below the level of her heart. Identify the snake if you can. If you have killed the snake, carefully place it in a container and bring it with you to the emergency department for identification.
- Be alert to signs of post-traumatic stress disorder, which can occur after a traumatic event like a bite. Long after the physical wound has healed, these children may continue to have emotional difficulties associated with the bite. They may feel fear about being bitten again. They may withdraw or cling to their parents. They may resist going outside to play, have trouble sleeping, have nightmares, or wet the bed. To help the healing process, give your child extra attention when you sense she needs it. Some children with post-traumatic stress disorder may require treatment by a mental health professional.

## Treatment

- If the wound is very large, or you can't stop the bleeding, continue to apply pressure to it. Call your pediatrician to find out where to take your child for treatment. If is the wound is so large that its edges won't come together, it may need to be sutured (stitched). Although this will help reduce scarring, in an animal bite, it may increase the chance of infection, so your pediatrician may prescribe antibiotics.
- Your pediatrician may prescribe an antibiotic to prevent bacterial infection in an open wound that's moderate or severe, if the wound has punctured the skin, or if the wound has penetrated a bone, tendon, or joint. Antibiotics may also be required if your child experiences a facial bite, a hand or foot bite, or bites to the genital area. Children who have weakened immune systems or no spleen often receive antibiotics too.
- If there is any risk of rabies, your pediatrician will tell you the procedure to follow. Rabies is a rare viral infection that can cause high fever, trouble swallowing, convulsions, and death. Your pediatrician can determine if your child's risk for rabies is high. If possible, the animal should be captured and examined. If you find a bat in a room where your child has been sleeping or playing, you should report it right away to your pediatrician, even if you don't find a bite mark.

## Burns

Burns are divided into 4 categories, according to severity. *First-degree burns* are the mildest and cause redness and perhaps slight swelling of the skin (like most sunburns). *Second-degree burns* cause blistering and considerable swelling. *Third-degree burns* may appear white or charred and cause serious injury not just to the surface but also to the deeper layers of the skin. *Fourth-degree* burns involve underlying subcutaneous tissue, tendons, or bones. Hot liquids, including drinks and tap water, are the most common causes of burns in children. Children may also incur serious burns from the sun and from everyday household items, such as irons, hair appli-

ances, cleaning products, and barbecue grills. Burns are painful; they also carry a high risk of infection. Severe burns may be life-threatening and can cause permanent injury and scarring.

## Prevention

Most burn injuries happen in the home. The following are tips to help prevent your child from getting burned:

- Keep matches, lighters, and ashtrays out of the reach of children.
- Cover all unused electrical outlets with plastic plugs or other types of outlet covers.
- Don't allow your child to play closely to fireplaces, radiators, or space heaters.
- Replace all frayed, broken, or worn electrical cords.
- Never leave barbecue grills unattended.
- Teach your child that irons, curling irons, barbeque grills, radiators, and ovens can get very hot and are dangerous to touch or play near. Never leave these items unattended. Unplug and put away all appliances after using them.
- Keep electrical cords from hanging down where children can pull on them or chew on them. Mouth burns can result from chewing on an extension cord or a poorly insulated wire.

See "Fire Injury Prevention," page 243.

### What You Can Do

- Soak the burn in cool water right away. Run cool water over the burn long enough to cool the area and relieve the pain immediately after the injury. Don't use ice on a burn; it may delay healing. Also, don't rub a burn; it can cause blistering.
- Cool smoldering clothing immediately by soaking it with water and removing it from the burned area, unless it's stuck firmly to your child's skin. In that case cut away as much clothing as possible.
- If the injured area isn't oozing, cover the burn with a sterile gauze pad or a clean, dry cloth.
- If the burn is oozing, cover it lightly with sterilized gauze, if available, and immediately seek medical attention. If sterile gauze isn't available, cover burns with a clean sheet or towel.

- Never put ointment or medicine on a burn, unless your pediatrician tells you to do so.
- Never put butter, grease, or powder on a burn; these home remedies can make the injury worse.
- When caring for a burn at home, call your pediatrician if you see signs of infection, such as increased redness or swelling, a discharge, or unpleasant odor.

### Treatment

- For anything more serious than a superficial burn, or if redness and pain continue for more than a few hours, talk with your pediatrician. All electrical burns and burns of the hands, mouth, or genitals should receive immediate medical attention. Chemicals that cause burns also may be absorbed through the skin and cause other symptoms. Call Poison Control at 800/222-1222, or your pediatrician, after washing off all of the chemicals.
- Call 911 or your local emergency number if the burn is large and your child is becoming ill from it.
- If your pediatrician thinks you can manage the burn at home, he or she will tell you how to take care of it with medications and dressings.

*Most pediatricians will admit a child to the hospital:*
- When burns are third-degree
- When burns cover 10% or more of the child's body
- When the burns involve the face, hands, feet, genitals, or a moving joint
- If the child is younger than 6 months of age, fussy, and too difficult to treat initially at home

## Cold Injury

Children who are exposed to cold temperatures may experience hypothermia or frostbite. Hypothermia develops when a child's temperature falls below normal due to exposure to cold. This condition often occurs when a child is playing outdoors in extremely cold weather without wearing proper clothing. As hypothermia sets in, the child may shiver and become lethargic and clumsy; his speech may become slurred, and his body temperature will decline.

Frostbite occurs when the skin and outer tissues become frozen. This condition tends to occur on extremities like the fingers, toes, ears, and nose, which may become pale, gray, and blistered. At the same time, the child may complain that his skin burns or has become numb.

### Prevention

- Make sure children are properly clothed for winter sports.
- Dress your child in several lightweight pieces of clothing, which provide more protection against cold. Use hats and cover ears.
- Limit time outside during periods of low temperature and high wind chill.
- Provide warming drinks at the end of outdoor play in the winter.
- Take your child into a warm environment when she complains of feeling cold.

### What You Can Do

- Take your child indoors immediately if you suspect frostbite or hypothermia. Remove any wet clothing, and wrap him in blankets or warm clothes.
- While still outside, cover your child's frozen parts with clothing or any available cloth. Tuck his frostbitten fingers in your armpits while carrying him to shelter.
- Once inside place the frostbitten parts of his body in warm (not hot) water; you can apply warm washcloths to the frostbitten nose, ears, and lips. Don't rub the frozen areas. After a few minutes dry and cover him with clothing or blankets. Give him something warm to drink. If the numbness continues for more than a few minutes, call your pediatrician.
- If water isn't available, wrap the frostbitten part in a blanket or other warm material. Don't use a heat lamp, hot water bottle, or heating pad. Ask your child to move his fingers or toes as soon as they feel warmer.
- If your child becomes lethargic and clumsy, or his speech is slurred, call 911 or your local emergency number right away. He may have hypothermia.

- Separate frostbitten toes or fingers with sterile gauze dressings.
- Don't place your child near a hot stove or radiator; the frostbitten part may be burned before feeling returns.
- Don't break blisters.
- Stop the warming process when your child's skin becomes pink and feeling begins to return.
- Seek medical attention right away.

**Treatment**
- A child who has suffered hypothermia or frostbite should be examined by a pediatrician.

## Convulsions

A rapid rise in body temperature may trigger convulsions or seizures in young children. Most seizures are brief, lasting only a minute or less, but they can be frightening. Febrile seizures tend to occur in children between 6 months and 5 years of age, but they occur most often around 12 to 18 months of age. Most children who have one episode never have another. Febrile seizures usually stop on their own and don't require emergency medical attention. A small percentage of these children develop epilepsy or non–fever-related seizures (also see "Seizures," page 134).

**Prevention**
- You may consider giving your child acetamino-phen or ibuprofen to make her more comfortable, but it won't prevent future seizures.
- Seizures due to a chronic condition such as epilepsy can usually be well controlled by anti-convulsant medication, which must be taken regularly and never stopped abruptly.
- If your child has epilepsy, make sure her friends, teachers, and caregivers are educated about it.

**What You Can Do**
- Place a convulsing child on her side with her hips higher than her head so he won't choke if she vomits. Don't place anything in his mouth.

- If the convulsion doesn't stop after 5 minutes, or is unusually severe (ie, trouble breathing, choking, blueness of the skin, having several in a row), call 911 or your local emergency number for medical help. Don't leave your child alone.
- When the seizure stops, call your pediatrician right away, and arrange for your child to be seen in the office or the nearest emergency department. Also, call your pediatrician if your child is on an anticonvulsant medication. This means that the dosage may need to be adjusted.

**Treatment**
- If your child has fever, your pediatrician will probably wish to examine her to find and treat the source of the fever.
- If there is no fever, and this was your child's first convulsion, your pediatrician will try to determine other possible causes by asking if your family has a medical history of seizures or if your child has had any recent head injuries.
- If your child has had seizures before and is on anticonvulsant medication, your pediatrician may adjust the dosage.

## Cuts and Scrapes

Most minor cuts and scrapes can be treated by gentle, thorough cleansing with water and soap followed by an antiseptic, antibiotic cream, or ointment and reassurance.

*Keep your child's immunizations, including the tetanus shot, up-to-date. If your child isn't fully immunized or it's been more than 5 years since his last tetanus shot, ask your pediatrician if a booster is needed.*

**Cuts**
Cuts, or *lacerations,* penetrate the tissues beneath the skin. Because the injury is deeper than a scrape, problems such as bleeding are more likely, and damage to nerves and tendons is possible.

### Prevention

Active, curious children suffer minor cuts and scrapes in the course of their explorations. Parents can't expect to prevent every mishap, but they can take sensible measures to reduce the numbers of cuts and scrapes and reduce the risk of serious injury.

- Keep potentially dangerous items (such as sharp knives) and breakable items (such as glassware) out of young children's reach. When she gets old enough to use knives and scissors, teach her how to use them properly, and insist that they be used safely. Warn her never to run while carrying breakable objects or sharp instruments such as pens, pencils, and scissors.
- Keep toys and outdoor play equipment, such as swings and climbing frames, in good repair. If toys can't be repaired, discard or dismantle them. Don't let unsupervised children play on hazardous equipment, such as swings or climbing bars.
- Make sure children wear protective pads and helmets for sports that involve hazards, such as skateboarding, bicycle riding, and in-line skating.

### What You Can Do

- Press firmly on the wound with clean gauze or cloth for 5 or 10 minutes or until bleeding stops (Figure 4-1). Resist the urge to look at the wound too soon; you may allow the bleeding to start again.
- If the wound bleeds again after 5 minutes of continuous pressure, reapply pressure, and call your pediatrician. Don't apply a tourniquet unless you've had special training; it can cause severe damage.
- Stay calm. The sight of blood frightens many people, but it's an important time to stay calm. You'll make better decisions, and your child will be less likely to get upset.

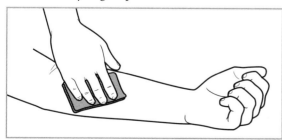

**Figure 4-1.**

- When bleeding stops, gently wash the wound with plain water, and examine it to make sure it's clean (Figure 4-2).
- Treat short, minor cuts at home provided the edges come together by themselves.

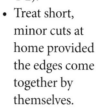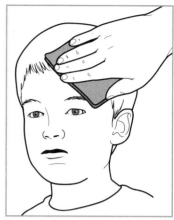

**Figure 4-2.**

- Apply an antibiotic ointment, such as bacitracin, then cover it with a sterile dressing or Band-Aid.
- It's safe to wash the wound with soap and water at least daily after the first 24 hours. Dry gently but thoroughly. Avoid using hydrogen peroxide or alcohol repeatedly as they can delay wound healing.
- As the wound heals, look for increased redness and swelling or pus drainage, which may signal infection. If these symptoms are present, call your pediatrician.

### Treatment

- Call your pediatrician if the laceration is more than half an inch deep or gaping, even if bleeding isn't severe. Deep cuts should be examined to find out if there is injury to tendons or nerves. Deep cuts may also require treatment to close the skin.
- Seek your pediatrician's attention for cuts to the face, chest, and neck, or for long lacerations. For best results wounds should be stitched within 8 hours.
- Ask your pediatrician to examine a laceration if there is any possibility that foreign matter, such as glass or dirt, may be trapped in it or if your child is too distressed to let you examine the wound thoroughly. Your pediatrician can administer a local anesthetic to make examination, cleaning, and treatment easier.

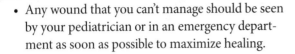

# BASICS OF FIRST AID

- Any wound that you can't manage should be seen by your pediatrician or in an emergency department as soon as possible to maximize healing.

## Scrapes

Most minor injuries in children are scrapes, or *abrasions,* which literally means the outer layer of skin is scraped off. If the abrasion covers a large area, it may appear to be very bloody, although the actual amount of blood lost is small. Properly cared for, abrasions quickly form a protective scab and heal without further treatment. They must be kept clean to prevent infection.

### What You Can Do

- Rinse the wound under cool running water to flush away contaminants and debris. Then wash the wound gently with soap and warm water. Use clean tweezers to remove any remaining debris.
- Apply an antibiotic cream or ointment, such as bacitracin, if the wound is large or oozing. Lightly cover it with a sterile dressing. The antibiotic cream or ointment will prevent the wound from sticking to the dressing.
- Make sure that dressings and adhesive tapes around your child's fingers and toes are loose enough to allow free circulation.
- Change the dressing routinely each day or whenever it becomes wet or dirty. If the dressing sticks, soak it off in warm water. Most wounds require a dressing for only 2 or 3 days, but your child may be reluctant to stop applying bandages that quickly; small children often regard bandages as badges or medals. You can leave the area loosely covered as long as you keep the bandage dry and clean and check the wound daily.
- If left alone, most abrasions will form a scab over them quickly. This was once thought to be the best natural remedy, but scabs actually slow the healing process and can lead to more scarring. If a scab forms, don't pull it off. You may apply an antibiotic ointment such as bacitracin to keep the scab moist.

- Be alert for pus, increased redness and tenderness, or fever, which may indicate that infection is present. If an infection develops, contact your pediatrician.
- Call your pediatrician if you need help cleaning a wound or if the injury occurred against a highly contaminated surface.

## Dental Emergency

Whether it's a toddler bumping into a table face-first or an older child engaged in a rigorous game of football, children can experience injuries to their teeth. A loosened tooth may bleed a little from the gums but often tightens up and heals on its own. A displaced tooth is usually pushed inward. Sometimes a tooth may be chipped or fractured. In some cases a tooth may be knocked out, which is an emergency if it's a child's permanent tooth.

### Prevention

- Provide properly fitted helmets with face and mouth guards for children involved in contact sports such as hockey, lacrosse, and football.
- Take household safety precautions: use gates at the top and bottom of stairs, remove trip hazards like cords or loose rugs, and consider padding hard surfaces like the coffee table or fireplace hearth.

### What You Can Do

- If a baby tooth is knocked out or broken, apply clean gauze to control bleeding, and call the pediatric or family's dentist.
- If a permanent tooth is knocked out, handle the tooth by the top and not the root (the part that would be in the gum). It's important not to let the tooth dry out. Place the tooth in milk in a small plastic bag, and place the bag in a cup of milk. You can also put the tooth in a cup of milk. Transport the tooth with your child when you seek emergency care. Call and go directly to the pediatric or family's dentist or an emergency department.
- Stop the bleeding using gauze or a cotton ball in the tooth socket, and have your child bite down.
- Have your child hold his jaws together gently but firmly to keep the pad in place and stop the bleeding.

- Place a cold cloth or ice pack on the lip to relieve swelling and pain.
- Give acetaminophen or ibuprofen if your child is in pain.
- If a tooth is broken, save the pieces in milk, and call the pediatric or family's dentist right away.

### Treatment

- A child who has sustained a heavy blow to the face or jaw may need to be x-rayed to determine the extent of the damage.
- Your dentist will try to re-implant the tooth if possible.

## Electrical Injury

When the human body comes into direct contact with a source of electricity, the current passes through it, producing what's called an electric shock. Depending on the voltage of the current and the length of contact, this shock can cause anything from minor discomfort to serious injury (even death).

Young children, particularly toddlers, experience electric shock most often when they bite into electrical cords or poke metal objects such as forks or knives into unprotected outlets or appliances. These injuries can also take place when electric toys, appliances, or tools are used incorrectly or when electric current makes contact with water in which a child is sitting or standing. Christmas trees and their lights are a seasonal hazard.

### Prevention

The best way to prevent electrical injuries is to cover all outlets, make sure all wires are properly insulated, tuck wires away from your child's reach, and provide adult supervision whenever children are in an area with potential electrical hazards. Small appliances are a special hazard around bathtubs or pools. For more information, see "Childproofing Your Home," page 231.

### What You Can Do

- Disconnect the power supply before you touch an injured child who is still receiving current; pull the plug or turn off the main switch.

- Never touch a live wire with your bare hands. If you have to lift a live wire from a child, use a dry stick, a rolled-up newspaper, thick clothing, or another sturdy, dry, nonmetallic object that won't conduct electricity.
- Move the child as little as possible because severe electric shock may have caused a spinal fracture.
- If you can't remove the source of the current, try to move the child, but don't use your bare hands. Insulate yourself with rubber or with any of the nonconductive items suggested for lifting a live wire so that the current doesn't pass from the child's body to yours.
- Once the current is off, quickly check the child's breathing, pulse, skin color, and alertness. If the child isn't breathing or there is no heartbeat, begin CPR immediately (see "Choking/CPR" chart appropriate to your child's age, page 215 or 216) while someone else goes for medical help.
- Once the child is safely removed from the current, check him for burns and call 911, your local emergency number, or your pediatrician right away.

### Treatment

- A child who has received an electric shock should be seen by a pediatrician because shock may cause internal damage that can't be detected without a medical examination.
- Your pediatrician will clean and dress surface burns and order tests for signs of damage to internal organs.
- Mouth burns (such as from biting an electric cord) are often much deeper than they appear. Your child may require surgery after the initial healing. Parents must be alert to the possibility of bleeding from mouth burns hours or even days after the injury. If bleeding occurs, apply a clean pad and call your pediatrician immediately.
- If a child has severe burns or any sign of brain or heart damage, she will need to be placed in a hospital.

## Fractures

Although the word *fracture* may sound serious, a fracture is just another name for a broken bone. Broken bones are a common childhood injury. Falls cause most of the fractures in this age group, but the most serious breaks are usually the result of automobile crashes. Because children's bones are more flexible and have a thicker covering than those of adults, they absorb shock better and heal more quickly. Children's fractures rarely require surgical repair. They usually just need to be kept free of movement, most often with the use of a molded cast.

It's not always easy to know if a child's bone is broken, especially if he's too young to describe what he's feeling. Ordinarily with a fracture you'll see swelling, and your child will clearly be in pain and unable—or unwilling—to move his limb; however, just because your child can move his bone doesn't necessarily rule out a fracture. Any time you suspect a fracture, notify your pediatrician immediately.

### Prevention

- Make sure your child has properly fitted footwear, headgear, and protective pads for sports such as baseball, skating, and hockey.
- During all car rides, preschoolers must be properly strapped into approved car safety seats or booster seats in the rear. All children should ride in the rear seat, properly buckled into safety belts or car safety seats. The risk of fractures or any other injuries is lowest when children ride rear-facing; if your child hasn't reached the manufacturer's weight or height limit for rear-facing, this is the safest way to ride. Many children can ride rear-facing well past the second birthday.

## What You Can Do

- If your child has a neck or back injury, call 911 or your local emergency number immediately. Don't move her yourself because it may cause serious harm to the spinal cord.
- Call your pediatrician at once if you suspect a broken bone. It can be difficult to recognize a fracture, especially in infants and toddlers. Look for swelling, pain, limping, and loss of movement. Your child may also guard others from touching it. A bone may be broken even though a child can move her limb.
- If your child has a broken leg, call an ambulance and let the paramedics supervise her transportation; don't try to move her yourself.
- If the hand or foot below the injury is blue or cold, call 911 or your local emergency number immediately.
- If an injured extremity is painful, swollen, or deformed, or if motion causes pain, wrap it in a towel or soft cloth, and make a splint with cardboard or another firm material to hold the arm or leg in place. Don't try to straighten the extremity. Apply ice or a cool compress wrapped in thin cloth for no more than 20 minutes. If there is a deformity, seek emergency care.
- If there is a break in the skin near the fracture, or you can see the bone, cover the area with a clean bandage, make a splint (Figure 4-3), and seek emergency care. Don't try to put the bone back in place.
- Don't give drinks or pain relievers to your child without asking your pediatrician first; if your child requires immediate surgery or another treatment, fluids may increase the risk of anesthesia, and pain relievers may interact with other necessary medications.
- For an older child, place a wrapped ice pack or cold towel over the injury for no more than 20 minutes to relieve pain. Don't use ice on infants and toddlers; extreme cold can lead to further injury.
- In the days after a fracture has been treated, watch your child for signs of fever, which may signal infection.

- While your child's limb is in a cast, call the physician who applied the cast immediately if your child complains of pain, numbness, or pale or blue fingers or toes; this may indicate severe swelling underneath the cast and means your child needs more room under the cast. If the cast isn't adjusted, the swelling may press on nerves, muscles, and blood vessels, which can produce permanent damage. To relieve the pressure, your doctor may split the cast, open a window in it, or replace it with a larger one.
- Call the doctor who applied the cast if it breaks or loosens.

### Treatment

- Your pediatrician will order x-rays to assess your child's injury and may recommend an orthopedic consultation.
- A plaster or fiberglass cast, called a *splint*, will be applied to keep the bone in place; surgery may be needed for extremely complicated fractures.
- If the bone has broken through the skin surface, a child may need to take an antibiotic.

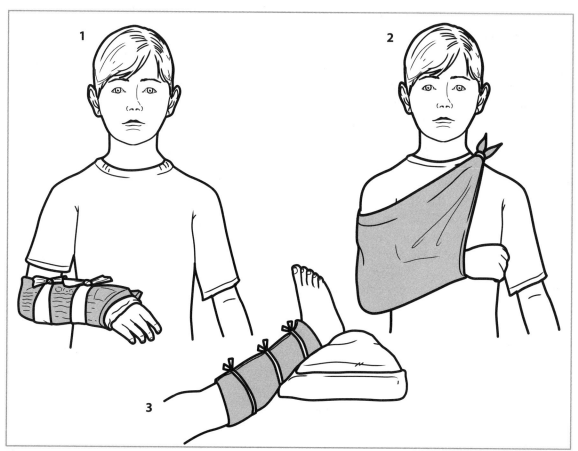

**Figure 4-3.** Protect the limb from unnecessary movement by using a rolled-up newspaper, magazine, or similar object for a splint (1) and then fashioning a sling from a scarf, torn sheets, or other material (2). An injured leg should be immobilized and elevated until your pediatrician or emergency physician can see the child (3).

## Head Injuries

It's almost inevitable that your child will hit his head every now and then, especially when he's a toddler. These blows may upset you, but your anxiety is usually worse than the bump. Most head injuries are minor and cause no serious problem. Even so, it's important to know the difference between a head injury that warrants medical attention and one that needs only a comforting hug.

If your child suffers a hard blow to the head, she will need to be evaluated by a physician. Even without loss of consciousness, if your child has significant memory loss, disorientation, altered speech, visual changes, or nausea and vomiting after a head injury, call 911, your local emergency number, or your pediatrician. A concussion is any injury to the brain that disrupts normal brain function on a temporary or permanent basis. A concussion requires careful evaluation and monitoring by your pediatrician to ensure that symptoms have completely resolved before clearing your child to resume full activities (both school and sports related).

### Prevention

- Always use restraints when using baby equipment such as carriers, strollers, and high chairs.
- Always keep one hand on your baby when he's lying on a changing table. Never leave your baby unattended on a changing table, bed, sofa, or chair. Put your baby in a safe place such as a crib when you can't hold him.
- Don't place bouncing chairs or infant seats on raised surfaces (ie, counters, tables, or other furniture).
- Don't use baby walkers; they're especially hazardous around stairs.
- Pad fireplace hearths, and keep your home free of hazards that could trip an inexperienced walker.
- Install window guards, and place gates at the top and bottom of all steps until your toddler has mastered them under your supervision.

- Stabilize items of furniture like dressers, floor lamps, or bookshelves by securing them to the wall or the floor. Secure TVs by strapping them to the wall or to a low, stable stand that's designed to hold them.
- Make sure young baseball players and other athletes wear properly fitting helmets.
- Never allow children to ride bicycles unless wearing helmets that meet US safety standards. Set an example by wearing a bike helmet while riding.
- On all car rides, make sure to place your child in approved car safety seats or booster seats. All children should ride in the rear seat, properly buckled into safety belts or car safety seats.

### What You Can Do

- Don't move a child who may have a serious head, neck, or back injury. This may cause further harm.
- Clean and dress superficial wounds. Apply a cold compress to reduce swelling. Keep an eye on your child for 24 to 48 hours to make sure there are no signs of more serious injury. Give children's acetaminophen or ibuprofen if your child complains of headache.

### *Call 911 or your local emergency number if your child*

- Loses consciousness
- Has a seizure
- Has muscle weakness, clumsiness, or inability to move a body part
- Has bleeding or watery discharge from the nose or ears
- Has abnormal speech or behavior
- *Call your pediatrician if your child has a head injury and any of the following:*
  - Drowsiness
  - Difficulty being woken up
  - Persistent (won't go away) headache or vomiting

### Treatment

- If you think your child may have a neck or back injury, or serious head injury, don't move him. Call 911 or your local emergency number for transportation to the hospital.

CHAPTER 5

# Guide to Safety and Prevention

## INTRODUCTION

Preventable injuries are the leading cause of death in children older than 1 year. Injuries often occur when a parent's or other caregiver's attention is diverted. The likelihood of injury increases during times of family stress (eg, an illness, a death in the family, a pregnancy or birth, change in environment). Children are also more vulnerable to injuries during the summer months, when they are out of school.

Of course, injuries vary in severity. Minor scrapes and spills go along with a child's exploration and learning process. Your child must touch, taste, feel, smell, and investigate to learn. Hazards that adults avoid by second nature, such as a hot stove or a sharp knife, are especially threatening to children, who are just learning to navigate a potentially perilous world and may not understand these dangers. Remember, to a small child, everything is new and equally interesting. Sharp is no different than dull, hot than cold, heavy than light, and dangerous than safe. Installing and implementing childproofing measures reduces the chances of an injury to your child by making her environment as safe as possible.

## GENERAL SAFETY GUIDELINES

Making your home safe should begin even before the birth of your baby. Once your baby gets older and starts to become more mobile, you will soon get in the habit of searching the floor for small objects, putting breakables away, and latching doors shut.

Certainly, by the time your child can sit on his own and use his hands for exploration (about 6 months of age), your home should be completely child-proofed. Reassess your safety measures as your child grows. How far and fast he can move, the heights he can reach, and the objects that attract his attention will change constantly. But here are some general guidelines.

- *The first few months.* As soon as a baby masters the ability to put things in her mouth, she will use this method to learn about objects. Toys should be big enough so that they can't fit entirely in her mouth. They should also be nontoxic and durable, without small or pointed parts or ribbons and strings. Check the toy's label or packaging to find the recommended age range, and choose toys that are labeled for your infant's age. Never hang a pacifier or anything else around a baby's neck. A string or ribbon could catch on something and strangle an infant.

- *Six to 18 months.* Your baby's improved coordination, ability to sit on his own, and rapidly increasing mobility require increased and constant watchfulness. Frequent room-by-room checking for possible hazards is extremely important at this age. Your baby's curiosity has extended beyond himself to the world around him, and his ability to explore that world grows daily. Be aware of the environment in which your child is playing. Your child should never be able to get hold of objects that you would not trust him to be alone with. If you would not be OK with your child being alone with something, he should not be able to get it. When your baby grabs for an unsafe object such as your purse, offer him a permitted object such as a book as a distraction.

- *Toddlers.* A toddler's mobility and curiosity, and the fact that a child at this stage will eat or drink even the worst-tasting substances, make poison prevention a critical priority. (See "Poison Prevention".) For any danger, remove the hazard or keep your child away from it, if possible. Use a firm "no" for dangerous situations, such as a hot radiator, and explain why ("No! The radiator is HOT!") At the same time, physically remove the dangerous object or move your child to reinforce the idea that the situation or object is not negotiable.
- *The preschool years.* Make safety rules, repeat them often, and apply them consistently. Explain why these rules must be obeyed, but stay vigilant about supervising your child and preventing access to hazardous situations.

## Poison Prevention

Every day, 300 children between the ages of 1 and 19 years are treated in emergency departments for poisoning, and 2 die. Personal-care products, cosmetics, and household cleaning products are common causes of childhood poisoning, with over-the-counter medications at the top of the list. Although they are generally safe for adults, over-the-counter products such as vitamin and mineral supplements (especially those with iron), aspirin, acetaminophen, and laxatives cause serious, even life-threatening, reactions in children because of their smaller size and the tendency for children to ingest the entire bottle. Here's what you need to do to keep your child safe from hazardous products.

- Keep all medications and vitamins safely locked up high out of sight and reach. Put them away right after use. Don't leave medicines in purses or pockets, and keep your child away from other people's purses and bags. Children have an uncanny way of finding potentially poisonous items, even in unusual places.
- Buy and keep medications in their own containers with child safety caps. Remember that these caps are child-resistant, not childproof, so keep them in a locked cabinet.
- Do not take medicine in front of small children; they may try to imitate you. Never call medicine or vitamins "candy" when giving them to your child to get her to take them. Check the label every time you give medication to make sure you are giving the right medicine in the correct dosage.
- Read labels on all household products before you buy them. Try to find the safest ones for the job, and buy only what you need to use right away.
- Many cosmetics and personal-care products are potentially toxic. Store them out of reach of children in childproof cabinets.
- Alcohol should be kept up high in locked cabinets. Glasses should be emptied and rinsed right away after a party at which alcohol is served.
- Never smoke near a child, whether in a house, car, or restaurant. Secondhand smoke is harmful to children and raises their risk for ear infections, asthma, headaches, and other health problems. You also create a risk for fires and burns to children and others. Keep in mind, too, that you are a role model for your child. If your child sees you smoking, she may want to try it as well. If you do smoke, make sure cigarettes and other tobacco products are out of a child's reach. Almost any amount of tobacco product may poison a child who eats it. This includes cigarettes, cigars, smoked butts, pipe and chewing tobacco, snuff, and nicotine gum, patches, and sprays.
- Never store cleaning products or detergents under the kitchen or bathroom sink unless they are in a cabinet with a safety latch that locks every time you close the cabinet. You can buy safety latches in many stores. Laundry detergents should be stored in a high or locked cabinet, not on top of

the washer or dryer. Single-use detergent packets must be kept out of sight and reach of children in a child-resistant container. While safety latches are effective in preventing children from accessing potentially hazardous things, they are not perfect and are never a substitute for careful supervision.

- In the garage, make sure to keep all paints, varnishes, thinners, pesticides, petroleum products, and fertilizers up high in a locked cabinet or locker. Store these substances in their original labeled containers. Store tools in a safe, out-of-reach area and locked. Be sure power tools are unplugged and locked in a cabinet when not in use. Discourage your child from playing near the garage. Be careful using the garage door opener, and make sure the automatic reversing mechanism is properly adjusted.
- Post the phone number for Poison Help (1-800-222-1222) near every telephone in your home and in your cell phone, along with other emergency numbers. Be sure that your child care provider and anyone else caring for your child knows when and how to use these numbers.

## CHILDPROOFING YOUR HOME

To see the world through your child's eyes, get down on your hands and knees and search for small objects, dangling cords, electric sockets, breakable objects, and dangerous corners. You will have a better idea of potential hazards that could hurt your child. By making your home childproof, you will give your child greater freedom to explore and play. Here's what you need to do.

- Install smoke and carbon monoxide detectors on every floor and outside all bedrooms. Check them every month to make sure they are working. It is best to use smoke detectors with long-life batteries, but if these are not available, change the batteries annually on a date you will remember. Develop a fire escape plan and practice it so you'll be prepared if an emergency does occur.
- Put safety plugs that are not a choking hazard in all unused electric outlets so your child can't stick her finger or a toy into the holes. If your child

won't stay away from outlets, block access to them with furniture. Keep electric cords out of reach and sight.

- To prevent slipping, carpet your stairs where possible. Be sure the carpet is firmly tacked down at the edges. When your child is just learning to crawl and walk, install safety gates at the top and bottom of stairs. Avoid accordion-style gates, which can trap an arm or a neck.
- Keep a fire extinguisher in the kitchen and one by each stairwell. Practice your fire escape plan every few months. Have your children practice "stop, drop, and roll" in case clothing catches fire.
- Certain houseplants, such as philodendrons and peace lilies, are toxic. Check with Poison Help (1-800-222-1222) to find out which plants are safe around small children. Potting soil may contain fertilizer that could be dangerous if ingested. Teach children never to sample wild berries and other plant parts unless an adult says they are safe. You may want to forego houseplants for a while or at the very least, keep all houseplants out of reach.
- Check your floors constantly for small objects that a child might swallow, such as coins, buttons, beads, pins, magnets, batteries, and screws. This is particularly important if someone in the household has a hobby that involves small items or if there are older children who have small items.
- If you have hardwood floors, be careful not to let children run around in their socks. Socks make slippery floors even more dangerous.
- Test the stability of large pieces of furniture, such as floor lamps, bookshelves, and television stands. Put floor lamps behind other furniture and anchor dressers, bookcases, and television stands to the wall. Deaths and injuries can occur when children climb onto, fall against, or pull on large pieces of furniture. Televisions should be anchored to the wall or low, sturdy furniture that is designed to hold them. Straps to anchor televisions and other furniture are inexpensive and can be purchased at baby stores.

- Attach cords for window blinds and drapes to floor mounts that hold them taut, or wrap these cords around wall brackets to keep them out of reach. Use safety stop devices on the cords. Cords with loops should be cut and equipped with safety tassels. Children can strangle on them if they are left loose. The US Consumer Product Safety Commission (CPSC) strongly recommends cordless window coverings in homes with children.
- Pay attention to doors between rooms. Glass doors are particularly dangerous because a child may run into them, so fasten them open if possible. Swinging doors can knock down a small child, while folding doors can pinch little fingers. If you have either, consider removing them until your child is old enough to understand how they work.
- Check your home for furniture pieces with hard edges and sharp corners that could injure your child if she fell against them. (Coffee tables are a particular hazard.) If possible, move this furniture out of traffic areas, particularly when your child is learning to walk. You can also buy cushioned corner and edge protectors that stick onto the furniture.
- Keep computers out of reach so that your child cannot pull them over on himself. Cords should be out of sight and reach.
- Open windows from the top if possible. If you must open them from the bottom, install operable window guards that only an adult or older child can open from the inside. Never put chairs, sofas, low tables, or anything else a child might climb in front of a window. Doing so gives her access to the window and creates the risk for a serious fall. Many stores sell metal or mesh window guards that can prevent falls as well.
- Never leave plastic bags lying around the house, and don't store children's clothes or toys in them. Dry-cleaning bags are particularly dangerous. Knot them before you throw them away so that it's impossible for your child to crawl into them or pull them over his head.

- Consider the potential hazard of anything you put in the trash. Any trash container that has dangerous items in it, such as spoiled foods or discarded razor blades, should have a child-resistant cover or be kept away and out of a child's reach.
- To prevent burns, check your heat sources. Enclose radiators, woodstoves, and kerosene heaters in screens so that your child can't get near them. Check electric baseboard heaters, radiators, and even vents from hot-air furnaces to see how hot they get when the heat is on. They too may need to be screened. Glass-fronted fireplaces can get extremely hot and must be screened to prevent unintended contact.
- The safest home for a child is one without a gun. If you must have a gun, you can reduce the risk of injury or death by storing it unloaded in a locked container, with the ammunition locked in a separate place. If your child plays in other homes, ask if guns are present there, and if so, how they are stored.
- Keep all alcoholic beverages in a locked cabinet and remember to empty any unfinished drinks right away. Alcohol can be very toxic to a young child.
- Keep a list of emergency numbers next to every phone. Include the number of your pediatrician, Poison Help (1-800-222-1222), hospital emergency department, next-door neighbor, and a responsible relative or friend. Be sure to list any numbers your babysitter might need, such as work or cell phone numbers.

## Preventing Choking

- Young children should always be seated and supervised closely while eating. Cut or break food into child–bite-size pieces, and encourage children to chew food thoroughly. Don't let children eat while playing or running; teach them to chew and swallow before talking or laughing.
- Any food that is firm or minimally compressible, such as hot dogs, nuts, or grapes or other fruits and vegetables, must be chopped into small

pieces. Peanut butter must be spread thinly, as large globs can block a child's airway. Encourage your child to chew thoroughly.

- Don't give young children hard, smooth foods such as nuts or raw vegetables that must be chewed with a grinding motion; children can't chew this way until about age 4 years, so they may try to swallow the food whole.
- Choose toys and playthings carefully. According to government regulations, toys sold for children younger than 3 years cannot have parts smaller than 1¼" wide and 2¼" long. If there are older children in the household, make sure that toys with small parts, such as construction kits, are well out of a toddler's reach. Follow the age guidelines printed on toy packaging.
- Keep your child away from objects and foods that have been associated with choking. These include latex balloons, baby powder, safety pins, coins, marbles and small ball-like magnets, pop-tops from beverage cans, pen caps, hard candy, vitamins, grapes, and popcorn.
- If you're not sure whether an object or food item could be harmful, purchase a standard small-parts cylinder at stores that sell child safety products and see if the object or food item fits inside the cylinder. If it fits inside, the object or food item is not safe.

## Baby's Room

Your baby will sleep and play in the nursery, so it should be extra safe. You should invest in a new crib that meets the current safety standard, which was implemented in 2011 (see "Crib"). If you must use an old one, check to see if it was recalled by the Consumer Product Safety Commission. Test construction and stability and regularly inspect furniture for hazards caused by wear and tear. All fabrics in your baby's room—pajamas, sheets, curtains—should be flame retardant.

## Crib

Extra care should be used when selecting a crib.

- There should be no more than 2⅜" between the slats.
- The mattress should fit snugly within the crib and be very firm. It should not sag when your baby is on it. The top crib rail should be at least 26" from the top of the mattress; continually lower the mattress as your baby grows.
- New cribs will no longer have a side drop rail. If your crib has a side rail, do not use it. Always check that the side-rail release mechanism is locked and cannot be released unintentionally. Never leave your baby in the crib when the side rail is lowered.
- The headboard and footboard should be solid with no cutouts. Any corner posts that can catch clothing should be removed.
- Place the crib away from windows where sunlight and drafts can make your baby uncomfortable and cords and drapes are a strangling hazard.
- Do not place comforters, blankets, stuffed animals, bumper pads, or pillows in the crib with a baby. These can cause smothering.
- Mobiles and crib gyms should be removed once your baby is able to pull herself to her hands and knees.
- As your baby gets bigger, do not place large toys or stuffed animals in the crib because they can make it easy for your baby to climb out.
- Once your child is about 3 feet tall, she should start sleeping in a bed.

## Changing Table

- Choose a sturdy, stable changing table with a 2" (5-cm) guardrail around all 4 sides. The top of the changing table should be concave so that the middle is slightly lower than the sides.
- Buckle the safety strap, but don't depend on it alone to keep your child secure. Never leave a child unattended on a changing table, even for a moment, and even if he is strapped in.

- Keep diapering supplies within your reach—but out of your child's reach—so you don't have to leave your child's side to get them. Never let your child play with a powder container. If she opens and shakes it, she's likely to inhale particles of powder, which can injure her lungs.
- If you use disposable diapers, store them out of your child's reach and cover them with clothing when he wears them.

## Bunk Beds

Although bunk beds are extremely popular, they pose several serious dangers. The child on the top bunk can fall out, and the child on the lower bunk can be injured if the top bunk collapses. If bunk beds might be improperly constructed or assembled, there could be dangerous structural flaws. Similarly, a mattress that doesn't fit properly could entrap your child. If you still choose to use bunk beds, take the following precautions:

- Don't allow a child younger than 6 years to sleep in the upper bunk. She won't have the coordination she needs to climb on and off safely or to stop herself from falling out.
- Check to make sure the beds are sturdy and well-constructed with strong supports under the top bunk. Wires or slats should be directly under the mattress and fastened in place at both ends. A mattress that is supported only by the frame of the bed or unsecured slats could come crashing down.
- Place the bed in a corner of the room so there are walls on 2 sides. This provides extra support and blocks 2 of the possible 4 sites for falling out. Do not place bunk beds near a window.
- Attach a ladder to the top bunk. Put a night-light by the ladder for middle-of-the-night bathroom trips.
- Install a guardrail on the top bunk. The gap between the side rail and guardrail should be no more than 3½" (8¾ cm). Be sure your child can't roll under the guardrail when the mattress on the top bunk is compressed by the weight of his body. If his head gets stuck under the guardrail, he may

suffocate or be strangled. You may need a thicker mattress to prevent this.
- Don't allow jumping or climbing on either bed.

## Playpens

- Use a playpen that meets current safety standards. Older playpens may have unsafe design features or may have been recalled.
- Make sure all 4 sides are upright and fully locked at all times. The holes of the mesh should be too small for a finger, toe, or button to get caught. Make sure the mesh does not have holes or tears in it.
- If the playpen has slats, they should be no more than 2⅜" apart so your child's head doesn't get caught between them.
- Never leave your child in the playpen when the drop side is down.
- When your child can pull himself to a standing position, remove all boxes and large toys that he could use to help him climb out.
- Remove the raised changing table when your child is in the playpen so he doesn't get entrapped in the space between the changing table and the side rails of the playpen.
- Never use circular enclosures made from accordion-style fences. Children can get their heads caught in the diamond-shaped openings and the V-shaped border at the top of the gate.

## Bathroom

The bathroom is a fascinating place for a child, but it's also an extremely dangerous place. The easiest way to prevent an injury in the bathroom is to make it inaccessible to your child. Place a latch on the door at adult height so your child can't get into the bathroom when you aren't around. If that's not possible, you'll need to take precautions to keep your child safe in the bathroom.

- Never leave a toddler unattended in the bathroom or bathtub. It takes only a few inches of water and 1 or 2 minutes for a child to drown.
- Install no-slip strips on the bottom of the bathtub. Put a cushioned cover over the water faucet so your child won't be hurt if he bumps his head against it.

- Close the lid of the toilet, and use a lid lock. A curious toddler who tries to play in the water can lose her balance and fall in.
- Set the water heater so the temperature at the faucet is no more than 120°F (48.9°C), which will prevent scalding. When your child is old enough to turn on the faucets, teach him to start the cold water before the hot.
- Keep medicines, cosmetics, razors and other sharp objects, and toiletries inside a locked medicine cabinet. Shampoo, conditioner, and other liquid products should be placed up high out of reach.
- If you use electric appliances in the bathroom such as hair dryers and razors, always unplug them and store them in a cabinet with a safety lock when they aren't in use. It's better to use them in another room, where there is no water. An electrician can install special bathroom wall sockets (ground-fault circuit interrupters [GFCIs]) that can reduce the likelihood of electrical injury if an appliance falls into water.

## Kitchen

For most families, the kitchen is where all the action takes place, and your child will want to be there with you. But the kitchen is filled with so many dangerous objects and appliances that experts often recommend making it off-limits to young children. A safer strategy is to keep your child in a high chair or playpen so he can watch you and others in the room. He should be securely strapped in and within your vision. Keep a toy box or drawer with safe play items in the kitchen to amuse him. You can eliminate most dangers by doing the following:

- Store dangerous items, including cleaning products, plastic bags, and sharp utensils, in a high cabinet, locked and out of sight and reach of children. If you must store items under the sink, use a child safety lock that refastens automatically every time you close the cupboard. (Most hardware and department stores have them.) Never put dangerous substances into containers that look as if they might hold food because it might tempt your child to taste them.
- Separate knives, forks, scissors, and other sharp instruments from "safe" kitchen utensils in a latched drawer. Keep sharp cutting appliances such as food processors out of reach of children in a locked cabinet.
- When cooking, use back burners whenever possible. Turn pot handles inward so that they do not stick out over the edge of the stove, where your child can reach up and grab them.
- When shopping for an oven, choose one that is well insulated to protect your child from the heat if she touches the oven door.
- If you have a gas stove, turn the dials firmly to the off position. If they're easy to remove, do so when you aren't cooking. If they're not, use child-resistant knob covers.
- Unplug and put away appliances when they are not in use. Be sure cords are tucked safely out of reach and sight of children so your child can't tug on them.
- Be aware of where your child is when you are carrying hot liquids. Never carry your child in one arm and a hot liquid in the other. A trip could cause a nasty burn.
- Never warm baby bottles in a microwave oven. The liquid heats unevenly, so there may be pockets of milk hot enough to scald your baby's mouth when he drinks. Also, some bottles have exploded when removed from the microwave.
- If your child shows interest in opening the doors to the refrigerator or freezer, consider purchasing a locking device. Small children can be injured by pulling out heavy items or even get trapped inside.
- Keep a fire extinguisher in your kitchen. (If your home has more than one story, mount an extinguisher in a place you will remember on each floor.)
- Do not place small refrigerator magnets where your child can reach them. Your toddler could choke on them.

## Preventing Falls

### High Chair

High chairs can be dangerous. Be especially wary of restaurant high chairs, which often do not have a suitable restraint system.

- Select a chair with a wide base so it can't tip over easily.
- If the chair folds, be sure the locking device is secure each time you set it up.
- Always strap your child in securely using the waist and crotch straps.
- Never leave your child unattended in the high chair.
- Do not begin using a high chair until your child can sit securely on his own and is eating solids.
- Position the high chair away from walls and tables so that your toddler cannot reach them and push off. Avoid placing it near a counter or table or within reach of a hot or dangerous object.
- If you plan to use a portable high chair that attaches to a table, choose one that locks onto the table. Be sure the table is heavy enough to support your child's weight without tipping. Also, check to see whether your child's feet can touch a table support. If she can push it, she may be able to dislodge the seat from the table.
- Make sure all caps or plugs on chair tubing are firmly attached and cannot be pulled off. They could be choking hazards.

### Walkers

The American Academy of Pediatrics (AAP) does not recommend the use of infant walkers. Children in walkers are more likely to fall down stairs, and head injuries are common. Walkers are associated with increased risk of burns and poisonings because they make it easier for babies to access hazards that may otherwise be out of reach. Walkers do not help a child learn how to walk and in fact have been shown to delay normal motor development. A stationary play center is a better choice. These do not have wheels but seats that rotate and bounce.

You may also want to consider a sturdy wagon or an "activity walker." Be sure the toy has a bar she can push and that it's weighted so it won't tip over when she pulls herself up.

## Basement, Laundry Room, and Utility Room

- Store the iron unplugged with the cord tucked away out of reach of children.
- Iron on a well-balanced board.
- Never leave the iron unattended when in use. Put it on a firm surface.
- Be sure all electric appliances are well vented and properly grounded.
- Keep cleaning supplies and tools locked up high out of the reach of children.
- Never leave clothes to soak in pails or basins if you have young children.
- Empty all buckets, fluid containers, and sinks right after finishing a task. Don't leave buckets unattended.
- Don't reuse 5-gallon, straight-sided, flat-bottom chemical containers as cleaning buckets.
- Store detergent, cleaning agents, bleach, and other laundry items safely out of children's reach.

## Avoiding Lead Poisoning

Nearly 1 million children in the United States still have unacceptably high levels of lead in their blood. Without early treatment, accumulated lead can cause learning, language, attention, memory, aggression, antisocial, and behavioral problems. Young children accumulate high levels of lead because they have a tendency to put objects in their mouths, including items contaminated by dust, bits of old paint, or dirt that contain lead. They may also breathe lead in the air. Common sources of lead include the following:

- Paint in homes built before 1978
- Soil around homes, which may be contaminated with flaking paint as well as with the lead that was formerly added to gasoline

- Drinking water from plumbing systems with pipes lined or soldered with lead
- Imported ceramic dishes
- Mini blinds made outside the United States before July 1997
- Stained glass, paints, hobby soldiers, and fishing weights
- Children's jewelry

Lead was allowed in house paint before 1978, so it may be on walls, doorjambs, and window frames of older homes. As the home ages, paint may come off in chips or as dust. Even if the house has since been repainted, the lead is still there.

If you suspect your home may be contaminated, contact a lead safety inspector. If you rent, your landlord is responsible for all maintenance, including repainting. Do not remove lead paint yourself; it is often more dangerous to remove than to live with it. Have a professional do the work and relocate your family, especially small children and pregnant women, during the process. Renovation projects that remove lead paint require the skills of someone trained in lead-safe work practices. You can find someone through your local or state health department. A few safety precautions you can take right away include

- Clean up paint chips and dust with disposable cloths or paper towels, water, and detergent. Wear gloves during cleanup and use garbage bags for all refuse. Keep children away from the cleaning process.
- Wash children's hands often, especially before eating and napping.
- Keep floors, window sills, toys, pacifiers, stuffed animals, and all surfaces clean.
- Do not vacuum paint chips because the vacuum will only spread the dust out through its exhaust.
- Remove shoes before entering to avoid tracking in lead from soil.

If you think your child has lead poisoning, talk with your pediatrician, who may order a blood test. Children who have lead poisoning should be removed from the home where they are being

exposed. They may require treatment with a drug that binds the lead in the blood. In rare cases, treatment may involve hospitalization. Children with lead poisoning will need to have their health, behavior, and academic performance monitored for many years. For more information on lead and its removal or management, contact the National Lead Information Center at 800/424-LEAD (5323) or www2.epa.gov/lead/forms/lead-hotline-national-lead-information-center.

## OUTSIDE THE HOME

Outside the home, your child's environment is more difficult to control. Young children must be constantly supervised to ensure their safety.

When your child is outdoors, make sure to apply sunscreen with a sun protection factor (SPF) of at least 30. Apply it at least 15 to 30 minutes before going out, and make sure to reapply frequently. Dress youngsters in comfortable, lightweight clothing that covers the body, including hats that shade the face and ears. Sunglasses with ultraviolet protection are a good idea too.

### Yard

As soon as your child is old enough to play outdoors, the yard should be childproofed as carefully as the inside of your home.

- If you don't have a fenced-in yard, teach your child the boundaries within which she should play. Always have a responsible person supervising your child.
- When you cook food outdoors, screen the grill so that your child cannot touch it, and explain that it is hot like the stove in the kitchen. Store propane grills so your child cannot reach the knobs. Be sure charcoal is cool before you dump it.
- Check your yard for poisonous plants. Remove mushrooms, poison ivy, and other hazardous plants as soon as they appear. Teach your child never to eat things he finds in the garden unless you tell him it's safe. Common poisonous plants found in the garden and yard include buttercups,

daffodil bulbs, English ivy, holly, mistletoe, tomato leaves, potato vines, rhododendrons, and rhubarb leaves. Brightly colored berries are especially attractive to young children, but many are poisonous. Be on the lookout for them.

- Teach your children to recognize and stay away from poison ivy, oak, and sumac.
- If you use pesticides or herbicides on your garden or lawn, read instructions carefully. If you or your neighbors use these products, make sure children are indoors when they are applied. Do not allow children to play on the lawn for at least 48 hours after treatment.
- Don't use a power mower to cut the lawn when young children are around. Never let a child ride with you on a riding mower. It is safest to keep children indoors when the lawn is being mowed.
- Never allow your child to play unattended near traffic. Do not allow her to cross the street by herself, even if it just to go to a waiting school bus.

## Playgrounds and Outdoor Play Equipment

- Keep children younger than 5 years on equipment separated from older children.
- Make sure there is sand, wood chips, or rubberized matting under swings, seesaws, and jungle gyms and that these surfaces are of proper depth and well maintained.
- Wooden structures should be made of all-weather wood, which is less likely to splinter. Examine surfaces periodically to be sure they are smooth. Metal structures can get extremely hot in the summer.
- Make sure your child always wears shoes on the playground.
- Do a periodic inspection of equipment. Look for loose joints, open chains that could come loose, and rusted cotter pins. Make sure there are no protruding pieces that could hook a child's clothing. Check for rusted or exposed bolts, and cover them with protective rubber. Report problems to the appropriate authorities if you see poor conditions on public equipment.

- Check that swings are light but strong. The seat should be made of plastic or rubber. The set should be fenced in to keep small children from running close to swings.
- Don't allow children younger than 4 years to use climbing equipment that is taller than they are without close supervision.
- Don't allow children to climb up slides. Make sure they use the ladder. Teach your child to leave the slide as soon as she is at the bottom.
- Children between 3 and 5 years of age should not play on seesaws unless they are with children of comparable age and weight.
- Do not allow children to use trampolines. About 100,000 children are injured on trampolines every year, and injuries include broken bones, head injuries, spinal cord injuries, and sprains. Older children should use them only in training programs for competitive sports such as gymnastics or diving, and only when supervised by a professional.

## In the Car

Each year, more than 5,000 children, teens, and adults younger than 21 years die in a motor vehicle crash. Many more children are injured; for every child who is killed, 18 are hospitalized and 400 receive medical treatment. With proper safety precautions, many of these injuries could be prevented.

From the moment you take your baby home from the hospital, it's critical to use a car safety seat that meets current standards. To keep your child safe in a car, keep these tips in mind.

- Always place a child younger than 13 years in the back seat of a car. It's the safest place for him to be.
- When installing a car safety seat, follow the manufacturer's directions carefully. Once you've finished installing a car safety seat, check that it is secure. If you can move the seat at the belt path more than an inch from side to side or front to back, it's not tight enough. Check that the seat is firmly anchored with the seat belt or LATCH (Lower Anchors and Tethers for Children) straps before each trip. If you lose the directions or

need to find out about car seat recalls, contact the manufacturer. In many cases, you can download installation instructions from the manufacturer's Web site.

- All children should be properly secured in car safety seats, booster seats, or shoulder/lap belts correct for their age and size.
- All infants and toddlers should ride in a rear-facing car safety seat until they are at least 2 years of age or until they reach the highest weight or height allowed by the manufacturer of their car safety seat. This may be well past the second birthday. Rear-facing is the safest way to ride, so children should ride that way as long as possible. Children who have outgrown a rear–facing-only seat can usually continue to ride rear-facing in a convertible seat.
- Children who have outgrown rear-facing seats should ride in a forward-facing car safety seat with a harness for as long as possible, up to the highest weight or height allowed by the manufacturer. Options include a convertible seat, combination seat, 3-in-1 seat, or forward–facing-only seat. Your pediatrician or a Child Passenger Safety Technician (CPST) can help you make the best choice for your child and vehicle. Find a CPST in your community at http://cert.safekids.org.
- When your child reaches the highest weight or height allowed for her car safety seat, your child needs a belt-positioning booster seat. Booster seats should be used until the vehicle's lap/shoulder seat belt fits correctly. This means that the shoulder belt lies across the shoulder, not the neck, and the lap belt fits low across the hips, not the abdomen. For most children, the seat belt will fit properly at around 4' 9" in height and between 8 and 12 years of age.
- Always wear your own seat belt; setting a good example will help your child form a lifelong habit of buckling up.
- *Never, ever* leave your newborn, infant, or child alone in the car. A moment is all it takes for a child to lock himself in, shift gears, release emergency brakes, burn himself on a cigarette lighter,

or become overheated. If you see a young child alone in a car, call 911; young children can over-heat quickly and die of hyperthermia even when the weather outside is mild.

## Strollers

A sturdy stroller is worth the value. Look for safety features such as a wide base that prevents the stroller from tipping over and a 5-point harness that can keep your child safe. Then follow these precautions.

- Use the brakes whenever you are stopped, and be sure your child can't reach the release lever. A brake that locks 2 wheels provides an extra measure of safety.
- Keep your child at a safe distance when you open and close the stroller. Make sure the stroller is securely locked open before putting your child in it. Children's fingers can get caught in the hinges that fold the stroller as well as stroller wheels.
- Do not hang bags on the handles of the stroller. This can cause the stroller to tip over.
- If you buy a double stroller, be sure the footrest goes all the way across both sitting areas. Separate rests can trap little feet.
- If you buy a stroller that allows an older child to sit or stand in the rear, pay attention to weight guidelines and make sure the child in back doesn't become overly active and tip the stroller.

## Swimming Pools and Water Safety

Water is one of the more ominous hazards your child will encounter. Drowning is the second leading cause of unintentional injury death in children aged 1 to 14 years in the United States, with the highest risk in children between ages 1 and 4 years. Nonfatal drowning episodes can cause hospitalization and permanent brain injury.

Extra safety precautions around water are essential because drowning happens quickly and silently. Everyone should know how to swim and follow basic safety rules.

Because water can be so dangerous, the AAP believes strongly that parents should never—even for a moment—leave children alone near open bodies of water such as lakes or swimming pools or near water in homes such as bathtubs, backyard pools, and spas. Whenever a young child is in or near water, a responsible adult should be within arm's reach providing "touch supervision." Parents should learn cardiopulmonary resuscitation (CPR) and keep emergency equipment such as life preservers and phones near the pool at all times. Here are other safety tips.

- Don't be lulled into a false sense of security because you think your child can swim.
- Children should wear safety-approved life jackets on boats at all times, even when sleeping.
- Do not take a baby in a pool until he is able to control his head, and never fully submerge a baby in water. Young children who are repeatedly immersed in water may swallow so much of it that they develop water intoxication. This can result in convulsions, shock, and even death.
- Children should learn to swim. The AAP supports formal swimming lessons for children aged 4 years and up, and for children aged 1 to 3 years who are ready to learn how to swim. Children develop at different rates, so parents should consider factors like frequency of exposure to water, emotional maturity, physical coordination, and health concerns related to swimming (eg, swallowing water, exposure to pool chemicals) when making a decision. While some swim programs claim to teach water survival skills to infants younger than 12 months, evidence shows that these programs are not effective in preventing drowning. Swim lessons do not provide "drown-proofing" for children of any age, so close supervision and other layers of protection are always necessary.
- Be alert to small bodies of water including fountains, buckets, and rain barrels. Because toddlers have large, heavy heads, they can overbalance, fall in, and be unable to lift their heads out of the water. To be safe, empty containers of water as soon as you're done with them.

- Make sure your child is supervised whenever he swims, preferably by someone who knows CPR.
- Do not allow running, rough play, or riding bikes near the pool. Do not allow glass or breakable dishware in the pool area.
- Make sure the deep and shallow ends of a pool are clearly marked in any pool your child swims in. Do not allow him to dive into the shallow end.
- Don't allow your child to use a spa or hot tub.
- Make sure your child wears a life jacket whenever she swims or rides in a boat. A child younger than 5 years should wear a flotation collar to keep her head upright and face out of the water.
- Adults should minimize distractions while supervising children near water. Avoid drinking alcohol, talking on a cell phone, or working on a computer.

## Home Pools

- Surround your home pool completely on all 4 sides with a fence that is at least 4' high. The fence should completely separate the pool from the house and the rest of the yard. Install a self-locking and self-latching safety gate and keep it locked at all times, even in the winter.
- Consider additional layers of protection, like rigid pool covers or pool alarms. These are not a substitute for a proper fence but may offer additional protection.
- Keep a portable or cell phone with you at all times near the pool.
- Have a safety ring with a rope and a pole that does not conduct electricity beside the pool at all times.
- Empty or securely cover wading pools when not in use.
- Learn CPR. (See Chapter 4, "Basics of First Aid," pages 215–216.) Research shows that poolside CPR can save lives—even if you don't do it perfectly.
- Use only battery-operated radios and other appliances by the pool; electric appliances are never safe near water.

## Preventing Injury From Animals

Children are more likely than adults to get bitten by an animal. It's important to be especially cautious when you're bringing a new baby into a home with a pet. Do not leave your baby alone with the animal for the first 2 or 3 weeks. Observe your pet carefully—feelings of fear or jealousy should give way as your pet gets used to this new relationship. If you have a child and are getting a pet, wait until the child is mature enough to handle and care for the pet (usually about age 5 or 6 years).

- Look for a pet with a gentle disposition. An older animal is often a good choice, but do not choose an older animal raised in a home without children. Puppies and kittens are more likely to bite out of friskiness.
- Teach your children to pet their dogs and cats gently on the back, not on their face, head, or tail. Don't allow your child to tease a pet by pulling its tail or taking away a toy or bone.
- Make it a firm rule never to disturb an animal when it is eating or sleeping.
- Don't leave small children alone with a pet. They may not recognize when the animal is getting upset or excited.
- Have all pets immunized for rabies and other diseases.
- Follow leash laws and keep your pet under control at all times.
- Teach your child not to approach an animal other than his own pet. Even if the owner gives permission, the animal may not want a stranger petting it.
- Instruct your child not to run, ride her bike, kick, or make threatening gestures if she is approached by a strange or barking dog. Your child should face the dog and back away slowly until she's out of reach.
- Teach children to observe wild animals from a safe distance. Wild animals can carry very serious diseases that can be transmitted to humans. If you see a wild animal that is injured or acting sick, strangely, or overly friendly, do not approach it. Instead, call your local animal control center or health department.

## TRAVELING WITH YOUR CHILD

Children can make great traveling companions, but planning before a trip is essential. Make sure you know in advance how you'll get from place to place and where you will stay. Try to plan age-appropriate outings; a backpacking vacation, for example, is probably not the best choice for a 3-year-old. If you have a newborn or an infant, try to plan the day's activities around her schedule. It is not wise to go sightseeing at her usual nap time. Teenagers may enjoy having a friend along on the trip.

- Childproof your accommodations, whether a friend's or relative's house, hotel room, or campsite, as soon as you arrive.
- Check that your hotel caters to children. Some have reliable babysitting services, allow children to stay in parents' room for free, or have special childproof rooms complete with cribs and changing tables. Check that the hotel crib is sturdy and safe before using it.
- In a hotel room, make sure the in-room bar is securely locked and keep the key out of children's reach.
- Try out any new equipment, such as baby carriers, at home.
- Before traveling outside the country, check with your pediatrician that your child's immunizations are up-to-date and whether supplemental immunizations are needed. Keep in mind that conditions at hotels in foreign countries may not be as safe as those in the United States, vehicles may not have adequate seat belts, and pools may not have safe, modern drainage systems. Be prepared to take steps or make your own rules to prevent injuries.
- Children often become restless or irritable when on a long road trip. Keep them occupied by pointing out interesting sights along the way and bringing a variety of snacks; soft, lightweight toys; and favorite music for a sing-along.
- Plan to stop driving and give you and your child a break about every 2 hours.

- Before allowing your child to swim in the ocean, check the water temperature and pollution levels. Check with local authorities about beaches with dangerous undertow (the current beneath the water surface). Make sure the water is free of jellyfish and other marine hazards.
- Encourage your child to wear beach shoes to avoid scratches from rocks, coral, and shells.

## Plane Travel

- Allow extra time to get through airport security. Let your child know what to expect in the screening process.
- A child is best protected when properly restrained in a car safety seat appropriate for the age, weight, and height of the child until the child weighs more than 40 pounds and can use the aircraft seat belt. The car safety seat should have a label noting that it is US Federal Aviation administration (FAA)–approved. Belt-positioning booster seats cannot be used on airplanes, but they can be carried on board or checked as luggage (usually without baggage fees) for use in rental cars and taxis.
- Although the FAA allows children younger than 2 years to be held on an adult's lap, the AAP recommends that families explore options to ensure that each child has her own seat. If it is not feasible to purchase a ticket for a small child, try to select a flight that is likely to have empty seats.
- To decrease ear pain during the descent, encourage your infant to nurse or suck on a bottle. Older children can chew gum or suck on a straw.

## Bicycles

Cycling is a great way for children to get outdoor exercise, increase coordination, and develop self-confidence and independence. However, it can be dangerous. Children and teens younger than 14 years are involved in more than 500,000 bicycle injuries each year. Many of these injuries could be avoided with proper safety measures.

- Parents who enjoy biking often consider purchasing a baby carrier that attaches to the back of the bicycle. But even with the best carrier and safety helmet, your baby is at risk for serious injury. This can occur when you lose control on an uneven road surface or if you happen to strike or be struck by another vehicle. Never put a baby younger than 1 year on a seat on the back of your bike. A much better choice is for your baby to ride in a bicycle-towed trailer. But do not use trailers on the roadway because they are low and may not be visible to drivers.
- Never let your child ride on the handlebars or place a seat there.
- Wait until your child is physically able to handle a tricycle before buying one. He should also be mature enough to follow your rules about when and where to ride. Buy a tricycle that is built low to the ground and has big wheels. This type of bike is safer and less likely to tip over.
- Insist everyone in your family wear a properly fitting helmet, and teach your child to wear one every time she rides.
- Most children don't have the balance and coordination to ride a bicycle until about age 7 years.
- Never let your child listen to headphones while biking; they're distracting and block out traffic sounds. Set a good example by not using them yourself.
- Make sure your child's bike is in good repair.
- Teach your child the rules of the road. Obey traffic signals and regulations. Ride with, not against, traffic. Stay to the far right or in a bicycle lane. When cycling in groups, ride single file.

## Fire Injury Prevention

Protecting your home against fire involves planning. There are precautions you can take that can help you protect you and your family.

- Never leave small children alone in the home, even for a minute.
- Install smoke detectors in furnace and sleeping areas. Check batteries once a month.
- Plan several escape routes from the house. Plan a place to meet right after leaving the house. Do home fire drills. Consider escape ladders for second- or third-story bedrooms.
- Do not smoke in bed. Always dispose of cigarette butts, matches, and ashes with care.
- Keep matches and lighters away from children.
- Use GFCI outlets in the bathroom and kitchen. An electrician can install GFCI outlets at a low cost.
- Be sure your gas water heater is off the ground. Spilled flammable liquids will be ignited by the pilot light.
- Do not clean clothes with flammable liquids.
- Place a barrier around open flames.
- Do not wear loose-fitting clothing near a stove, fireplace, or open space heater.
- Have your heating system checked and cleaned yearly. If you are a renter, ask your landlord to have this checked yearly.
- Check electric appliances and cords regularly for wear or loose connections.
- Use only 15-ampere fuses for lighting circuits. Never use a substitute for a fuse.
- Place fire extinguishers around the home where the risk of fire is greatest—in the kitchen and furnace room and near the fireplace.
- If you do have a fire, get everyone out as quickly as possible. Do not stop to get dressed or put out the fire. Call the fire department from a neighbor's house.

## FINDING CHILD CARE

Because today's family often includes a single parent or 2 working parents, finding reliable child care is a necessity. It's also a process that often leaves parents emotionally exhausted. It is helpful to talk with friends and relatives to see which child care facilities they recommend or if they can recommend reliable babysitters. The following tips can help ensure your child's safety and your peace of mind:

## Babysitters

Children thrive when they're cared for in a safe, healthy environment by supportive adults who are warmly affectionate and help children learn, interact, and work out solutions while helping them avoid choices that can cause harm. Here's what to do when hiring a child care provider to come to your home.

- Request references and the names and phone numbers of former employers. Perform a background check, if possible. Ask for documented work experience (preferably as far back as 5 years).
- Ask the babysitter specific questions. For example, ask about her approach to discipline, scheduling, feeding, comforting, and providing appropriate activities. Determine if her approach matches your style of child rearing and is appropriate for your child. Make sure the babysitter shares your philosophy about how to react to excessive crying, an accident, or an unwillingness to sleep.
- Emphasize your views on discipline. Explain your policies on smoking and drinking around your child, and make clear your policy on having visitors at the house.
- Spend time with the sitter and your child and watch how they interact.
- Show the sitter where all fire exits, first aid kits, flashlights, and emergency phone numbers are located. Ensure that he knows how to administer CPR and knows what to do in case of a choking emergency.

- Show the babysitter where all baby supplies are kept. Go over the proper way to feed, pick up, change, and comfort your baby. Also describe your child's schedule and any special preferences your child may have, such as listening to a story before napping.
- Arrange a week when you can be home to watch the sitter work under your supervision.
- Monitor the performance of the person you hire. Consider making unannounced visits, especially if your child does not yet speak.
- Treat your babysitter as a professional; draw up a contract that includes a job description, hours, salary, and overtime pay, if any.

## Child Care Centers

Child care centers typically provide care for children in a nonresidential building with classrooms of children in different age groups. Of the 12 million children in child care in the United States, about 9 million are in licensed facilities. The rest are in unlicensed centers that are unregulated. Centers demonstrate a higher commitment to quality by participating in the accreditation process.

- Be sure the center is licensed. Ask whether a background check is done on all employees. Inquire at social service agencies to see if any reports or complaints have been filed. Find out if children are required to provide health and immunization reports.
- Inspect the center. Is it clean? Is it free of hazards? Are there enough toys and books for children? Is there an area with hand-washing facilities for changing diapers? Where are diapers disposed? Make sure all of the childproofing tips in this chapter are followed by the center.
- Ask about food service. If your child will be bringing food, check if there is proper storage or refrigeration. If food is prepared on-site, make sure the food preparation area is clean and secure from wandering children.

- Ask about the goals of the program. Some are organized and try to teach new skills. Others are more relaxed and let children develop skills on their own. Still others are in between.
- Look at the employee-child ratio. The younger the child, the more adults there should be in his group. Designated ratios vary from state to state.
- Ask about staff rules. Are staff prohibited from smoking, even outside? Are staff immunizations required?
- Find out what happens on a typical day. Ideally, there should be a mix of physical activity and quiet times. Some activities should be group-oriented and others individualized. Time for meals and snacks should be set aside. While some structure is desirable, there should be room for free play and special events too.
- Spend time at the center to see if the children look happy and how they are treated. Be wary of centers that do not allow parents to drop in.
- Make sure staff follow steps to reduce the risk of sudden infant death syndrome (SIDS) by placing infants on their backs to sleep. Make sure they place your baby to sleep on a firm sleep surface that is free of bumpers, blankets, and other soft items. Doing so will reduce the risk of SIDS.
- Gather information on policies on sickness, payments, and meals and snacks. You should also find out about administration of medication and first aid, napping arrangements, transportation of children on field trips, and how parents may contact staff. In addition, find out about security procedures.
- Child Care Aware has information for parents about quality child care and links to find child care close to home (www.childcareaware.org).

## Home Alone

Making the decision to leave a child home alone hinges on the age of the child and her maturity. Most states do not have laws about the ages at which kids can be home alone. In general, most kids in fourth or fifth grade are ready to be left alone for brief periods, but make sure your child isn't afraid to be left alone.

Before children are left alone, it's best to do a practice run. Show and tell them what to expect and what to do if the phone rings or the power goes out. Let them talk you through what they'd do. Make sure they know how to use the phone (landline and cell), how to shut off the alarm system, and where flashlights are kept.

Make sure they know their name and address (as well as when to give it out and when not to!). When you are both comfortable, start out with brief periods alone—a run to the grocery store or bank, for example—and gradually extend the time apart. Some good guidelines include

- Have your child call you when he gets home. He can e-mail or text you too. This establishes a routine and helps give parent and child some peace of mind.
- Establish rules about what's acceptable in your absence. As children get older, it becomes even more important to make rules about what's acceptable, such as having other kids over and how many can visit.
- Set limits on television viewing.
- Post emergency numbers as well as numbers of neighbors and family members near the phone. Keep your work and cell phone numbers handy too. Make sure your child knows how to dial 911 or your local emergency number.
- Remind your child not to tell callers that you are not home. Rehearse something with your child that he can say to a caller. Explain to your child that he should not answer the door for visitors when you are not home.

## Protecting Children From Abduction

Many parents worry about keeping their child safe in and around the neighborhood. Fortunately, child abductions are rare, although they understandably get plenty of media attention when they occur. Most abductions occur when children are taken by noncustodial parents (parents who do not have custody of the children), although a smaller number of stranger abductions do take place each year. Here are some suggestions to help keep your child safe.

- When you're shopping with your child, keep an eye on him at all times, as he can move out of your line of vision in an instant.
- When choosing a preschool, ask about safety issues. Make sure a policy is in place in which your child can be picked up only by his parent or someone else you designate.
- Although your child should be supervised by a trusted adult at all times, it is still important to teach her to never get into a car or go along with someone unfamiliar to her. If a stranger tells her something like, "There's a lost puppy in my car. Come into the car for a minute and see if you know him," your child should emphatically say, "No." In fact, tell her to run away as fast as possible from dangers like this and to yell very loudly and find a trusted adult in any situation in which she feels threatened.
- When hiring babysitters, always check references and ask for recommendations from friends and family members.
- For more information, contact the National Center for Missing & Exploited Children at 800/THE-LOST (843-5678) or www.missingkids.com.

# Resources

The following organizations and Web sites offer more information on the symptoms in this book. Rather than being all inclusive, this list is simply a way to help you get started on your search for more information. Make sure your pediatrician knows your questions and concerns. Remember, you and your pediatrician are partners in your child's health.

Please note: Listing of resources does not imply an endorsement by the American Academy of Pediatrics (AAP). The AAP is not responsible for the content of the resources. Phone numbers and Web sites are as current as possible but may change at any time.

## AMERICAN ACADEMY OF PEDIATRICS RESOURCES

### American Academy of Pediatrics

**www.aap.org**
**847/434-4000**

The AAP is a professional medical organization of more than 62,000 pediatricians dedicated to the physical, mental, and social health and well-being of infants, children, adolescents, and young adults.

### HealthyChildren.org

**www.HealthyChildren.org**

The official AAP Web site for parents features hundreds of informational articles on various aspects of children's health, from infancy through the teenage years.

### Centers for Disease Control and Prevention

www.cdc.gov
800/CDC-INFO (232-4636)

Offers information about numerous illnesses and health problems as well as advice on healthy living, emergency preparedness, environmental health, injury prevention, and immunizations

### Health.gov (From the US Department of Health & Human Services)

www.health.gov

Provides information on health topics by age and sex as well as guidelines on healthy eating and physical activity

### MedLine Plus

www.nlm.nih.gov/medlineplus

Provides information on symptoms, illnesses, health and wellness, diagnoses, and different systems of the body

### National Institute of Diabetes and Digestive and Kidney Disorders

www.niddk.nih.gov

Offers information on illnesses that affect the endocrine system, the digestive tract, and the urological system

### National Institutes of Health

www.nih.gov

Offers information on medical research and health problems as well as advice on healthy living

### National Institute of Mental Health

www.nimh.nih.gov

An in-depth site on common mental health disorders, with information specific to children and teens

### National Institute of Neurological Disorders and Stroke

www.ninds.nih.gov

Offers information on developmental delays and various brain disorders

## US Department of Agriculture

www.usda.gov

Offers information on nutrition, including the Web site ChooseMyPlate.gov, as well as details on food safety, first aid, and emergency preparedness

## US Food and Drug Administration

www.fda.gov

Offers up-to-date information on food and nutrition and medical devices and drugs as well as news on general health

## GENERAL AND PEDIATRIC HEALTH WEB SITES

## American Academy of Family Physicians

www.familydoctor.org

Offers information for the whole family, from infancy to seniors, on illnesses and health problems, prevention and wellness, and medications

## Cleveland Clinic

www.clevelandclinic.org

Provides an A to Z guide on assorted health information and information about healthy living, diagnostics, medical devices, and drugs and supplements, including newsletters

## KidsHealth.org (From the Nemours Foundation Center for Children's Health Media)

www.KidsHealth.org

Provides perspective and advice about a wide range of physical, emotional, and behavioral issues that affect children and teens

## Mayo Clinic

www.mayoclinic.com

Offers information on illnesses and health problems, drugs and supplements, tests and procedures, and healthy living

## Merck Manual Home Health Handbook

www.merckmanuals.com

Features symptoms, first aid, drug information, and resources

## American Academy of Allergy, Asthma & Immunology

www.aaaai.org
414/272-6071

## American Academy of Child & Adolescent Psychiatry

www.aacap.org
202/966-7300

## American Academy of Dermatology

www.aad.org
866/503-SKIN (7546)

## American Academy of Orthopedic Surgeons

www.aaos.org
847/823-7186

## American Academy of Pediatric Dentistry

www.aapd.org
312/337-2169

## American Association for Pediatric Ophthalmology and Strabismus

www.aapos.org
415/561-8505

## American College of Allergy, Asthma & Immunology

www.acaai.org
847/427-1200

## American Hair Loss Association

www.americanhairloss.org

## American Heart Association

www.heart.org
800/AHA-USA-1 (800/242-8721)

## American Optometric Association

www.aoa.org
800/365-2219

## American Psychological Association

www.apa.org
800/374-2721

## Arthritis Foundation

www.arthritis.org
404/872-7100

## Autism Speaks

www.autismspeaks.org
888/288-4762

## Common Sense Media

www.commonsensemedia.org
415/863-0600

## Epilepsy Foundation

www.epilepsyfoundation.org
800/332-1000

## Food Allergy Research & Education

http://foodallergy.org
800/929-4040

## The International Dyslexia Association

www.interdys.org
410/296-0232

## National Center for Learning Disabilities

www.ncld.org
888/575-7373

## National Sleep Foundation

www.sleepfoundation.org
703/243-1697

# Index

Hyperventilation syndrome, 181
Hypoglycemia, 189
Hypothalamus, 86
Hypothermia, 45
Hypothyroidism, 93
Hypotonia, 173

**I**

Ibuprofen, 52, 86, 144
Idiopathic kyphosis, 127
Idiopathic thrombocytopenic purpura, 43
Immune suppression, 86
Impetigo, 139
Inborn heart condition, 101
Incontinence
    daytime, 160
    urinary, 160–161
Indigestion, 102–103
Infantile spasms, 135
Infants. *See* Babies
Infections
    bacterial, 105
    breast, 49
    ear, 3, 15, 76–79, 87, 133
    fungal, 106, 208
    herpes virus, 75, 119, 139, 145
    HIV, 204, 206
    kidney, 35
    mouth, 119
    parasitic, 23, 71, 91
    respiratory, 15, 87
    sexually transmitted, 204, 206
    sinus, 133
    streptococcal, 21, 29, 75, 97, 118, 128
    tonsillar, 145
    upper respiratory, 29
    urinary tract, 21, 29, 37, 87, 162
    viral, 21, 75, 105, 113, 118
    yeast, 106, 118, 165
Infectious bacterial diarrhea, 71
Infectious diarrhea, 7, 91
Infectious gastroenteritis, 87
Infectious mononucleosis
    appetite loss and, 29
    fatigue and, 191
    sore throat and, 145
    swollen glands and, 155
    weakness and, 173
Infectious viral gastroenteritis, 71
Inflammatory bowel disease, 23, 93
Inflammatory polyps, 129
Influenza, 59, 87
Inguinal hernia, 153
Inhalants, 212
Insect repellent, 40

Insects
    bites and stings of, 78, 107
    in ear, 78
Insomnia, 210
Intertrigo, 107, 208
Intestinal blockage, 3, 21, 25, 55
Intoeing, 46–47, 170
Intussusception, 43
Iritis, 83
Iron-deficiency anemia
    fainting and, 188
    fatigue and, 190, 191
    paleness and, 124, 125
Irritability, 104–105
Irritable bowel syndrome, 23, 71, 103
Isolation
    avoiding normalization of, 184–185
    problems of, 174

**J**

Jaundice, 10–11
    breast milk, 11
    physiologic, 10, 11
    treating, in newborns, 10
Jellyfish venom, 41
Jock itch, 106, 107, 208
Joint pain, 108–109
Joint swelling, 108–109
Juvenile idiopathic arthritis or lupus,
        53, 109, 113, 127
Juvenile polyarthritis, 113

**K**

Kawasaki disease, 87
Keloid, 141
Kidney disease, 193
Kidney infection, acute, 35
Kitchen, safety in, 235
Knee injuries, preventing, 194
Knee pain, 194–195
Knock knee, 46–47
Kyphosis
    idiopathic, 127
    postural, 127

**L**

Labial adhesions, 163
Labyrinthitis, 73
Lactase, 26
Lactose, 26, 90
Lactose intolerance, 22, 26, 91, 103
Language milestones, 146
Laryngomalacia, 176
Laryngotracheal malacia, 15
Laryngotracheobronchitis, 51, 177
Laundry room, safety in, 236
Lazy eye, 60, 61

Lead poisoning, 23, 125
    avoiding, 236–237
Learning difficulty, 111, 157
Learning disabilities, 183
Learning problems, 65, 110–111, 201
Legg-Calvé-Perthes disease, 109
Lesbian, gay, bisexual, transgendered,
        questioning (LGBTQ),
        204, 205
Leukemia, 25, 42, 43, 125
Lice, 140
Lichen simplex, 139
Life, responding to stressors in, 176–177
Lifesaving techniques, 213
Lightheartedness, 72
Limb/leg pain, 112–113
Lisp, 147
Longevity, 191–193
    peer pressures and, 191–193
Long QT syndrome, 189
Love, compromised ability to feel, 180–181
Low blood sugar, 189
Lumps on the wrist, 152
Lung disorder, 45
    collapsed, as cause of chest pain, 52
Lupus, 109
Luteinizing hormone (LH), 202
Lyme disease
    bites and stings and, 40, 41
    fever of, in babies and children, 87
    joint pain and, 109
    limb and leg pain and, 113
    preventing, 108
Lymphatic system, 154
Lymphocytes, 154

**M**

Malabsorption, 25, 71, 148, 149
Malaria, 40
Mallet finger, 109
Malnutrition, 92
Manic depression, 183, 199
Marijuana use, 212
Mastoiditis, 78
Masturbation, 114–115, 204
Meatal stenosis, 163
Meckel diverticulum, 129
Media overuse, 116–117, 196–197
Medications
    side effects of, 119
    sleep and, 143
    teens, media, and, 211
Meningitis, 97, 169
Menstrual cycle, 204
Mental health challenges, vulnerability to,
        175

Metabolic disorder, 186
Methemoglobin, 44
Methemoglobinemia, 44
Methicillin-resistant *Staphylococcus aureus* (MRSA), 139
Migraine headaches, 23, 96
Mild trauma, 97
Milia, 13
Mini-puberty, 48
Moles, 139
Mongolian spot, 13
Monilial, 165
Mononucleosis, 87
Moodiness, temperament and, 198–199
Mood swings, 198–199, 200
Moral imagination of violence, 172–173
Motion sickness, 73, 169
Motor development
    normal, 57
    slow, 57
Motor problems, 111
Mouth infection, 119
Mouth pain, 118–119
Muscle cramps, 121
Muscle pain, 120–121
Muscle strain or spasms, 112, 121
Muscular disorder, 65
Muscular dystrophy, 171, 172, 173
    diagnosing, 172
Myasthenia gravis, 173, 191
Myopia, 166
Myositis, 120

**N**
Narcolepsy, 190, 191, 210
Navel, swelling around, 24
Neonatal acne, 13
Nephrotic syndrome, 25
Nettles, 107
Neural tube defects, 64
Neurogenic bladder, 161
Neurologic disorder, 65, 99
Neuromuscular problems, 73
Neuromuscular weakness, 171
Nevus flammeus, 13
Newborns. *See also* Babies
    caring for your, 1
    treating jaundice in, 10
Nightmares, 85
Night terrors, 85, 134
Nocturnal emissions, 204
Nocturnal enuresis
    primary, 36, 37
    secondary, 36
Nocturnal myoclonus, 159
Nodulocystic acne, 207

Noisy breathing, 176–177
Nonfatal drowning, 217
Nonspecific diarrhea, 71
Normal motor development, 57
Nosebleeds, 42, 122–123
Nostril, foreign object in, 133
Nursemaid's elbow, 109
Nystagmus, 61

**O**
Obesity-related hypertension, 193
Obsessive-compulsive disorder (OCD), 180
    tics as signs of, 158
Obstructive sleep apnea, 210
Oral thrush, 118
Orthostatic hypotension, 188
Osgood-Schlatter disease, 195
Osteochondritis dissecans, 195
Osteomyelitis, 113, 120
Otalgia, 76
Otitis externa, 78, 79
Otitis media, 72, 76, 78, 79
Outdoor play equipment, 238
Out-toeing, 170
Overeating, 103
Overfeeding, 81, 175
Overheating, 8
Oversleeping, 191
Overstimulation, 3, 17
Overuse cyst, 195
Overuse injuries, avoiding, 112

**P**
Pacifiers, 2
    keeping your baby happy with, 4
Pain
    acute abdominal, 20–21
    back, 34–35
    chest, 52–53
    chronic abdominal, 22–23
    functional, 22
    joint, 108–109
    knee, 194–195
    limb/leg, 112–113
    mouth, 118–119
    muscle, 120–121
    rectal, 128–129
    urinary, 162–163
Paleness, 124–125
Panic attacks, 181, 188
Panic disorder, 180
Parasitic infection, 23, 71, 91
Parent-child relationship as exceptional, 183–184
Paroxysmal coughing, 134

Partial seizures, 135
Patellar maltracking, 195
Pediatric autoimmune neuropsychiatric disorder associated with streptococcal infections (PANDAS), 158
Peer pressures, longevity and, 191–193
Penis, inflammation of, 163
Peptic ulcer, 53, 103
Perianal abscess or fistula, 129
Perianal dermatitis, 55, 129
Periorbital cellulitis, 83
Personality change, 200–201
Petechiae, 42
Phobias
    school, 85, 181
    social and specific, 180
Physiologic jaundice, 10, 11
Pigmentation disorders, 138
Pinworms, 107, 128, 129
Pityriasis rosea, 140, 208
Plane travel, 242
Plantar wart, 140, 153
Playgrounds, 238
Playpens, 234
Pneumonia
    aspiration, 51
    breathing problems and, 50, 51
    chest pain and, 52, 53
    wheezing and, 177
Pneumothorax, 52
Poisoning
    actions to take, 218
    lead, 23
        avoiding, 236–237
    prevention of, 218
    treatment of, 218
Poison ivy, 107
Poison oak, 107
Poison prevention, 230–231
Poison sumac, 107
Pollack, William, 181
Polyps, 123
Port-wine stains, 13
Positive reinforcement, 38
Poststreptococcal glomerulonephritis, 25
Post-traumatic stress disorder (PTSD), 85, 180
Postural kyphosis, 127
Posture defects, 126–127, 172
Post-viral cerebellar ataxia, 73
Precocious (early) puberty, 203
    breast swelling and, 48, 49
    growth problems and, 93
Pregnancy, 189, 191, 205
Premature breast growth, 48

The Big Book of Symptoms

Strabismus, 60–61
Stranger anxiety, 84
Strangulated hernia, 21
Strep throat, 87, 144, 145
Streptococcal throat infection
    abdominal pain and, 21
    appetite loss and, 29
    drooling and, 75
    headache and, 97
    mouth pain and, 118
    rectal pain and, 128
Stress, 159
Stress injury, 113
Stridor, 176
Strollers, 239
Stuffy nose, 132–133
Stuttering, 147
Styes, 82, 83
Subconjunctival hemorrhage, 83
Substance use and abuse, 211–212
    depression and, 183
    fatigue and, 191
    personality change and, 201
Sucking blisters, 118
Sudden infant death syndrome (SIDS),
        14, 244
Suicide, teenage, 200
Swellings, 152–153
    around navel, 24
    breast, 48–49
Swimmer's ear, 78, 79
Swimming pools, water safety and,
        239–240
Swollen glands, 154–155
Sydenham chorea, 158, 159
Synovitis
    toxic, 108
    transient, 108
Systemic illness, 29

**T**

Tall stature, 93
Tear duct, blocked, 82
Teenagers. *See* Adolescence
Teen sleep quandary, 209
Teething, 63
Telogen effluvium, 94, 95
Temperament, 104
    moodiness and, 198–199
Temperature, taking rectal, 9
Temper tantrums, 31, 110, 130, 156–157
Tension headache, 97
Thalassemia, 125
Thelarche, premature, 48, 49
Third-degree burns, 220
Thoracic (rib cage) asymmetry, 137

Thrush, 145
Thumb-sucking, 63
Thyroid disorder, 173, 191
Thyroid problems, 136
Tibial torsion, 46, 47
Tibia vara, 47
Ticks, 108
    identification of, 40
    removal of, 40
Tics/spasms, 158–159
    as signs of obsessive-compulsive
        disorder, 158
"Time-in," 38
Tinea capitis, 95
Tinea cruris, 208
Tinea pedis, 140, 208
Toddlers, shoes for active, 171
Toilet training, steps to, 36–37
Tonsillar infections, 145
Tonsillitis, 75, 155
Tonsils, 144
Tooth, 63
Topical calcineurin inhibitors, 106
Torsion, 21
Torticollis, 137
Torus fracture, 88
Tourette syndrome, 147, 159
Toxic alopecia, 95
Toxic synovitis, 108
Tracheobronchitis, 59
Tracheomalacia, 176
Transgender, 206
Transient synovitis, 108
Transient tic, 159
Trauma
    abusive head, 4
    mild, 97
Traveling with your child, 241–242
Trichotillomania, 95
Troubled relationships, problems of, 174
Truancy, 201
Tularemia, 40
Tumors
    dizziness and, 73
    headache and, 97
    high blood pressure and, 193
    knee pain and, 195
    personality change and, 201
Tympanostomy tubes, 77

**U**

Ulcerative colitis, 23, 71, 93, 103
Ulcers, 52
    aphthous, 118
    peptic, 53, 103
    ulcerative, 23, 71, 93, 103

Umbilical hernia, 24
Upper respiratory infection, 29
Urethra, soap in, 163
Urinary incontinence, 160–161
Urinary pain/difficulty, 162–163
Urinary tract infections (UTIs), 21, 29, 37,
        87, 162
    preventing, 162
Utility room, safety in, 236

**V**

Vagina, foreign object in, 163, 165
Vaginal itching/discharge, 164–165
Varicella, 141
Vasovagal syncope, 189
Vernix, 12
Verruca, 140, 153
Vertigo, 72
Violence, moral imagination of, 172–173
Violent entertainment, appetites for, 176
Viral hepatitis, 149
Viral infection
    abdominal pain and, 21
    irritability and, 105
    leg pain and, 113
    of the mouth, 75
    mouth pain and, 118
    of the throat, 75
Viral pharyngitis, 87
Vision problems, 166–167
Vitiligo, 138
Vomiting, 14, 168–169
Von Willebrand disease, 42, 43
Vulvovaginitis
    itching and, 106, 107, 165
    preventing, 164

**W**

Walkers, 236
Walking problems, 170–171
Wandering eye, 60–61
Warts, 140, 153
Wasp sting, 41
Weakness, 172–173
Weight gain/loss, 174–175
Wet dreams, 204
Wheezing/noisy breathing, 176–177
Wilms tumor, 163
Wolff-Parkinson-White syndrome, 189
Wrist, lumps on, 152
Wryneck, 127, 137

**Y**

Yard, safety in, 237–238
Yeast diaper rash, 165
Yeast infections, 106, 118, 165